W9-BRD-303

Hospital Planning Handbook

"Planning is not merely the process of determining the most efficient way to achieve certain goals. It is a process in which we keep asking whether the goals are valid. It is a process in which we keep raising the possibility of alternate goals to meet the needs of a rapidly changing world where yesterday's goals may no longer be valid."

John C. De Boer

HOSPITAL PLANNING HANDBOOK

REX WHITAKER ALLEN
ILONA VON KÁROLYI

The Hugh Stubbins/Rex Allen Partnership
Cambridge & San Francisco

A Wiley-Interscience Publication

JOHN WILEY & SONS

New York • Chichester • Brisbane • Toronto

Library of Congress Cataloging in Publication Data:

Allen, Rex Whitaker.
  Hospital planning handbook.

  "A Wiley-Interscience publication."
  Bibliography: p.
  Includes index.
  1. Hospitals—Planning. 2. Hospitals—Design
and construction. I. Karolyi, Ilona von, joint
author. II. Title.

RA967.A43   362.1'1   75-30599
ISBN 0-471-02319-1

Printed in the United States of America

10 9 8 7 6 5 4

This book is dedicated to Hugh Stubbins and his associates and to the staff of The Rex Allen Partnership, without whose combined support and patience it could not have been written.

Preface

I am telling you what happened, rather than what ought to have happened. The
preparation of the plans for the rebuilding of St. Thomas' Hospital has been a tremendous muddle from the beginning, and will not serve as a model for any other body....

G. H. Bateman
St. Thomas' Hospital

We hope that this handbook will help the busy professional avoid some
of the muddle that typically surrounds the preparation of a program for new
hospital construction—what is sometimes called "the brief to the architect."
It often happens that the architect becomes involved in the preparation of
the brief himself, and this book is thus directed to him as well as to the
hospital administrator, who needs to know what it is the architect will need
to know. We deal with design factors only in passing—design comes later
in the process. What we have tried to do is provide an outline of process and
methodology that will enable the preliminary work to be done with some confidence and dispatch. We have not provided answers, nor have we attempted
to ask all possible questions. Aware of the danger of treating complex problems simplistically on the one hand, and the equal danger to decision
making of too much information, we have tried to mark out a reasonable and
realistic level of analysis. We have chosen certain areas of hospital activity
that seemed to us to be particularly difficult or sensitive as examples for full
exploration and have passed more lightly over the areas where there is a
full body of literature. Because outpatient services seem to us to be a major
area of development in the near future, particular emphasis has been placed
on planning for outpatient clinics and emergency services.

Planning for physical facilities requires an understanding of the amount
and nature of activities and their interrelationships and impacts on each
other. Before the architect can begin his work many decisions must be made,

but such decisions are difficult and may have been postponed until the architect appears on the scene. Even in a profit–making organization responsible people find decision making difficult: In a voluntary organization, where goals, attitudes and organizational structures are diffuse and changeable, it is even harder. For this very human reason it often devolves upon the architect to organize the decision making structure and process, to ask the controversial questions, and to cajole, bully, and lead the way towards the goal that he and the institution presumably share: to get something done.

Politics is a part of this process and cannot be ignored. We have tried to indicate the kinds of political issues that are likely to prove troublesome, both internally within the institution and outside in its relation to the larger community.

But the hot political issue of one year may be dead the next—it is necessary to assess very carefully the reality of political questions and to try to distinguish between a passing fashion and a real issue. Medicine is not less subject to fashion than any other field of human endeavor, although the swing from one area of concern to another may take a little longer.

We would like to express our appreciation of the director and staff of the Countway Library of Medicine at Harvard for providing us access to the library's resources; to Tim Laput for his drawings and graphics; to C. Michael Daley for his invaluable editorial assistance; to the several patient typists who managed to put all the pieces together; and finally, to the Stubbins/Allen Partnership, which made the whole venture possible.

REX WHITAKER ALLEN
ILONA VON KÁROLYI

The Hugh Stubbins/Rex Allen Partnership
Cambridge, Massachusetts
and San Francisco, California
June 1975

Contents

Hospital Planning Handbook

Introduction

1. THE NEED FOR PLANNING

The need for planning an institution is so obvious as not to be an issue—although, judging from the results, even a number of new institutions have suffered from inadequate planning, and long-range planning for older institutions is often neglected.

Many hospitals in this country (especially in its eastern part and among its oldest and most distinguished institutions) occupy outdated buildings that are located on crowded sites with little space for expansion. Over the years courtyards have been filled in, wings have been joined to old buildings, or stories built on top of them. In many hospitals change is continuous—something is always in the process of being added, remodeled, or moved. Every addition or change brings with it a whole chain of shifts as vacated space is filled—and very little of this kind of change occurs within the frame of any sort of long-range plan. Most moves are made in response to immediate pressures, and generally not until the pressure has become urgent. Frequently, too, space is assigned or reassigned not because of the rationalized needs of a department but because of the reputation or political muscle of the chief of a service or the head of a department. The result is that functions are split and fragmented, spaces are unsuited to their functions, and circulation patterns become so complicated that even long-term employees are bewildered. While no plan is likely to eliminate entirely this kind of ad hoc change, a well-thought-out development plan, fully circulated among staff members, can help. Simply the fact that there *is* a plan, and that the staff *knows* there is a plan, means that requests for additional space or objections to proposed changes will have to be more fully justified and documented than would otherwise be the case.

Anyone who has participated in any sort of facilities planning will be able to confirm that trying to plan a single additional unit generates both interest in, and need for, planning of related and even apparently peripheral areas. In fact it is almost impossible, and certainly unwise, to plan a single part without to some degree planning the whole. Often the need

1

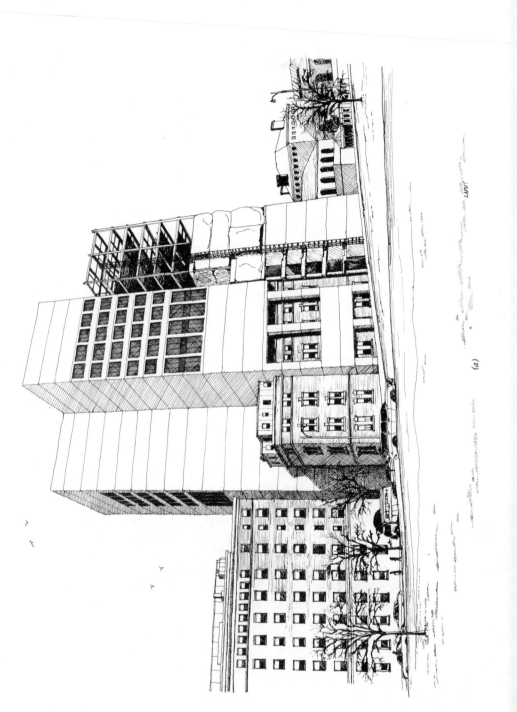

(a)

2

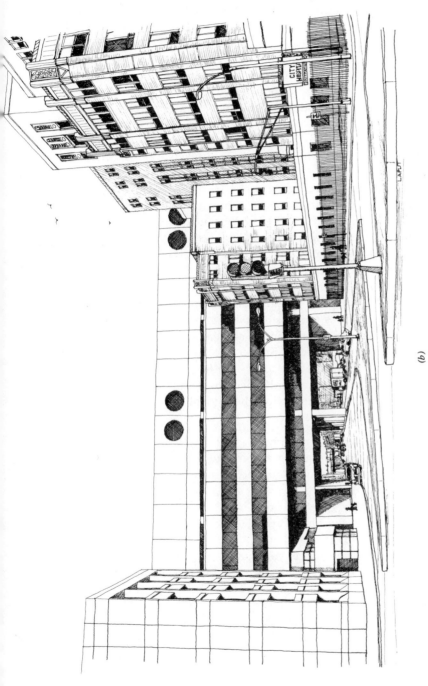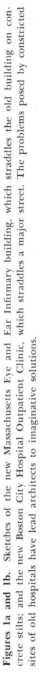

(b)

Figures 1a and 1b. Sketches of the new Massachusetts Eye and Ear Infirmary building, which straddles the old building on concrete stilts; and the new Boston City Hospital Outpatient Clinic, which straddles a major street. The problems posed by constricted sites of old hospitals have lead architects to imaginative solutions.

3

to plan for a specific facility provides the impetus for a total planning effort; and this is as it should be. If it is possible to get the long-range, broad-brush planning underway before specific and detailed planning begins, a great deal of time, effort and money will have been saved.

Planning is a dynamic process that defies static documentation. However, planning is necessary for orderly development. It can be carried out at many levels of detail and in many time frames. At the outset it is necessary to determine what level of detail will be of value at a given time. Frequently, excessive detail is documented too early. A department head may be asked to develop a list of space needs room by room long before any means have been established for fulfilling his requirements. Such premature requests can only prove frustrating to the department head and result in an eventual lack of cooperation when the proper time for such programming arrives. Even too detailed a definition of equipment at the inception of an immediate project may be premature. Chances are that in a large construction project such equipment will have have been superseded by a new model by the time the building is ready to receive it. Conversely, it is necessary to have available adequate information at each stage of planning and to provide sufficient lead time for certain stages such as purchasing, fabrication or roughing-in utilities so that the project can proceed in an efficient manner.

To assure a smooth, orderly project the first step in the planning process is to establish a schedule for the entire project. Since conditions for each project will vary, the order, length of time, and need for each step will be different. The following checklist of steps, however, may be helpful:

- Preplanning schedule.
- Determination of community need for health care.
- Evaluation of existing conditions (including seismic hazards and other possible restraints).
- Demographic survey of service area.
- Statement of goals and objectives related to community needs.
- Capital financing plan.
- Operational program to meet goals and objectives.
- Master development plan as a framework, including gross departmental area allocations, schematic plans, and construction staging.
- Cost analysis.
- Detailed space program of first stage for construction.
- Equipment list.
- Design of first stage.
- Construction of first stage.

• Evaluation of operation and feedback to preplanning schedule and master plan.

2. PREPLANNING SCHEDULE

The preplanning step should outline the level of detail required for each subsequent step and the anticipated time when each step should be completed. Such a schedule should be continuously updated and refined and become increasingly detailed as the design and construction process progresses. Until recently a bar chart was the principal tool used for scheduling. Although it can indicate what should be done when, it is unable to show the interrelationship and interdependency of tasks. For increasingly complex projects something more was needed. Several systems have been developed to assist the planner in organizing and dovetailing the myriad tasks necessary for rational planning. One of these systems is the Program Evaluation and Review Technique (PERT) developed by consultants to the U.S. Navy for the Polaris atomic submarine project, and another is the Critical Path Method (CPM) developed for E. I. DuPont. Both these systems use network analysis as their basic tool. They differ in that PERT places emphasis on method and the probability of completing a project in a stated time period, whereas CPM is used to organize the process in the least time commensurate with the lowest cost. In many respects the systems overlap. Generally, for the procedures outlined in this book either system is equally applicable as it is not necessary to go beyond network analysis on which both systems are based.*

Network analysis starts with a listing of the tasks or activities necessary to achieve a predetermined objective. An estimate is made of the duration of each activity, that is, how much time it will take to complete. The inception and termination of each task is a point in time that is referred to as an event. Except for the first and last events, events generally comprise two or more simultaneous occurrences, the end of at least one activity and the beginning of at least one other. Once this listing has been completed, a preliminary attempt should be made to place the activities in chronological order. This will simplify the task of determining which activities are dependent upon the completion of other activities or, conversely, which activities must precede the start of other activities. One way to arrive at such an order is to write each activity on a separate card and arrange the cards on a table or pin them to a wall in the most logical sequence (1-1).

---

* Should the reader want a more detailed discussion there are many reference works available on the subject (see Bibliography).

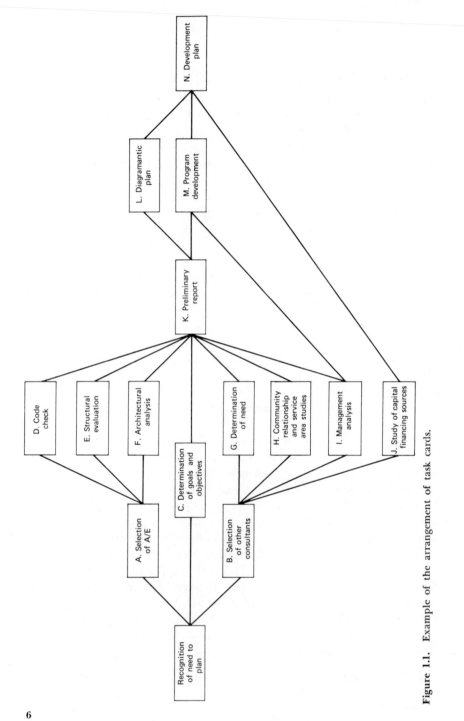

Figure 1.1. Example of the arrangement of task cards.

Task No.	Task or Activity	Responsibility of	Duration (wks)	Directly Follows	Directly Precedes	Start	Finish
				Order		Event No.	
A	Selection of/Architect/Engineer	Owner	4	—	D,E,F	1	2
B	Selection of Other Consultants	Owner	4	—	G,H,I,J	1	3
C	Determination of Goals and Objectives	Owner	12	—	K	1	6
D	Code Check	A/E	4	A	K	2	4
E	Structural Evaluation	A/E	6	A	K	2	5
F	Architectural Analysis (including mech. and elect.)	A/E	9	A	K	2	6
G	Determination of Need	Consultant	6	B	K	3	6
H	Community Relationship and Service Area Study	Consultant	8	B	K	3	7
I	Management Analysis	Consultant	8	B	M	3	8
J	Study of Capital Financing Sources	Consultant	10	B	N	3	10
K	Preliminary Report	A/E	2	C,D,E, F,G,H	L,M	6	8
L	Diagrammatic Plans	A/E	6	K	N	8	9
M	Program Development	A/E	8	I,K	N	8	10
N	Development Plan	A/E	4	J,L,M	—	10	11

Figure 1-2. Example of Task Schedule

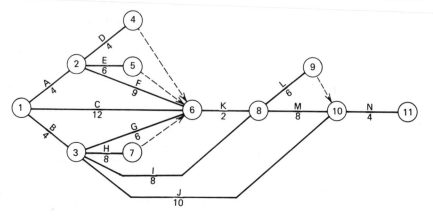

Figure 1.3. Example of network analysis.

When precedence and dependency have been determined, this information can be tabulated (1-2) and a network diagram established (1-3).

Responsibility for each task and estimated duration should also be entered in the table and then each event should be numbered. Note that concurrent tasks that should terminate in the same event are given separate inception or terminating event numbers that are connected to each other by dotted lines representing dummy activities. These dummies have no duration. Their only purpose is to eliminate ambiguity and permit the tasks or activities to be identified by unique starting-finishing events. Using this information, it becomes a matter of simple arithmetic to determine early and late start times, early and late finish times, and float time for each activity (1-4). This in turn can be related to calendar dates so that a bar chart can be drawn to a graphic time scale (1-5). Thus both network diagram and bar chart have value: the network to illustrate interdependency and to identify critical activities (those with zero float time); the bar chart to represent graphically elapsed time. In an extremely complex job or one where new tasks or activities will need to be added as the work progresses, it may be advantageous to use data processing equipment to understand the effect of changes, to model alternatives, and to determine the optimum course of action. Basically, however, the greatest benefit will derive from the organizational process itself, listing tasks and establishing their interdependency.

There are other benefits that can be derived from the network analysis system. As is suggested in Fig. 1-2, it is usually advisable to establish responsibilities, at first in a generalized way—owner, consultant, and so on—and perhaps later by specific individual. Also, man-hours or man-

Activity No.	Duration (Wks.)	Start Early	Start Late	Finish Early	Finish Late	Float	Calendar Earliest Start	Calendar Latest Start	Calendar Latest Finish
1-2	4	0	0	4	4	0	Jan. 1	Jan. 1	Jan. 29
1-3	4	0	1	4	5	1	Jan. 1	Jan. 8	Feb. 5
1-6	12	0	1	12	13	1	Jan. 1	Jan. 8	Apr. 2
2-4	4	4	9	8	13	5	Jan. 29	Mar. 5	Apr. 2
2-5	6	4	7	10	13	3	Jan. 29	Feb. 19	Apr. 2
2-6	9	4	4	13	13	0	Jan. 29	Jan. 29	Apr. 2
3-6	6	4	7	10	13	3	Jan. 29	Feb. 19	Apr. 2
3-7	8	4	5	12	13	1	Jan. 29	Feb. 5	Apr. 2
3-8	8	4	7	12	15	3	Jan. 29	Feb. 19	Apr. 16
3-10	10	4	11	14	23	9	Jan. 29	Mar. 19	Apr. 9
6-8	2	13	13	15	15	0	Apr. 2	Apr. 2	Apr. 16
8-9	6	15	17	21	23	2	Apr. 16	Apr. 30	Jun. 11
8-10	8	15	15	23	23	0	Apr. 16	Apr. 16	Jun. 11
10-11	4	23	23	27	27	0	Jun. 11	Jun. 11	Jul. 9

Figure 1-4. Example of Network Schedule

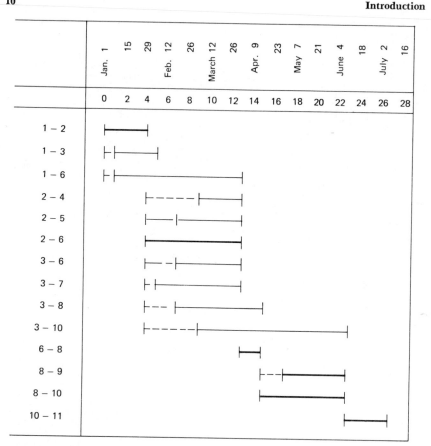

Figure 1.5. Example of a bar chart.

weeks of work to complete each task can be estimated to determine costs, both for the owner and for the professional adviser or consultant (see Fig. 1-6). It should be noted that man-weeks are used instead of man-hours because overtime can be worked if necessary to maintain the schedule. Obviously, however, if overtime is anticipated for any task, an adequate contingency should be built into the original budget. Finally, by establishing a logical sequence and dependency of events it is possible to determine which activities are critical to completion on time, which are on the critical path, and which should have the greatest attention. Also, such a procedure establishes how much leeway or float time there is for the other activities. Such information improves communication between all participants in the planning process and as a result the overall effectiveness of management.

Task No.	Task	Avail. Wks.	Avail. Hrs.	Manpower Cate-gory	Manpower % of Time	Rate Per Hr.	Cost	Totals
D	Code Check	4	160	B	0.75	40	$4,800	
	Direct Costs and Total						—	$4,800
E	Structural Evaluation	6	240	A	0.05	60	720	
				B	0.50	40	4,800	
				C	0.33	20	1,600	
	Direct Costs and Total						—	7,120
F	Architectural Analysis of Existing Buildings (including mechanical and electrical systems)	9	360	A	0.05	60	1,080	
				B	0.50	40	7,200	
				C	0.33	20	2,400	
	Direct Costs and Totals						—	10,680
K	Preliminary Report	2	80	B	0.50	40	1,600	
				C	0.50	20	800	
	Direct Costs and Totals						500	2,900
L	Diagrammatic Plans	6	240	A	0.05	60	720	
				B	0.75	40	7,200	
				C	0.50	20	1,600	
	Direct Costs and Totals						500	10,820
M	Program Development	8	320	A	0.10	60	1,920	
				B	0.67	40	8,530	
				C	0.25	20	1,600	
	Direct Costs and Total						200	12,250
N	Development Plan	4	160	A	0.10	60	960	
				B	0.75	40	4,800	
				C	0.50	20	1,600	
	Direct Costs and Total						1,500	8,860
	Subtotal							$57,430
	Contingency—10%							5,740
	Total							$63,170

Figure 1-6. Example of Professional (A/E) Fee Estimate to Program a Development Plan

3. ORGANIZATION OF THE PLANNING TEAM

Essential to a successful planning effort is the way those involved work
together and make decisions. There is no one best structure for a planning
team. Each institution will require a setup unique to its particular
method of operation. What is important is that careful thought be given
to finding the most appropriate organization at the inception of
planning. Generally, it is desirable to funnel information through as
small a group as possible with one person assuming primary responsibility for organization, scheduling, and record keeping and for providing
the necessary leadership to keep the process in motion. This person may
be a full-time staff member or an outside professional. He should obviously have competent backup to provide continuity should he cease to be
available. Other members of the team may have permanent assignments
or be brought in for specific responsibilities or advice.

4. DECISION MAKING

Nothing is more detrimental to planning or more frustrating to the
planner than "buck-passing" in decision making. It is, therefore, essential
that policies be adopted that clearly define at what level which decisions
are to be made. The sequence of decisions, like the levels in planning,
should also be carefully organized—broad decisions first and more detailed ones as the planning process progresses. A concern for details too
early will almost inevitably result in errors of judgment that may invali-
date the entire process.

Decisions can be reached more readily if information is organized as
follows:

1. Definition of problem.
2. Definition of goal.
3. Presentation of alternatives to reach goal.
4. Description of courses of action.

Graphic displays can often be helpful in transmitting recommendations
to decision-makers. Such displays can be simple tabulations of pros and
cons, an evaluation matrix or a listing of problems, objectives, alternative solutions, and plans of action.

It is also well to recognize that "decisions of the kind the executive
has to make are not made well by acclamation. They are made well only
if based on the clash of conflicting views, the dialogue between differing
points of view, the choice between different judgments. The first rule in

decision making is that one does not make a decision unless there is disagreement."*

5. THE PLANNING PROCESS

It is well to realize from the beginning that planning for an institution as complicated as a hospital is likely to be an extraordinarily difficult and often frustrating task. It is sometimes necessary to analyze an existing operation in far more depth and detail than appears warranted for the early planning stages. On the other hand, it may also prove necessary apparently to oversimplify in order to get anything accomplished. Which way to tip the scale in a particular situation is a matter that can be left only to the judgment of the individual who is charged with doing the work at a particular institution, with a particular group of officials, doctors, administrators, trustees, and perhaps patients. It may be worth pointing out that the need to go into excessive detail generally results from having to prove to a vested (and possible defensive) interest why requirements may be less than the interested party had anticipated or demanded. It is likely to result from political rather than actual problems.

An excellent guide to the process of planning for voluntary organizations is a book by John C. De Boer entitled *Let's Plan* (Pilgrim Press, Philadelphia, 1970):

The planning system requires that the policy base be touched at every planning stage so that the planners may be sure that they are working on a concern that is important to the organization, not merely to the planner . . . the role of the planning group is not to make policy; it is to advise the policy makers. . . . At regular intervals, probably no farther apart than six months, the planning committee should get out the long-term plan, study it afresh, undertake any new research that seems called for, and update the plan. In effect the process of long-term planning is always occuring.

6. THE STAGES OF PLANNING

No single part of the planning process can be isolated. The process is circular and repetitive. For all kinds of planning—functional, financial, physical—the process starts with a broadly outlined program and in succeeding stages becomes more clearly defined and specific. If for each kind of planning the levels of detail can be made congruent, the process will be considerably more efficient than if, for example, a detailed physical

* Drucker, Paul, *The Effective Executive*, Grove Press, New York, 1964.

plan is prepared without equivalently detailed planning of operations and financing. A complete congruence can perhaps rarely be achieved, but it can and should be approximated. A physical plan will be a wasted effort if it is not based on a realistic estimate of financial and personnel resources available. It should also reflect as accurately as possible a projection of the activities to be accommodated.

Since this handbook deals primarily with physical facilities—or perhaps more accurately, with the functional and programmatic considerations necessary to arrive at an estimate of physical space requirements—the levels of detail are outlined briefly in physical planning terms. These levels can be simplified and defined roughly as follows:

Stage One—Feasibility

In very broad outline, the anticipated numbers of inpatients and outpatients are determined. Hospital-wide gross area planning standards are applied on the basis of numbers of beds or hundreds of outpatient visits. Such standards can be derived from a cursory analysis of existing facilities of similar type and size (such as E. Todd Wheeler's summary in his book, *Hospital Modernization and Expansion,* or the American Hospital Association's annual summaries) without breaking the space down by department or function. This very general level of planning will be sufficient to determine the probable adequacy of a proposed site or to make a rough estimate of construction costs.

Stage Two—Master Program and Plan

Here a reasonably thorough analysis of projected functions, operations, and utilization is needed. While still of a general nature, the analysis is sufficiently detailed to outline the requirements of major functions or departments of the hospital with some degree of accuracy. The requirements for space indicate the particular orientation of the institution and are a reflection of its specific character. It is with this level of programming that this handbook deals.

The programming process, in the sense in which it is being dealt with here, consists of the following steps:

1. Making lists of questions to be resolved.
2. Letting everyone concerned know what is in the lists, and why.
3. Asking everyone concerned to review and revise the lists and to make lists of their own.
4. Simplifying all the lists, translating them into consistent terms, and making them digestible.

5. Letting everyone review everyone else's list.
6. Drawing conclusions from all the lists.
7. Letting everyone concerned review and revise the conclusions.
8. Making new lists.

Repeat as needed.

While this is an obvious oversimplification it is nevertheless a useful outline of the process. The principle factors needed for a successful planning effort are clear definitions and good communication. The planner's work consists largely in reducing vast amounts of information to manageable proportions and making it digestible. It is essential that planning at this stage be presented in a form that will allow the assumptions and calculations on which the plan was based to be retraced and revised over a period of time: Since change is inevitable, and many factors are only doubtfully predictable, any plan, no matter how well prepared, will require regular and frequent updating and revision. To keep the plan flexible and thus useful, it must be possible to make changes logically and consistently.

The information gathered and presented at this level of planning will be sufficient to draw up a physical master plan, and to provide the basis for an estimated operating budget.

Stage Three—Detailed Programming and Planning

Within the context of a well-prepared master program and plan, the development of plans for a specific facility will follow with a minimum of difficulty. The general outlines of functional and financial feasibility will have been determined, and the problem will merely be how most effectively to allocate resources, the limits of which have already been defined. Two distinct steps will be needed: a final definition and quantification of the workload (patients, beds, visits, procedures), of the level of sophistication of facilities and equipment, of the numbers of personnel, and of anticipated utilization factors; and then more or less detailed descriptions of spaces and the relationships between spaces. When these two steps are taken, design of the first increment of construction can begin.

1

Health and Hospital
Planning Considerations

1.1. DEFINITION OF SERVICE AREA

Prior to determining a community's needs for health care, it is necessary
to define the community or service area. This may vary from an easily
identified demographic entity to an international area for specialty
service. An example of the former is a community hospital in a small
isolated metropolitan area with a population of 50,000. An example of
the latter is a large hospital, probably a teaching institution, with a
recognized specialty such as cardiac transplant that may draw patients
from any part of the world. It is essential then that the scope of service
be analyzed to determine whether the service area extends beyond
normal geographic boundaries.

Normally people tend to go to hospitals recommended by their
physicians; this is to a lesser degree true with facilities for other types of
nursing care. It is understandable that convenience for the physician is
often the determining factor in the choice of institution. Physicians'
offices tend to be located at the centers at which people ordinarily shop
and trade and have social, educational, and religious ties. Increasingly,
the hospital serves as a similar center for health care and health education. The service area of the institutions, therefore, is apt to reflect the
pattern of usage of the shopping center and the location of patient resi-
dences. Sources of information that may help in determining the limits
of a service area include:

    a.   Existing health care institutions—addresses of patients.
    b.   Physicians' offices—addresses of patients.
    c.   Stores, banks, and newspapers—addresses of customers.

d. Utility companies—addresses of consumers.

e. Schools, post offices, and churches—areas served.

f. City, county, and state planning traffic departments.

When the service area has been thus defined a survey of the area should be made; it probably will include examination of official census figures, vital statistics, and special population estimates to arrive at:

a. Total population.

b. Age distribution of population in at least the following categories: Under 15, female 15 to 44, and over 65.

c. Mortality and mortality trends.

d. Income distribution and home ownership.

e. Occupational distribution, particularly in regard to industrial hazards.

f. Seasonal variations.

g. Insurance coverage.

In addition, information should be assembled about existing medical services and facilities, including data on the availability of professional personnel. The inventory of facilities should include a list of beds by category of occupancy and a detailed statement of the extent of ancillary services.

If planning is being done for an existing facility, one of the first tasks will be to evaluate existing conditions (see Chapter 2). Simultaneously, it is necessary to determine needs. Determination of need at a time when methods of delivering health care are in a state of flux is on of the most difficult yet essential requirements for rational planning. Concurrently, an institution should develop a statement of goals and plot a course of action to achieve them. Establishment of an operating policy for each of the several disciplines in an institution is equally important. This book will provide only peripheral guidance in these areas, as its main purpose is to assist in determining projected need and in translating that need into a program for reasonable and functional physical space.

To best determine need, two procedures are necessary: to divide the need into categories of care and to make rational projections of future requirements for each category. Perhaps at this point it should be mentioned that it is advisable to distinguish between need and demand. There can often be demand in excess of need, or need in excess of demand. Need is a measure of services required to maintain well-being in a designated population. Demand is the sum of individually expressed health service requirements. Demand can generally be measured by an examination of existing patterns. Need, on the other hand, requires a more detailed analysis of a defined service area, its present and future shortcomings.

Health care can be categorized in many ways. For physical planning purposes it is convenient to subdivide it as follows:

- Prevention—public health programs, immunization, and public education.
- Diagnosis—physiological and psychological examination.
- Therapy—emergency, intensive, acute, extended, minimal, home, and ambulant.
- Rehabilitation—physical and mental restoration to a state of well-being.
- Education (medical and public) and research.

At this time in the United States no overall system exists; therefore, it is necessary to treat each of these categories independently.

1.2. PREVENTION

The two extremes of health care—prevention and rehabilitation—have been receiving new emphasis in an attempt to reduce the need and, therefore, the cost, in both human and economic terms, of diagnosis and treatment. For years public health programs have concentrated on environmental problems—quality of water, immunization against communicable diseases, and so forth. Now not only are these areas of concern expanding because of environmental issues, but also there is increasing emphasis on immunology and new programs are being developed to detect early the onset of illness. One of the first of such detection programs on an organized basis was the Kaiser multiphasic clinic. Subsequently, several such programs have been developed both in connection with hospitals and as independent units, some as part of prepayment plans and others on a referral basis. There is currently insufficient evidence to determine their efficacy in reducing the incidence of acute illness; however, the theory and the potential for application of sophisticated hardware to monitor both variations from the norm and variations from prior individual examinations make it appear as though the prospects for success are excellent. Should this be the case, demand will develop rapidly and for many years to come demand for preventive facilities will far exceed supply. Translation of this demand into physical facilities will only depend on economic limitations and the development of clearly stated functional programs. A variety of solutions are possible, depending upon the organization of the service team and the extent to which data processing equipment is utilized. The development of a program can follow the guidelines set up for comparable therapy departments in subsequent chapters of this book. Particular attention should be given to variations in duration of examination procedures and to the development of an orderly progression through the clinic both for the convenience of the public and of the medical staff. For example, from a psychological point of view it is far better to fill gaps between procedures with a self-answerable questionnaire than to leave a person waiting idly for the next examination. Obviously those examinations whose results may suggest some immediate follow-up should be scheduled first.

1.3. REHABILITATION

At the other end of the spectrum the need is almost equally unfilled. Only minimum attention has been given to the social and humanitarian aspects of rehabilitation. In general, after the illness has been cured, little thought has been given to the problems of postconvalescence. Often these can be stupendous. Economic drain due to cost of care and loss of income can cause psychiatric problems. Physical handicaps may require extensive retraining. It is increasingly recognized that the cost of neglect is far greater in human and social terms than the cost of well-organized rehabilitation programs. Again the need exceeds availability of services so that the construction of facilities is only limited by the availability of staff, capital improvement funds, and adequate repayment programs.

1.4. DIAGNOSIS AND THERAPY

Projection of need for facilities for diagnosis and therapy is a far more complicated and difficult process. A great number of statistical approaches have been proposed. Reduced to the simplest terms, an evaluation of existing levels of care in a service area defined by geography (or other definable category, such as ethnic community that may be necessary if there are language barriers), a determination of deficiencies, and a prognosis of trends in a reasonably predictable period of time should result in an acceptable statement of future need. Statistical documentation of the existing pattern of care is usually no problem and population projection is also relatively easy. Difficulties arise when evaluating deficiencies (need versus demand) and when attempting to interpret the effect of innovative programs for providing care on the need for physical facilities. However, "as the pace of technological and social change accelerates, the need for timely and accurate forecasts is correspondingly increased."*

* Howarth, William J., "The Role of Operational Testing in Forecasting Health Services Trends" in *Health Services Research,* Vol. 8, No. 3, Fall 1973.

Therefore, it is essential that some process be adopted that results in reasonably accurate projections.

A general analysis of need for diagnositc and therapeutic services may serve to obtain a broad perspective on current status of care. But to obtain a more accurate appraisal and to look to future need it is necessary to break diagnosis and treatment into subcategories and also to examine various levels of care. The following are recommended basic subcategories that are most likely to need consideration in facility design:

- Medical.
- Surgical.
- Obstetrical/Gynecological.
- Pediatric.
- Orthopedic.
- Psychiatric/Alcoholic.

For programming purposes these categories should be evaluated at the following levels of care:

1. Ambulant/Outpatient/Primary.
2. Emergency.
3. Intensive/Coronary/Burn Unit.
4. Acute.
5. Skilled Nursing: Extended, Long Term, or Chronic.
6. Self/Independent/Minimum.
7. Home.

Finally, because there is growing recognition of the need to avoid duplication of increasingly expensive services, each institution has a responsibility to consider its role in the community. Actually, any voluntary organization has a similar responsibility, as can be seen in the following quotation from *Let's Plan* by John De Boer:

In the light of what *other* organizations are prepared to do or not do with respect to this concern, what should *this* organization be prepared to do? Thus questions like the following need to be asked by the planning group:

- Is this concern *our* concern, or is it more properly some other group's concern?
- Is this concern our concern *alone,* or should it be shared by others?
- Is this a concern that is important to us *now,* or would it be better to postpone consideration to a later time?
- Is the apparent concern the *real* concern, or a symptom of a deeper underlying problem—or of a different but related problem?

1.5. PROJECTIONS

As has been stated, statistical documentation of existing patterns of care in existing institutions should serve as a basis for preliminary projections of future demand. An analysis of true need should follow; however, at the beginning it is a generally accepted practice to look back the same number of years that one attempts to look forward. The level of accuracy decreases with the extent of the projection.

At the inception of planning, statistics should be gathered from all existing institutions in a defined service area. Such statistics should be a yearly record of departmental operations at three or five year intervals. Monthly statistics for one or two years may also be valuable to indicate seasonal variations. The following is a checklist to suggest the data that will be required to make the projections outlined in subsequent chapters:

- Population characteristics (by age, sex, and income).
- Outpatient visits and emergency procedures.
- Number of available beds.
- Inpatient admissions or discharges (medical/surgical; obstetric/gynecological; pediatric; orthopedic; psychiatric/alcoholic).
- Patient days (by similar categories).
- Surgical procedures (major and minor).
- Births (normal and caesarian).
- X-Ray procedures (by type, if available).
- Isotope procedures.
- Radiotherapy procedures.
- Laboratory procedures (by type, if available).
- Special procedures (by type; see Chapter 5).

Some of the above information can be assembled from the *Guide* issues published annually by the American Hospital Association, from the various state plans for hospitals, and from publications of the U.S. Census Bureau.

Useful Formulas

Patient days = Average daily census (ADC) $\times$ 365
$\qquad$ *or:* Admissions $\times$ average length of stay

Percent occupancy = $\dfrac{\text{Average daily census}}{\text{available beds}}$

$\qquad$ *or:* $\dfrac{\text{Patient days per year}}{365 \times \text{available beds per year}}$

1.6. ANCILLARY AND AFFILIATED INSTITUTIONS, SERVICES AND FACILITIES

Without going into great detail, it may be worthwhile to summarize some of the kinds of facilities or services that are, might be, or should be associated with a hospital. The judgment as to which kinds of associated functions should be considered will have to be made on the basis of local conditions. From a long-range point of view it is valuable for the hospital to consider which of these might form part of the hospital's future.

Extended Care

This may be seen as care that goes beyond what is available at a nursing home but that does not require the routine access to physicians and the elaborate diagnostic and therapeutic services of the hospital itself. An extended care facility should be located near a hospital, however, and may in fact be joined to the general circulation system for easy transfer of patients in both directions.

Self or Minimal Care

This may be compared to a nursing or rest home, except that patients can perform most of their own care, including walking to a dining area, dressing, and so on. They require a minimal level of professional care— special diets and preparation for diagnostic or minor therapeutic procedures.

Terminal Care

As dying becomes a subject for open discussion, some experimental efforts are underway* to plan the care and treatment of the dying patient in a realistic and humane way, taking into account not only his needs but those of his family and the staff who work with him.

Doctors' Offices, Group Practices, or Health Maintenance Organizations

There is considerable value to physicians, patients, and the hospital itself if the doctor's offices and the places where patients receive their primary care are located near the hospital. It ensures a degree of coordination and joint use of certain facilities that makes sense both in convenience and in economic terms. Such facilities may be more or less integrated with the hospital itself.

* Several such programs exist in England. An example in the United States is Hospice, Inc. in New Haven, Connecticut at present programatically active and planning the development of a specially designed facility.

1.7. RESIDENTIAL FACILITIES

Staff

While the traditional nurses' dormitory may be a thing of the past, there may be sound argument for providing close-by, convenient, and moderately priced housing for several elements of the hospital's working population, including nurses, interns, residents, students of various kinds, and even supporting staff.

Patients and Relatives

Where public lodging facilities are absent, remote, or costly, it may make sense for the hospital either to build or to provide land for building an inn or motel for out-of-town patients and their relatives.

Candidates for Rehabilitation—Housing for the Handicapped

Often the handicapped are forced to live in nursing homes because traditional housing is unsuited to their needs. Housing especially designed for this group, close to a hospital, may help to rehabilitate patients who might otherwise become permanent invalids.

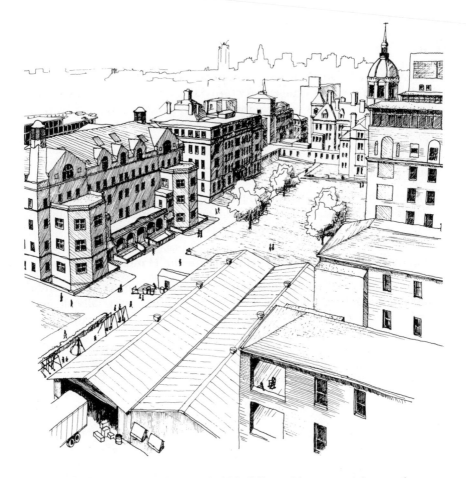

Figures X and Y. The replacement of old buildings with new ones does not have to mean the elimination of green space. In the proposed renewal illustrated in the second drawing, the amount of open space is actually increased. Travel times from one part of the hospital to the other are sharply reduced by providing enclosed cross-corridors raised above the ground level so as not to interrupt movement across the courtyard (Master Plan for Johns Hopkins Medical Institutions, Baltimore, Md.; Hugh Stubbins/Rex Allen Partnership, Architects).

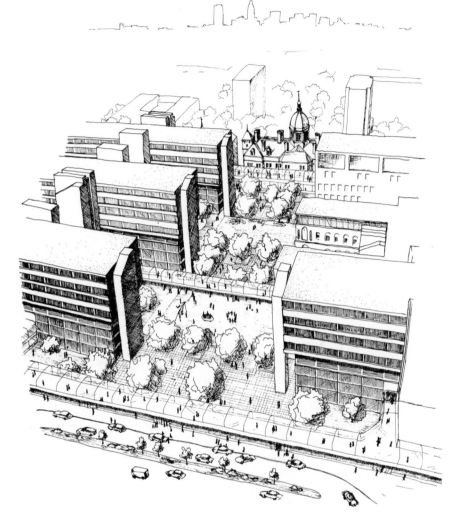

Figures X and Y (*continued*)

2

Analysis of Existing Conditions

2.1. BACKGROUND/DISCUSSION

In an existing institution an overall picture of current operations and facilities is the first step in planning. At a very broad level of planning such a summary may provide the basis for projection of future requirements. For the rather more detailed approach with which this book is concerned, a documentation of conditions at the time when planning begins is a necessary tool for succeeding efforts. As the work goes forward it will often be necessary to refer back to this early documentation and the data on which it is based, and it is, therefore, important that the working papers and tabulations be as consistent and complete as time and manpower allow. In planning for the future, people will always ask "but how does that compare to the way it is *now*?"—even though the way it is now may not be strictly relevant. Current conditions almost always provide a necessary basis for comparison.

The object of this portion of the work is a preliminary document that will do the following:

- Give a concise outline of the structure and organization of the institution, including all departments and major work units, and affiliations with other institutions.
- Provide a convenient summary of the locations and net or gross areas of all departments, including nursing units and work units, and if desired an analysis of the physical condition of all existing structures, including a check for code conformance, and of structural, mechanical, and electrical conditions.
- Provide a summary of personnel by category of work and department, corresponding to departments listed in the space summary.
- Provide an outline of the workload of major hospital functions.

In the process of discussing present deficiencies, projections, and future needs with departments at a later state of planning, it will be helpful to have the specifics—nuts, bolts, and numbers—readily available for reference. A grasp of general conditions will enable the planner to direct his questions to the main issues: It will also allow him to deal tactfully both with the problem of the department that makes grandiose plans and projections without much basis in fact and with the opposite problem of the department that has been working under such difficult conditions for so long that its director cannot see beyond the need for another technician or a new file cabinet.

2.2.   DISTRIBUTION OF FLOOR AREAS

Purpose

To prepare a matrix showing the distribution of areas by location. Areas may be either net areas if derived from an inventory or gross areas taken off plans.

Information needed

Floor plans or facility inventory.

Planning decision needed

What functional categories will be used to group and summarize departments? Will a gross area take-off from floor plans provide adequate information, or should assignable space be used?

Even among architects there is a certain amount of confusion about the definition of areas. AIA Document #D101 defines gross square feet (GSF) as "the sum of the areas of the several floors of the building, including basements, mezzanine and intermediate floored tiers and penthouses of headroom height, measured from the exterior faces of exterior walls." In this text net (or assignable) square feet (NSF) represents areas measured from the inside dimension of all assignable rooms (including toilets, janitors' closets, and mechanical rooms, but not including shafts, electrical closets, or interstitial space). Net areas are more suitable for programming as net square feet represents space that is assignable to a specific function. After listing all net areas for each department, the sum should be increased by 30 to 55% to arrive at gross departmental areas. This will account for walls, partitions, columns, and mechanical shafts. The wide variation in net to gross ratios is due to many factors, such as size and number of rooms in the department, size of the department, type and extent of mechanical systems, type of structure, and so forth.

Nursing, outpatient, diagnostic and treatment, and administrative services will require a high factor; supply, maintenance, and engineering services a lower factor. Finally, another 12 to 15% (the larger percentage being applicable in larger projects or where provisions are made in smaller projects for expansion) should be added to the total of gross departmental areas for general circulation: corridors, stairs, and elevators. Since determination of the correct ratio is a matter of judgment, the inexperienced programmer will do well to use conservative, high percentages to avoid an unexpected increase in gross area when plans are developed. An overall net to gross of 1.55 to 1.70 is considered quite acceptable. For example, if the total net assignable area is 60,000 square feet, the total gross should be between 93,000 square feet and 102,000 square feet.

In a detailed tabulation, only assignable space should be included, and general-use corridors, mechanical spaces, stairs, and elevators excluded. As the net-to-gross ratios of buildings are quite variable, only by considering net areas is it possible to obtain a true picture of how much space is required for a particular activity. However, even net area is not in itself adequate to describe the amount of space needed since the shape of space will also determine its usefulness.

Procedure

Tabulate and summarize rooms or spaces by building and floor level. Although floor-level summaries are not necessary for the programming planning stage, they will be needed for the design process, since both horizontal and vertical relationships are important. A format for tabulating space is illustrated in Table EC-1 and Table EC-2. Table EC-1 also provides a form for summarizing the condition of the building.

A final martix, listing all buildings and grouping departments into functional categories will serve to summarize existing space. This final tabulation can be analyzed in the traditional way by dividing each category of space by the number of hospital beds. This may be interesting for purposes of comparison with other hospitals and may give some measure of the extent of deficiencies.

2.3. WORK LOADS OF DEPARTMENTS

A brief summary of hospital statistics should be collected, including patient days, discharges, radiological procedures, clinical laboratory tests, number of outpatient visits, and so on. More detailed work will have to be done in all these areas later, but it will be convenient to have on hand whatever summary statistics are readily available.

Table EC-1. Space Summarized by Building

Building A	Floor	Department	NSF	Factor	GSF	Totals (GSF)
	Subbasement	General Stores	000	1.3	0000	
		Dietary-stor.	0000	1.3	0000	
		Radio Therapy	0000	1.5	0000	
	Floor Total				0000 × 1.15 =	00,000
	Basement	Dietary-kit.	000		000	
		Sterile Supply	000		000	
	Floor Total				0000 × 1.15 =	00,000
Building Total						00,000

The *Departmental Areas* header spans the NSF, Factor, and GSF columns.

Date of Construction:
Code conformance:
Condition of finishes:
Structural system and condition:
Utility systems:
Electrical systems:
Medical systems:

Table EC-2. Space Summarized by Floor Level

Floor	Department	Build. A	Build. B	Build. C	Totals (GSF)
S-B	Storage	000	0000	—	
	Dietary	0000	—	000	
	Radiology	0000	0000	—	
Floor Total					00,000
Basement	Dietary	0000	0000	—	
	Sterile Supply	0000	—	0000	
Floor Total					00,000

The *Departmental Gross Areas* header spans the Build. A, Build. B, and Build. C columns.

Table EC-3.   Space Summarized by Department

Department	Building	Floor	Net Area (NSF)	Totals-NSF
Radiology	Building A	SB	0000	
		1	0000	
		2	0000	
	Building Total			0,000
	Building B	B	0000	
		3	000	
	Building Total			0,000
Department Total				00,000

2.4. DISTRIBUTION OF BEDS

A matrix similar to that used for space analysis should be made to illustrate the distribution of hospital beds by location and service and by service and type of accommodation:

Table EC-4.   Distribution by Service and Floor

Floor	3	4	5	6	Total
Med/Surg.	—	48	64	64	176
OB	20	—	—	—	20
Ped.	—	16	—	—	16
Ortho.	20	—	—	—	20
Psych.	18	—	—	—	18
Total	58	64	64	64	250

Table EC-5. Bed Distribution by Service and Type of Accommodation

Type	Priv.	Semi-Priv.	4-Bed Ward	Total
Med. Surg.	12	152	12	176
OB	2	10	8	20
Ped.	2	10	4	16
Ortho.	—	12	8	20
Psych.	6	12	—	18
Total	22	196	32	250

Note that bassinets in post-partum nurseries are not included in the bed count, but bassinets in the pediatric nurseries should be included in the bed count.

2.5. PERSONNEL

Purpose

To summarize all personnel in the hospital by department, by category of work, by full time equivalency, by head-count, and by time of duty.

Information needed

- Lists of hospital personnel identified by department or work unit, time of duty, full-time equivalency, and type of work.
- Lists of other personnel who may be on duty in the hospital but are not included in hospital personnel lists. In the case of a teaching hospital, faculty, students, investigators, and reasearch support personnel may not be on the hospital payroll but should be accounted for. There may also be adjunct activities in the hospital whose personnel do not appear on a master list.

Procedure

Because it may be difficult to sort out overlapping categories of people, the first round of summarizing personnel will tend to be detailed. Much depends on how personnel records are maintained and how well the information is organized. If the lists are computerized, so much the better.

It may be simplest to sort out the lists by work shift first. The heaviest shift should receive the most attention, with the others summarized as necessary. Listing first every department and every category of worker, the departments and worker categories can then be grouped and summarized.

The personnel list may have separate categories of clerical workers, ranging from administrative assistants through secretaries to file clerks. These could all be grouped into one category of clerical workers. Nurses and nurses aides can be a single category, and all types of technicians can be grouped.

However, in designing the groupings, it should be kept in mind that the primary purpose of the listing has to do with space. A distinction should thus be maintained between workers who are associated with a distinct work area and those who float—cleaners and messengers, for example. The floating worker population may not need a work station for the performance of duties, but they will need to be counted to determine the level of such supporting services as employee health service, day care, cafeteria, washrooms, and lockers. Their numbers will also have an impact on traffic and parking.

It is helpful to list separately full-time and part-time personnel and to record both the headcount (HC) and the full-time-equivalency (FTE) of part-time workers. This should be based on departmental measures rather than on the number of hours worked by an employee: If a clerk works half-time in the radiology area and half time in the emergency room, the clerk may appear on personnel records as a full-time employee. For planning purposes it is more important to know that each of these functions needs a half-time person than it is to know that one person is working full-time.

A summary of personnel for each shift might look like this:

Table EC-6. Personal Summary by Department and Category—Dayshift

Depart-ment	Clerical			Technicians			Maintenance Messengers		
		Part time			Part time			Part time	
	Full time	FTE	HC	Full time	FTE	HC	Full time	FTE	HC
A	10	3	9	4	1	2	—	—	—
B	3	1.5	3	—	.3	1	2	2	3
C	2	—	—	3	4	6	—	.5	1
Totals	15	6	12	7	5.3	9	2	2.5	4

To find out how many people are actually on hand during the day, add up the full-time column and the headcount column of part-time employees. To determine the total of full-time equivalent workers, add up the full time, and the full-time equivalent column of part-timers. If shifts are staggered, a computerized listing may be needed to determine the maximum number of people in the building at one time. Overlapping shifts will affect the need for parking.

A further step, after a detailed listing such as the one illustrated has been made, will be to summarize the departments and categories of workers by function in the same way as was done for facilities in the first part of this chapter.

3

Outpatient Services

3.1. BACKGROUND/DISCUSSION

Until the turn of the century hospitals were charitable institutions for the care of the poor. It was not until medicine developed scientifically and technologically that the more affluent and their doctors made use of hospital inpatient services. In the case of hospital outpatient services, this trend did not make itself felt until much later. Only recently have several factors changed the nature of hospital outpatient services and made it necessary to consider them in a new light.

A major factor has been government provision of support for medical services to the poor, which has enabled this portion of the population to buy its care where it would, or could. In some cases this reduced the numbers of patients using large public or private hospital clinics, because these patients could now make use of the services of private physicians. However, in many of the larger metropolitan areas there were few alternatives to the large hospital clinic, and the utilization of their services remained the same or increased. Whatever the volume of visits, it became clear that the hospitals could no longer consider these patients medically indigent and that consequently the same quality of care would have to be provided as was given to private patients. Although it may continue in fact, a two-class system of care is no longer acceptable in principle.

Concurrently, with the ability of a larger part of the population to choose and pay for services, there have been decreases in the ability of the health care system as a whole to provide certain services even to those willing and able to pay for them. The decrease in the number of general practitioners is one factor: In 1965, 57% of all doctors in the United States were practicing primary care. By 1970 the proportion had gone down to 50.3%, and only two years after that it was down to 42.9%. Although attempts to mitigate the situation are being made from several directions, there is little evidence to suggest that the trend away from general pracice will be turned around as long as specialization continues to return so much greater dividends of status, financial security, and intellectual stimulation to the physician. It has become difficult for even the middle-class consumer to find a provider of primary care and a guide through the maze of specialization. The hospital-based clinic thus becomes a relatively attractive alternative.

From the physician's point of view also, the hospital has become increasingly attractive as a place to treat his ambulatory patients. As sophisticated and expensive technologies proliferate, it becomes less feasible for a doctor to provide his own diagnostic and treatment facilities. Group practice arrangements enable doctors to provide some of these, but there is no question that the availability of extensive supporting services gives the hospital a central role in the provision of all types of medical care. Questions of legal liability have also, perhaps, served to encourage the doctor to refer patients to hospital outpatient and emergency departments or to see them there. A study by the American Hospital Association (*Hospitals* V.47 No. 18, 1973, Research Capsule #11) shows that in the fifteen years between 1955 and 1971, while hospital outpatient visits as a whole (including clinic and emergency visits) increased by about 180%, referrals increased by about 250%.

Although it has been apparent for some time that third-party payment policies were encouraging unnecessary hospitalization and unnecessary emergency room visits, it is only relatively recently that a reasonable amount of documentation of this fact has been available and that substantial moves have been made to change reimbursement policies and to increase the availability of comprehensive health care. It will still be some time before a full range of preventive care services become available to the population as a whole and even longer before the effcts on the health of the population and on the health care field can be measured.

It can be argued that many of the factors that affect the utilization of hospital outpatient services, such as availability of professional manpower, the mobility of the population, and the means of payment for services, may be quite easily and significantly affected by unforseen circumstances and by social and political decisions. The one factor that appears unlikely to change is the continued demand for complex and expensive medical instrumentation and equipment, and it is this that appears to argue most definitively that hospital-based clinics are not a passing phenomenon. This is not to say that all clinic services will be centrally located in the hospital but to suggest that the hospital will increasingly be the organizational, clinical, and technical focal point of such services.

The modes in which preventive, comprehensive, primary, and specialty care are organized, provided, and paid for are undergoing so much discussion, experimentation, and change that even the vocabulary changes from one year to the next. It is thus impossible to describe all the possible permutations. What follows is an outline of some of the key distinctions that may be made in attempting to sort out those elements applicable to a particular situation, their interrelationships, and their impacts on each other.

Characteristics of the Patients and Their Behavior

- Their sexes, ages, and social, racial, and economic characteristics.
- Where they live, how they get to the hospital, and how long it takes them.
- Why they choose this hospital; how they are referred.
- How they present themselves; by appointment, by clinic schedule, on an emergency basis.
- The mechanism by which they pay for the services rendered them.

Characteristics of the Providers and Their Behavior

- Who provides the services—nurse, physician assistant, attending or staff physician, house officer, specialist, superspecialist.
- The times at which the provider is available.
- The mechanism whereby the provider is paid for his services.
- The mechanism by which the providers' services are organized and scheduled.
- The relationships among the providers, the hospital, the outpatient and emergency departments and the supporting departments.

Characteristics of the Service

- Preventive
- Diagnostic
- Therapeutic
- Managerial
- Follow-up
- Rehabilitative
- Consultive
- Scheduled
- Unscheduled

Characteristics of the Illness or Disability

- Episodic
- Chronic
- Emergency
- Urgent
- Noncritical
- Medical
- Surgical
- Psychiatric
- Etc.

These lists are clearly not exhaustive: They are provided merely to suggest a framework for organizing a complex subject.

Certain attitudes and decisions taken with regard to the relationships among the several parts of an outpatient service and between the outpatient services and the hospital as a whole will have a critical impact on the the hospital design process. The traffic generated by any but the smallest outpatient service is considerable; it is generally considered desirable to remove outpatient traffic from inpatient areas. It may, however, be considered desirable to locate the outpatient service near the emergency department or near certain supporting services which also serve inpatients. If so, consideration must be given to screening, both visually and auditorily, the ambulance entrance. It is the architect's problem to resolve these issues and arrive at an acceptable compromise if all criteria cannot be met—but it is the responsibility of the hospital to define its priorities. Some of the most important questions are outlined below.

- What attitude is to be taken towards the noncritical patients who use the emergency room as a replacement for the family doctor? Are these patients to be discouraged from this practice by education or other means? Or will some legitimate structure be provided to deal with them on the assumption that a felt need is being expressed for which the hospital can best provide a service? Will a walk-in primary care clinic be provided? Will this be an extension of the emergency department and its triage area?
- To what degree is integration of inpatient and outpatient services necessary or desirable from the standpoint of clinical practice or efficient utilization of supporting facilities? From an educational standpoint?
- What degree of autonomy will the outpatient department have, in both clinical and organizational terms? That is, who will control it and how?

What will the professional staffing be, and who will control these and how?

Distribution and Relationships Among Outpatient Services

To facilitate discussion of this complex subject, it is suggested that a diagram be drawn up, showing the flow of patients from one unit to another and indicating the impact on ancillary and supporting departments. In the example, only major elements are shown. Where more detailed data are available and needed, such a diagram can be expanded to show additional elements and secondary impacts.

In the example shown, 60,000 patients come through the emergency entrance in a year's time. Of these 40,000 or 67% are considered true emergencies and are dealt with in the emergency department or admitted to the hospital. Those who are not admitted may be treated and kept for observation, treated and dismissed without further referral, or referred for further treatment and follow-up care. The 15,000 patients in the latter category become part of the scheduled clinic work load. The 40,000 true emergency cases account for 74,000 radiology procedures.

The noncritical portion of the emergency work load is subdivided into two further categories: those who are treated and dismissed and those who are referred to the scheduled outpatient clinics for diagnosis or treatment. The 10,000 visits in the latter group, added to the 15,000 true emergency cases referred to the scheduled clinics, together account for 19% of visits to the general clinics and 20% of visits to the specialty and subspecialty clinics.

The scheduled clinics account for a total of 130,000 visits a year. The larger portion of these visits occur in the general clinics where 15,000 visits are the result of visits initially made to the emergency department. The balance of 65,000 visits are referred from outside by physicians, social agencies, or the patients themselves. The scheduled clinics account for 162,500 radiology procedures per year, or 61% of the total outpatient radiology work load. The balance of the work load comes from the emergency room (74,000 procedures) and from referrals by private physicians or other hospitals (30,000 procedures).

In the following sections outpatient services will be discussed separately according to the nature of their organization, that is, scheduled and unscheduled. This distinction is made because the way of calculating requirements depends on the degree to which demand is either controlable or predictable. The work load of scheduled clinics can be at least partly controlled: It is the hospital's choice how much service is to be provided and how it is to be organized. In the case of emergency and unsched-

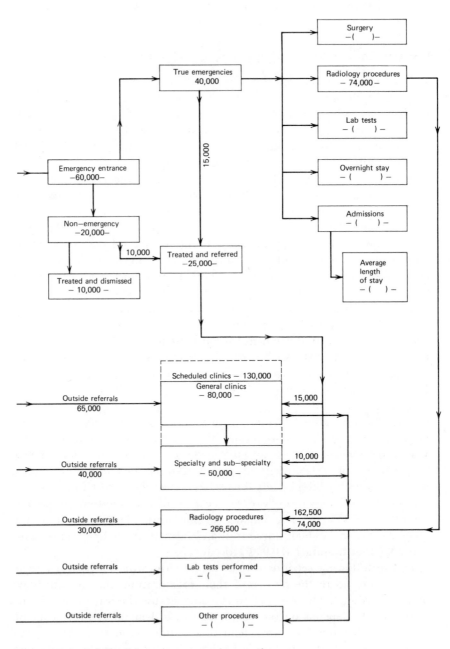

Figure OP-A Relationships among outpatient service.

uled services the rules are clearly quite different: Demand may be predicted but not controlled. And forces outside the hospital and its staff will have a much greater impact on the emergency department. The term "unscheduled services" is thus used to denote both emergency services and primary care or other clinic services, such as walk-in or evening clinics, which may be offered as an alternative to the emergency department on a nonscheduled basis.

It is perhaps appropriate to note at this point that statistics which are available about outpatient services suffer from serious problems of definition. There appears to be little agreement as to what constitutes an outpatient visit (some hospitals count a referral to the radiology department as an outpatient visit, and some do not); what is meant by a referral; and how a true emergency is to be defined. It will be important, therefore, that early in the planning effort all relevant terms be clearly defined so that all members of the planning team will be speaking in equivalent terms.

3.2. UNSCHEDULED AND EMERGENCY OUTPATIENT SERVICES

The kind of information that must be gathered in planning for the emergency department depends very much on local situations and on policies of the hospital and of local regulatory agencies. Some of the main considerations that should be discussed and clarified before beginning specific planning are suggested below.

General Planning and Policy Decisions Needed

1. What changes in the characteristics of the service area population are in prospect that may affect the volume and types of visits to the emergency department?

2. What is the attitude of the hospital to the different kinds of patients who make use of the emergency room? That is, will nonemergency patients be discouraged from using it and, if so, how? What procedures will be used to sort them out from the true emergency patients when they do appear at the emergency room? What alternative provision will be made for them?

3. In the light of current efforts to categorize emergency departments by the type of care they are equipped to deliver and to match this to local and regional needs, what role is the hospital likely to play in its particular region? What would be the impact on the hospital as a whole, and on the emergency department itself, of such categorization? That is, would services not currently available have to be added to bring the

emergency facilities up to a certain standard? Would this tend to increase the work load both for the emergency room and for other hospital services? Would it increase admissions to a significant degree? Conversely, if the emergency department fell into a lower category, would this lose patients for the hospital as a whole?

4.   What is the estimated peak load that the emergency room must be able to handle with reasonable ease? How is the estimate arrived at? What provision must be made for numbers beyond this in the event of major disasters?

5.   What arrangements will be made for medical staffing of the emergency department: for example, physician rotation, on-call assignments, full time medical director, group practice arrangement?

Answers to these general questions will dictate the level of detail and specific questions for planning. The steps outlined represent the kinds of procedures that may be needed for certain situations, but it would be impossible to cover all eventualities in a methodology of this kind. The planner will have to adjust the procedures to reflect the particular problem: If there is to be no attempt to sort out nonemergency patients from true emergency patients, for example, it would be wasted effort to analyze this characteristic of the work load.

Emergency Department—Current Conditions

Work Load: Step One

Purpose

To determine the net growth of emergency room visits over a selected period and, if possible, to determine changes in the nature of the visits. To determine changes in the ratio of emergency visits per 1000 population for the emergency service area.

Information needed

1.   Emergency department statistics for a selected period. Depending on how records are kept and what statistics are routinely developed, it may or may not be possible to determine changes in the ratio of true emergencies to total emergency room visits and the age, sex, and economic status of patients.

2.   Population data covering the same period for the hospital's emergency service area (which may or may not be the same as the general service area) indicating total population and population by age, sex, and economic condition, if a detailed analysis is to be done.

Procedure

If census data or estimates are available at 5-year intervals, the census years may be matched to the same year of emergency room statistics to estimate the emergency room visits per 1000 population for each period. The data may be tabulated as follows:

Table ER-1.

Year	Service Area Population	Emergency Visits	
		Total Visits	Visits per Thousand
Year 0	—	—	—
Year 5	—	—	—
Year 10	—	—	—

The analysis may be expanded by breaking down, for each year, the population by age, sex or other relevant factors for each year. A simple graph may help to illustrate the concurrent trends.

Work Load: Step Two

Purpose

If a simple projection of current patterns based on internal evidence and population trends is all that is needed, the preceding data will provide an adequate base. However, if there are plans either by the area hospitals or by government agencies to categorize emergency facilities or if the hospital itself wishes to examine and perhaps change its emergency service, it will be necessary to go beyond the basic analysis. How this is done will depend largely on the kinds of records that are kept and the kinds of analyses that may have previously been done by the hospital. Before beginning a more detailed analysis, therefore, it will be necessary to determine exactly what needs to be known about the emergency department's work load, what data is already available, and what amount of effort can be expended to collect additional data. The basic purpose of this step is to sort the emergency room visits by chosen categories and to determine their utilization patterns. Since patterns may provide clues to such questions as who the patients are and why they use the emergency room, work load and utilization should be studied together.

Planning decisions needed

1.   What categories of emergency room patients need to be identified? For example: true emergencies, primary care; surgical patients, medical patients; major surgical and minor surgical; major medical and minor medical; adult and pediatric; and so on.

2.   Once it has been determined what categories of patients or disabilities are pertinent, clear and concise definitions must be developed; for example: What constitutes a true emergency? What is the line between major and minor? At what age does a patient stop being a child and become an adult?

3.   Will it be necessary to determine historical trends with regard to the distinction of emergency visits, or will it be sufficient to study data from the immediately preceding year? The director and staff of the emergency department may be able to estimate whether or not the distribution of types of visits has changed significantly, and in what areas. These areas can then be studied in historical perspective.

Information needed

Depending on the detail required for the study, some or all of the following information may be needed:

1.   The types of patients by: residence; age and sex; economic status; how they were referred; how they arrived at the emergency room and when.

2.   The categories of visits broadly by degree of urgency: major emergency; urgent but not life threatening; nonemergency.

3.   Similar to above, the categories of visits in more detail by: trauma; medical emergencies (diagnosis); surgical emergencies (diagnosis); minor, urgent (diagnosis); general medical care—primary care—nonemergency.

4.   Characteristics of visits: patterns of utilization of the emergency room by month, day of the week, hours of the day or night; patients admitted for observation, acute care, or intensive care (by type); radiology procedures generated; laboratory procedures generated; other procedures generated.

Procedure

The arrangement of data will depend on which data have been selected as significant. The table below suggests how a matrix may be drawn to illustrate a hypothetical case at a minimal level of detail. If a historical trend analysis is to be done, a table of this kind can be drawn up for each year, or for each year at a 5-year interval, to correspond to Table ER-1.

Table ER-2. Distribution of Emergency Visits by Age and Visit Category (Years)

Characteristics of Visits	Patients by Age (or Other Characteristic)			
	0–14	15–64	65-up	Total
Trauma	—	—	—	—
Surgical Emergencies	—	—	—	—
Medical Emergencies	—	—	—	—
Nonemergencies	—	—	—	—

Peak Loads

Procedure

The data summarized in the table below may provide clues as to why the emergency department is used in the way it is. A regular heavy load of injuries on Friday and Saturday nights will suggest that the work load results from normal weekend celebration, but heavy loads of nonemergency visits in the daytime and early evening may suuggest that patients do not have an accessible source of primary care. Evening non-emergency visits throughout the week would tend to suggest the same and also that patients do not wish or are unable to contact their physicians at that time. The more specific the time categories are, the more useful the information; but this type of data may be hard to extract from records. To arrive at the numbers of visits for each day and time span, a typical week should be selected, or the data from several weeks may be averaged.

Table ER-3. Distribution of Visits by Time and Type

Day and Time of Visits	Characteristics of Visits				
	Total Visits	Trauma	Surgical Emergency	Medical Emergency	Non-Emergency
Weekdays					
9 am–5 pm	—	—	—	—	—
5–9 pm	—	—	—	—	—
Fridays					
8 am–5 pm	—	—	—	—	—
5–9 pm	—	—	—	—	—
9–2 am	—	—	—	—	—
Saturdays	—	—	—	—	—

Facilities

Purpose

To determine the overall adequacy of emergency facilities for the current work load and to identify any deficiencies in space or location.

Information needed

1.   A list of the major rooms used by the emergency department, their net areas, and their approximate capacities, for example, treatment room (four beds).

2.   Summary of physical relationships and means of access to major supporting areas such as operating rooms, intensive care, radiology facilities.

Procedure

Summarize the total area and major rooms available to the emergency department. A tabulation might look like this:

Table ER-4.   Summary of Facilities

Room Type	Number of Rooms	Capacity	Area NSF
Waiting	1	15 seats	300
Exam/Treatment	4	8 stations	800
Minor OR	2	2 stations	540
Resuscitation	1	1 bed	120
Observation	1	6 beds	500
Isolation	1	1 bed	150
Other	—	—	600
Total Area			3010

Utilization of facilities

Procedure

Using Table ER-4 and Table ER-3, which outlines typical utilization patterns, discuss with the emergency department's director and medical and nursing staff the adequacy of facilities as related to the average and peak work load. The impressions of the staff, who are familiar with the day-to-day operation of the facility, will be invaluable in estimating the extent of deficiencies and may provide suggestions for further analysis or directions for planning. They may suggest, for example, that their current space would be adequate if some other provision could be made for the nonemergency portion of the load; or that they could handle a work load of *x* number of cases on Friday nights if they merely had one more examination and treatment room and a bit more waiting space. The comments and suggestions of the department should be briefly summarized and a percentage estimate made of space deficiency under current work loads.

Impact of the emergency room on other departments

Purpose and information needed

To determine the amount of work load which the emergency room generates for other departments of the hospital. If data is available, this may be done on the basis of annual statistics. If not, a survey may be made of several typical days or weeks of activity. The data may be obtainable from the emergency department itself or from the records of other departments. The amount of data that will be needed depends on the particular project. In particular, plans for categorization of hospital emergency rooms will suggest that a full study be done in order to determine what the impact of decisions will be. (See Table ER-5).

Personnel

Purpose

To determine staffing patterns.

Procedure

A verbal statement should be obtained from the emergency department as to how coverage of the emergency department is arranged. Since in many departments a number of medical and nursing staff will be on call or working elsewhere with a priority for assignment to the emergency room when needed, it may be difficult to find out exactly how many man-hours are expended in the emergency department. The best approach appears to be to examine the work hours assigned during a typical week and extrapolate from that. (See Table ER-6). The same breakdown of hours should be used as was used for Table ER-3.

Emergency Department—Projections

Work load

Purpose

To determine the volume and type of visits to the emergency department at a target date.

Table ER-5. Work Loads Generated by the Emergency Department

Hospital Functions		Annual Number	
Admissions	Average Length of Stay of ER Admissions	Patient days	Number per 100 ER Visits
All admissions from ER	—	—	—
Acute care:			
Medical	—	—	—
Surgical	—	—	—
Psychiatric	—	—	—
Other	—	—	—
Intensive:			
Medical	—	—	—
Surgical	—	—	—
Cardiac	—	—	—
Other	—	—	—

		Procedures	Number per 100 ER Visits
Surgical Procedures:			
General surgery	—	—	—
Orthopedics	—	—	—
Etc.	—	—	—
Diagnostic Radiology:			
Procedure Type A	—	—	—
Procedure Type B	—	—	—
Etc.	—	—	—
Laboratory:			
Test Type A	—	—	—
Test Type B	—	—	—
Etc.	—	—	—
Human Function Diagnostic and Treatment:			
Pulmonary Lab	—	—	—
Hemodialysis	—	—	—
EEG	—	—	—
Pharmacy:			
Emergency prescriptions	—	—	—
Other orders	—	—	—
Referrals:			
Outpatient screening clinic	—	—	—
Other outpatient clinics	—	—	—
Follow-up referrals	—	—	—

Table ER-6.   Emergency Room Man-Hours per Week (FTE)

	Physicians	Nurses	Aides	Porters	Clerical	Other	Total
Weekdays	—	—	—	—	—	—	—
9–5	—	—	—	—	—	—	—
Etc.	—	—	—	—	—	—	—
Fridays	—	—	—	—	—	—	—
Etc.	—	—	—	—	—	—	—
Weekly Total	—	—	—	—	—	—	—

Information needed

1.   Projected population estimates for the emergency service area for the target date.

2.   Data from Table ER-1 showing the trend in the hospital's emergency load per 1000 population of its service area.

(*Note*: The preceding two elements may be considered as totals, or for more detailed projections broken down by age and other categories.)

3.   Data from Table ER-2 showing characteristics of visits by category of patient.

4.   Any operative regulations or directives with regard to the distribution or organization of emergency services that will have an immediate impact on planning.

5.   Information on other emergency resources available in the area.

Planning and policy decisions needed

1.   Assuming a constant rate of emergency visits per 1000 population, what adjustments should be made on the basis of increases or decreases in the *hospital's share* of emergency visits by the population as a whole?

2.   What are the national or regional trends in emergency visits per 1000 population that may make it necessary to adjust the visit/population ratio as a whole?*

3.   Should the questions outlined above be considered for the emergency department's total visit load?

4.   Should the nonemergency portion of the work load be projected separately?

5.   Are there any external factors, such as changes in third-party payment policies, changes in the characteristics of the population, reduction

* Between 1955 and 1970 the national figure of ER visits per 1000 rose from 64 to 212.

in the number of available family practice physicians, and so forth, which are likely to have a significant effect on the volume and types of visits? How can these be evaluated and quantified?

6. What effect will categorization of emergency facilities have on the hospital's emergency department? What category is the hospital likely to fall into? Would visits be increased or reduced, and by how much?

Summarize the projections on the basis of decisions made with regard to these questions.

Procedure

The detail to which projections are made will depend on particular circumstances. The procedure outlined below illustrates a general level, continuing the examples in the preceding section:

Table ER-7. Projected Emergency Visits

Category of Visits	Current Visits—Year 19			Projected Visits—Year 19			
	Popula-tion	Visits	Visits per Thousand	Popula-tion	Visits per Thousand	Visits	% Incr.
Surgical Emergencies	—	—	—	—	—	—	—
Medical Emergencies	—	—	—	—	—	—	—
Nonemergencies	—	—	—	—	—	—	—
Totals	—	—	—	—	—	—	—

Utilization patterns

Purpose

To project the numbers and types of visits for a typical week by day and time of day.

Information needed

1. Data from Table ER-7 above, indicating the distribution of visits by category.

2. Information from Table ER-3, showing the distribution of the current work load during a typical week.

Planning decision needed

Should it be assumed that the cuurrent distribution of visits by type and by time of day will continue? If not, how should it be adjusted?

Procedure

On the basis of percentage increases shown in Table ER-7 above for each category of patient, adjust the current pattern of visits (Table ER-3) to reflect the projection:

Table ER-8. Distribution of Visits by Time and Type—Projected

Day and Time of Visits	Characteristics of Visits			
	Surgical Emergency	Medical Emergency	Nonemergency	Total
Weekdays				
9–5 pm	—	—	—	—
5–9 pm	—	—	—	—
Etc.	—	—	—	—
Fridays				
9–5 pm	—	—	—	—
5–9 pm	—	—	—	—
9–2 am	—	—	—	—
Etc.	—	—	—	—

Distribution of facilities

Purpose

To determine alternatives and requirements for the relationships of major functions.

Information needed

Information collected in the analysis of current facilities, showing the amount and type of space currently available, relationships to other departments, and estimates of deficiency.

Planning and policy decisions needed—Emergency and Ancillary departments

1. How will the nonemergency portion of the patient load be handled? Will there be a triage area where patients are evaluated? What

disposition will be made of patients who are deemed to be nonemergencies? During the day, when clinics are in session? In the late afternoon and evening, and on weekends? Will there be a general medical or screening clinic associated with the emergency room to take care of these patients?

2. Should there be a separate entrance for emergency vehicles and patients who arrive by car or on foot?

3. What types of surgery (if any) with what types of anesthetic will be done in the emergency department itself? What relationship is required to the major operating suites? What ancillary surgical facilities are required in the emergency department?

4. What will be the relationship of the emergency department to radiology facilities? Will the emergency department have its own facility?

5. Will there be a 24-hour emergency laboratory near the emergency room? Is a laboratory required in the department itself?

6. Will there be a unit of short-stay observation beds for the emergency department itself, or shared with other departments? What will be the criteria for admission? Where should the unit be located?

Projected Space Requirements

Purpose

To make a rough estimate of space requirements.

Procedure

A straight projection of area requirements related to numbers of visits can be applied for general long-range planning *if* the types of functions and activities remain relatively the same and if there are no major changes in the distribution of types of visits or the pattern of visits in time. Using current visit data and current area, calculate the annual number of visits per net square foot after any adjustments have been made to correct deficiencies in area. For example: Assume that 40,000 visits a year are handled in an area of 5000 net square feet and that the space deficit is estimated at 15%. To operate effectively under the current work load a total of 5750 net square feet would thus be required. Dividing the annual visits by this area results in a planning guideline of seven visits per net square foot. Extrapolating from this, a projected annual visit load of 60,000 visits would require 8600 net square feet.

Procedure—To make a detailed estimate

On the basis of the work load projections summarized in Table ER-8 discuss with the emergency department's clinical and supporting staff

the numbers and types of facilities that will be required to handle the typical patient load at peak periods. Determine the number of casualty patients who will need to be accommodated in the event of a catastrophe and how they should or can be provided for.

This discussion should not focus on room sizes or groupings of beds at this stage of planning. Questions should be expressed in terms of numbers of beds or work stations that can be converted to square footage later. For purposes of comparison, the results of these space projections may be compared to existing facilities by using the visits-per-net-square-foot method previously described.

Personnel

Purpose

To estimate the man-hours needed to operate the emergency department at the target date, either by weekly total or by time period.

Information needed

1.   Data from Table ER-6 showing weekly man-hours by personnel category and time.
2.   Data from Table ER-3 showing visits by visit category and time.

Procedure

Match the number of man-hours to the number of visits to arrive at a ratio that can be used for projection. For example, if there were 800 visits during a typical week and 600 man-hours spent in the emergency room during that week, there would be 1.33 visits per man hour, or .75 man-hours per visit. Apply this ratio to the projected number of visits to determine the man-hours needed. This method assumes that the current staffing pattern will continue and that there will be no major changes in the distribution of visits by category, but it should be sufficiently accurate for general planning.

3.3.   SCHEDULED OUTPATIENT SERVICES

Background

A clinic consultation is an attempt to reproduce efficiently on a mass scale what essentially should be a private, unhurried and dignified personal consultation. *Mr. R. G. Main, Surgeon, Falkirk Royal Infirmary*

Scheduled clinics may be defined as that portion of outpatient activity for which there is sufficient regular and predictable demand so that it can be organized into a system. The level of activity may not be so great as to qualify as being "on a massive scale," but it must be great enough to warrant repetitive scheduling. Lack of efficiency in clinic operations will not have the devastating financial impact of unused hospital beds, but it is certainly in the interest of the hospital to develop a reasonable standard of efficiency in the utilization of clinic staff and facilities, not only for financial reasons but because increasingly the outpatient service will be the community's primary point of contact with the hospital. Several factors are important to efficient utilization: These are discussed briefly below. An initial awareness of the importance of these factors will enable the planner to be alert for weaknesses in the present system as he collects data on current conditions.

Organization and Utilization

Appointment systems

Many hospital clinics operate on what is called a block appointment system. The word "appointment" used in this context is misleading: The system merely calls for a certain number of patients to be present at a given time. The system is intended to provide a sufficient pool of patients so that the physician will at no time find himself idle and to limit the pool to the capacity of the waiting room. The system results in long waiting times for a majority of patients. For example, if twelve patients are told to arrive at ten in the morning and if each visit takes about 10 minutes with the doctor, the first four patients would experience a waiting time of 30 minutes or less. The rest would experience waiting times of between 30 minutes and 1 hour and 50 minutes. Knowledgeable patients may try to outwit the system by arriving late, but if, as often happens, the physician is also late they will still spend a long time waiting. Some studies suggest that patients can be relied upon to keep individual appointments with a reasonable degree of punctuality if it is demonstrated that the bargain will be kept from the clinic's side. Other studies suggest the reverse. It appears likely that this is a matter very much dependent on the attitudes, experiences, and customs of particular population groups as well as on local means of transportation, availability of parking, and so on. The advisability of using an individual appointment system is, therefore, something that should be explored in the light of local conditions.

Physician punctuality

More than one study has concluded that lack of physician punctuality may be more of a problem than lack of patient punctuality.

Use of examining and consulting rooms

The sequences of physician activity and patient activity during the visit can have a considerable impact on the use of examination and consultation rooms during the time the clinic is scheduled and thus on the turnover of patients. There are a number of configurations of rooms and sequences of activity in common use. One arrangement is for the doctor to have at his disposal a consultation room or office and two examining rooms. A patient is seen in the office, then goes to one of the examining rooms where he undresses and waits. In the meantime the doctor is seeing a second patient in his office. When the second patient is sent to the second examining room to undress and wait, the doctor examines the first patient. The first patient then dresses and waits while the doctor examines the second patient. While the doctor is giving instructions, prescriptions, or explanations to the first patient in the office consultation room, the second patient waits again. The purpose of this arrangement is to make the fullest use of the doctor's time, which is more precious, at least in this context, than the patient's. However, a British study showed that a physician who had a single room at his disposal—a combined consultation/examination room with a curtained cubicle behind which the patient could undress and dress—was able to make about 30% more effective use of his time; in addition he felt that he was able to give fuller attention to his patients and experienced a reduction in pressure. He could use the time during which the patient was undressing to complete his notes on the previous patient, and while the patient was dressing he could either write up that visit or answer the patient's questions through the curtain. And the patient spent no time waiting during the course of the examination itself. This finding would, of course, be inapplicable to clinics where a nurse or physician assistant is performing a part of the examination.

Effect of the efficiency of ancillary and supporting services

If appointments can be coordinated and results quickly obtained from radiology or laboratories, many long waits for patients or repeat visits can be avoided. Difficulties in obtaining medical records can also account for long waits.

Common or shared use of facilities

The greater the shared use of facilities, the more efficient scheduling of clinic sessions can be. If facilities are flexibly designed there is no reason why most clinics cannot use the same basic clinic module. In most cases only equipment differs. Certain types of treatment rooms are specialized, but most examination and consultation rooms are of similar design and configuration.

Scheduling of physician's time

If the clinic itself is in control of the doctor's time and can schedule him according to the dictates of demand and utilization of facilities, the clinic can function more efficiently than if scheduling is done at the convenience or availability of the physician. Thus, a clinic that operates on a contractual basis with the physician will be more efficient than one which operates less formally.

Location

The structure of outpatient services may interlock with the rest of the hospital in a range of modalities all the way from complete integration to an almost self-sufficient and separate facility. Some of the common arguments *for* separate facilities are:

- A separate organization can function more efficiently in terms of scheduling and communications and is easier for the patient to find his way around in.
- It removes outpatients from the central hospital where they present a traffic and control problem, and thus makes the circulation and access problems of both inpatient and outpatient sections easier to solve.
- It enables the outpatient department to develop a clear structure of its own and reduces the tendency of clinicians and administrators to regard it as a stepchild.
- It may be easier to expand.
- It may be more centrally located in relation to the population it serves.
- It may require a less expensive structure.

The arguments *against* separating include:

- Clinical standards may be lower because outpatient physicians will lose touch with their inpatient counterparts. Departmental affiliations may be weakened.
- Separate ancillary departments may be difficult to staff and may suffer from a lack of professional supervision.
- Distance between inpatient and outpatient facilities may be an inconvenience to doctors who have responsibilities in both areas.

- A separate facility may require duplication of certain services that could otherwise be shared.
- Some outpatient facilities require a relationship to the central hospital because of use by inpatients as well as outpatients.

The question may be asked: What types of activity are both inpatient and outpatient oriented, and what factors are controlling in each case? For example, facilities for rehabilitation may serve a larger number of outpatients than inpatients—but access by inpatients may be the controlling factor. A similar question may arise with regard to psychiatric outpatients. If a large portion of the outpatient load were the result of follow-up visits by patients who had originally been hospitalized it might be determined that, for clinical reasons, it would be desirable to provide continuity not only of staff but of environment and that, therefore, outpatients should be seen in the same place they were seen when they were inpatients.

Scheduled Clinics—Current Conditions

There are two parts to the study of existing conditions. The first is a compilation of data to show the characteristics of the work load and the utilization patterns of clinics; the second is an analyysis that will provide information necessary to the projection of facility requirements.

Work load

Information needed

Outpatient statistics, preferably for a period of not less than 5 years, which show the total number of annual visits for each clinic or specialty, the ratio of new to return visits for each, and the percent of total each group of visits represents. If only a general analysis is called for, the ratio of new and return visits may be omitted. If data are not available for individual clinics, it may be possible to obtain totals for groups of clinics. The information may be displayed as follows:

Table OP-1. Summary of Characteristics of Clinic Workload over an (X)-Year Period

| | Annual Visits | | | | | | | | | |
| | Year 1 | | | | | Year 2 | | | | |
Clinic	New	Return	Total	New:Old Ratio	Percent of Total Visits	New	Return	Total	New:Old Ratio	Percent of Total Visits
Clinic A	35,000	15,000	50,000	70:30	56	40,000	15,000	55,000	73:27	54
Clinic B	10,000	20,000	30,000	33:67	33	12,000	23,000	35,000	34:66	34
Clinic C	8,000	2,000	10,000	80:20	11	9,500	3,000	12,500	76:24	12
Total	53,000	37,000	90,000	59:41	100%	61,500	41,000	102,500	60,40	100%

From the same statistics, calculate the annual rate of change experienced by each clinic or group of clinics from one year to the next, and for the period as a whole:

Table OP-2. Changes in Clinic Visits for an (X)-Year Period

Clinic	Year 1	Year 2		Year 3		Year 4		Year 5		Percent Change over (X) Years
	Number	Number	Percent Change[a]	Number	Percent Change[a]	Number	Percent Change[a]	Number	Percent Change[a]	
Clinic A	50,000	55,000	+10%	—	—	—	—	—	—	—
Clinic B	30,000	35,000	+17%	—	—	—	—	—	—	—
Clinic C	10,000	12,500	+25%	—	—	—	—	—	—	—
Totals	90,000	102,500	+14%	105,000	+2%	108,000	+3%	120,000	+11%	+33%

[a] From preceding year

If planning is to be fairly detailed, it may be desirable to determine the level of fluctuation of visits on a monthly or daily basis or both. Cursory study of the statistics should indicate whether or not fluctuations are significant. If they are, the range of the deviation may be illustrated or summarized by a table comparing the averages, highs, and lows over a selected period:

Table OP-3. Typical Fluctuations in Visits by Days of the Week (or Month)

Day (Month)	Number of Visits over (X) Period		
	Average	High	Low
Mondays	—	—	—
Tuesdays	—	—	—
Etc.	—	—	—

Utilization

From clinic schedules for the preceding year determine the number of hours the clinic was in session. Determine or estimate the number of exam rooms* used per clinic session, and multiply the number of session hours by the number of exam rooms to arrive at the number of room-hours scheduled. If it is impossible to sort out the rooms used by a

---

* *Note on clinic planning method:* The examination room is used as the key in dealing with scheluled clinics because it is the factor common to all: Supporting facilities can be derived from the number of exam rooms after utilization assumptions for the latter have been decided.

given clinic, it may be necessary to recombine groups of clinics and match them to a group of exam rooms that they use in common. The information may be summarized thus:

Table OP-4. Summary of Annual Clinic Hours and Rooms

Clinic	Annual Clinic-Session Hours Scheduled	Number of Exam Rooms	Annual Exam-Room Hours
Clinic A	1389	24	33,336
Clinic B	—	—	—
Clinic C	—	—	—
Totals	—	—	—

Facilities

Find the net area assigned to each clinic if the clinic has exclusive use of the space. Where space is shared, the clinics may be combined and the space assigned to the group. The net area should include exam and treatment rooms, consultation rooms, nurses stations, utility rooms, individual clinic waiting areas, and clerical space and circulation within the department. Main waiting areas and circulation should be listed separately. Most of the information needed for this should be available from data collected earlier in the planning process and summarized according to the outline in Chapter 2. The types and numbers of major rooms may be listed, and the information summarized:

Table OP-5. Summary of Clinic Facilities

Clinic	Exam Rooms	Consultation	Treatment	Other	Total Net Areas
Clinic A	24	9	2	—	6624
Clinic B Clinic C	—	—	—	—	—
Totals	—	—	—	—	—

Personnel

List personnel by category. Part-time personnel should be listed by full-time equivalency (FTE) with the numbers of individuals represented shown in parenthesis. The total full-time equivalents and total individuals should be indicated:

Table OP-6.　Summary of Personnel

Personnel Category	Weekdays		All Nights		Saturdays		Total FTE	Total Individuals
	FT	PT	FT	PT	FT	PT		
Nurses	4	3(6)	—	—	2	2(4)	11	16
Etc.	—	—	—	—	—	—	—	—
Totals	—	—	—	—	—	—	—	—

Utilization analysis

Purpose

To analyze the data collected and presented in Part 1 in ways that will facilitate the projection of future requirements. Two methods of analyzing the information are presented; the first very simple, the second somewhat more detailed. The purpose of the second method is to explore the efficiency of the current utilization of facilities.

Procedure: Annual visits per net square foot

This method requires merely that the numbers of visits be divided into the net area available to them. As has been suggested in the previous section, it may be necessary to group the visits of clinics that use facilities on a common basis with other clinics. The figure of visits per net square foot, which is the result of this simple calculation, does, of course, reflect differences in utilization—but taken alone it does not provide enough information to allow for adjustments in future planning. The range of difference among clinics and among hospitals is so great that as a general planning standard it is only useful at the most general level. As a reflection of the status quo at a particular

Table OP-7.　Average Annual Visits per Net Square Foot

Clinics	Annual Visits	Net Area	Annual Visits per NSF
Clinic A	50,000	6624	7.5
Clinic B } Clinic C }	—	—	—
Central Facilities	—	—	—
Totals	—	—	—

institution it may be adequate, however. Using data from the immediately preceding year (Table OP-1 and OP-2) and the net area per clinic (Table OP-5) calculate the numbers of visits per net square foot for each clinic or for all clinics. For central shared facilities, use the total visits of all clinics, or apportion the area to the individual clinics on a pro rata basis.

Procedure: Average visits per exam-room hour

This method allows for future adjustment of the several factors, but it is based on averages and is, therefore, not sufficiently refined to be used for actual scheduling. The purpose of the method is to determine the relationship, in current practice, between numbers of visits and the room-hours scheduled to accommodate them. Room-Hours refers to the number of rooms used, multiplied by the number of clinic session hours scheduled. Average Visits Per Room Hours refers to the total number of visits divided by the total room-hours available; it does *not* refer to actual time used by visits. The figure incorporates whatever efficiency factor is currently operative. Average Minutes per Visit (60 divided by average visits per room-hour) is an alternate way of expressing the time factor.

Using data from Tables OP-2 and OP-4, calculate the visits per room-hour for each clinic or group of clinics and summarize as follows:

Table OP-8. Average Visits per Room-Hour—Year (and/or Average Minutes per Visit)

Clinic	Annual Visits	Annual Exam Room-Hours	Average Visits per Room-Hour	Average Minutes per Visit
Clinic A	50,000	33,336	1.5	40
Clinic B	—	—	—	—
Clinic C	—	—	—	—
Totals	—	—	—	—

If the figure of minutes per visit appears high, this is because of the problem of scheduling. There will always be times when the number of rooms available does not match the number of visits, and a room or two will stand empty part of the time. Clinics must be scheduled for a specific time and place, and no matter how flexible the facilities and efficient the appointment system, 100% efficiency of utilization cannot be achieved. If one could assume that on the average the patient actually spends 25 minutes in an exam room, the efficiency rate in the example would be 63% (25÷40).

Procedure: Determining efficiency of clinic facilities utilization

The utilization of rooms during the time that clinics are in session is only one factor in determining efficiency. In the same way that rooms cannot be filled all of the available time, so also clinics themselves cannot be scheduled 100% of the time. It will be useful, both in an assessment of current operations and for projections of future requirements, to determine the current level of efficiency of clinic utilization. This may be done by computing the percentage of time that clinics are scheduled as a ratio of the time they potentially could be scheduled. To do this, it will be necessary to decide on a figure that can realistically be considered as representing 100% efficiency. Such an ideal or potential figure might be 2500 hours a year per room (8 hours a day, 6 days a week) or 1560 hours a year (6 hours a day, 5 days a week). In the example below, 1820 hours has been chosen as a reasonable potential, representing 100% efficiency. The clinic efficiency rate in the example is 76% or the ratio between the actual 33,336 room-hours scheduled and the potential 43,680 room hours available. If data are available, the calculation should be made separately for each clinic.

Table OP-9.   Average Clinic Utilization—100% = 1820 Hours per Room

Clinic	Number of Rooms	Actual Room Hrs Scheduled	Potential Room Hours	Percent Clinic Efficiency Rate
Clinic A	24	33,336 (1389/room)	43,680 (1820/room)	76%
Clinic B	—	—	—	—
Clinic C	—	—	—	—
Totals	—	—	—	—

To summarize, the two steps outlined above provide a means of determining the efficiency of (a) room utilization and (b) clinic scheduling and utilization. While it is obvious that efficiency has a great effect on the planning of facilities, it may be well to illustrate how dramatic the effect can be on space requirements and building costs.

Example

Assume that a clinic currently meets 3 days a week for 5 hours a day, using 16
exam rooms. There are 18,720 visits a year. Scheduled room hours total 12,480
per year (780 hours per room times 16 rooms). Dividing the total visits by the
total room hours shows that on the average there are 1.5 visits per room hour,
or that each visit consumes 40 minutes of available time. The clinic efficiency
rate is about 43%, using 1820 potential room hours as representing
100% efficiency (780 ÷ 1820). Let us assume that space requirements for this clinic
total 9350 gross square feet. At $75.00 per square foot, the space required for
this clinic would cost over $700,000 to construct.

Keeping all other factors constant, how much space would be required to
accommodate this clinic if sessions could be scheduled 5 days a week, for 7 hours
a day? In this case each room would have a capacity for 1560 scheduled clinic
hours per year: at the rate of 1.5 visits per room hour each exam room could thus
handle 2340 visits per year. Dividing the annual visit load by the visit capacity
of each room shows that only 8 exam rooms would be needed (18,720 ÷ 2340 = 8).
The clinic efficiency rate would have increased to 86% (1560 ÷ 1820). Space requirement and construction dollars would similarily be reduced to half: The
space would cost only $350,000. It is probably safe to assume that operating cost
would also be considerably reduced.

The presentation of this illustration should provide some food for
thought about the question of space utilization. It must be cautioned,
however, that there may be factors far more important than efficient
utilization of facilities, and the illustration is not intended to suggest
that maximum utilization should be a controlling factor. It is merely
worth pointing out that the cost penalty of loose scheduling can be considerable. Whether or not the cost is justified is a different question
altogether.

Room utilization

Procedure: Actual time per visit

It may be desirable to determine the typical time required for patient
visits to different clinics. There may be clinical standards for the
amount of time an outpatient visitor should spend with a doctor; or
surveys may be made. Physicians and clinic staff may be able to make
good estimates. Whatever means are chosen, the clinical staff should be
the ones responsible for approving the estimates. The purpose of the
exercise is to provide a means of comparing actual exam room time
used to the average visits per room hour. Only the time that the
examination room is in use should be considered, but all of that time

should be included. New and return visits may be shown separately since there may be a considerable difference between the amount of time each consumes. The estimates or survey results may be broken down as follows:

Table OP-9.   Computed Time per Visit for New and Return Visits

Clinic	Undressing and Waiting	Time with Doctor	Dressing and Waiting	Other	Clean up and Preparation	Total Exam Room Minutes per Visit
Clinic A						
New visits	—	—	—	—	—	—
Return visits	—	—	—	—	—	—
Clinic B						
New Visits	—	—	—	—	—	—
Return visits	—	—	—	—	—	—

Procedure: Determining room utilization data

Using the estimates calculated in Table OP-9 and the ratio for each clinic of new to return visits (Table OP-1) compute the number of visits that *could* take place per room hour. This figure represents 100% utilization of the exam room during the time that the clinic is in session No vacancy factor is included in the figure. Using data from Table OP-8, which shows the average visits per room hour, compare the computed visits per room hour with the average visits per room. This ratio is the room utilization rate.

Table OP-10.   Estimated Room Utilization Rate—Computed Visits per Hour = 100%

Clinic	Computed Visits Per Room Hour	Average Scheduled Visits Per Room Hour	Percentage Room Utilization
Clinic A	2.5	1.5	60%
Clinic B	—	—	—

Personnel

Purpose

To determine the total man-hours per clinic visit for all clinic personnel excluding physicians.

Procedure

Multiply the total full-time equivalent personnel from the bottom line of Table OP-6 by the number of hours that are defined as FTE. If this is done by the year, for example, the FTE hours may be 2000. On a daily basis, if a normal work day is 8 hours and there are 10 full-time equivalent personnel on duty, the total man hours for that day would be 80. If these man-hours were spent in a clinic where 120 visits a day took place, the man-hours per visit would be .67. It is normally not necessary for this stage of planning to use detailed data: Totals should be sufficient.

Table OP-11.   Total Man-Hours per Clinic Visit

FTE Personnel	Hours per FTE	Total Man Hours	Total Visits	Man Hours per Visit
10	8	80	127	.67

SCHEDULED OUTPATIENT CLINICS—PROJECTIONS

Purpose

To determine the distribution of a given total of projected outpatient visits for a selected target date; the utilization assumptions that can be made to determine the physical requirements for these visits; and the numbers of personnel who will be needed. Certain basic planning and policy decisions will have to be made before specific planning procedures can begin.

General planning decisions needed

1.   On what basis are outpatient clinics projected? In most situations there is a mix of types of patients, and it will be necessary to determine in a general way the source of the demand for the several groups. In the case of a teaching hospital with a large community work load the demand may be based primarily on the needs of a population for general medical and surgical care. This group of patients may then generate a certain demand for specialty and subspecialty clinic services. Growth will in this case be a function of unmet needs and changes in population, limited by the capacity of the hospital and its staff to provide services. A second group of patients may be referred by their own physicians for consultations; these will usually place heavier demands on the specialties than on general medical and surgical clinics. The level of demand by these

patients will depend on alternatives in the area and on the numbers of physicians associated with the hospital, and will probably depend less heavily on population factors. The reputation of the hospital for excellence in a particular area may generate a demand from a wider area. The data that were summarized in Tables OP-1 and OP-2 may indicate historical trends of the activity of the department itself; the trends can confirm or lay open to question the basis of assumptions about growth.

2.   What trends can be observed in outpatient department statistics with regard to changes in the distributions of visits by specialty, and how are these to be evaluated? Are any controls to be placed on numbers of visits to particular clinics or groups of clinics?

3.   Are there any changes in third-party payment policies that may serve to change recent patterns? How can the effects of such changes be quantified?

4.   Will the clinics be operated for maximum efficiency or on the basis of physician availability? This question probably goes to the issue of whether physicians are salaried and on a full-time or regular part-time schedule; or in the case of a teaching hospital whether an effective rotation system can realistically be put into effect. This is not an easy question: It may be tempting to opt for efficiency and to assume that a way will be found to implement the aim, but the result of guessing wrong can be a serious underestimation of facility requirements.

5.   What is the projected number of total outpatient visits?

6.   What types of teaching programs are in prospect?

Work load

Information needed

Historical data summarized in Table OP-1, Table OP-2, and Table OP-3.

Specific planning decisions needed

1.   In light of trends indicated by changes in the distribution of visits to clinics, how should the projected total of clinic visits be distributed among the clinics?

2.   Within clinics, what changes may be expected in the ratios of new and return visits?

Distribution of visits

Purpose

To determine the number of visits each clinic is expected to have at a target date.

Procedure

On the basis of decisions made with regard to the total number of visits projected, and the distribution of visits by specialty or clinic, compute the number of visits anticipated at the target date for each clinic. Adjustments to the distribution of visits should be shown. Data from the preceding year may be included to allow for comparisons:

Table OP-12.

Clinic	Annual Visits—Existing		Annual Visits—Projected	
	19— Visits	Percent of Total	Adjusted Percent of Total	Projected 19— Visits
All visits	200,000	100%	100%	300,000
Clinic A	50,000	25%	35%	105,000
Clinic B	—	—	—	––
Clinic C	—	—	—	—
Clinic D	—	—	—	—

Changes in Ratio of New and Return Visits

The following more detailed analysis may be desirable under certain circumstances:

Purpose

To compute the estimated time required for each specialty or clinic, separately for new and return visits, and to adjust the ratio of new and return visits as needed.

Procedure

Calculate the number of new and return visits for the projected target date according to decisions made with regard to adjustment of new/return ratio. From Table OP-9 determine the amount of time required for each category and multiply the time per visit by the number of visits. The calculations may be summarized as follows:

Table OP-13. Projected Visit-Hours

Clinic	Projected New Visits per Year				Projected Return Visits per Year			
	Adjusted New:Return Ratio	Projected New Visits	Minutes Per Visit	Total Hours	Projected Return Visits	Minutes per Visit	Total Hours	Total Annual Visit Hours
Clinic A	65:35	68,250	20	22,750	36,750	12	7,350	30,100
Clinic B	—	—	—	—	—	—	—	—
Total	—	—	—	—	—	—	—	—

Room hours needed—Definition of terms

Visit time must now be adjusted to allow for those utilization factors that were discussed in the section on current conditions. Because the terms used may be confusing because of their similarity, a brief degression is made here in order to define the terms, to clarify the sense in which they are used, and to explain the method of calculating utilization factors.

Visit Hours. The time during which an examination room is in use, including dressing and undressing time, waiting time, time with the doctor, time with others, and clean-up and preparation time between visits.

Room Hours. The time that an examination room is scheduled and available for use, whether it is actually being used or not.

Room Utilization Rate. The proportion of room hours that is consumed by visit hours. A room that is scheduled for 6 hours but is actually used for only 5 has a room utilization rate of 83%.

Scheduled Clinic Hours. This represents the number of hours actually scheduled as clinic sessions and is comparable to the visit hours defined above.

Potential Clinic Hours. This is an assumed figure based on a realistically possible schedule of operations—for example, a 5-day week composed of 8-hour days.

Combined Utilization Factor. The product of room utilization rate and the clinic utilization rate.

Clinic Utilization Rate. The proportion of potential clinic hours consumed by scheduled clinic hours (comparable to the room utilization rate defined above).

Room Hours Needed. The number of room hours shown as needed at the chosen combined utilization factor to handle the projected number of visit hours.

Example
Assume: 40,000 annual visits

24 minutes per visit = 16,000 visit hours $\left(\dfrac{40,000 \times 24}{60} \right)$

1.5 scheduled visits per room hour, or 40 minutes per visit = 26,667 room hours

The room utilization rate = 60% $\left(\dfrac{16,000 \text{ visit hours}}{26,667 \text{ room hours}} \right)$

Assume: 780 scheduled clinic hours per room
          1820 potential clinic hours per room (7 hours × 5 days × 52 weeks)

$$\text{The clinic utilization rate} = 43\% \left(\frac{780 \text{ SCH}}{1820 \text{ PCR}} \right)$$

The combined utilization factor is 26% (60% RUR × 43% CUR)

Conclusions: The number of room hours needed is 61,538

$$\left(\frac{16,000 \text{ visit hours}}{26\% \text{ CUF}} = 61,538 \right)$$

The number of rooms needed is 33.8 or 34

$$\left(\frac{61,538 \text{ room hours needed}}{1820 \text{ potential hours per room}} = 33.8 \right)$$

Utilization decisions needed

If visit hours have been calculated as shown in Table OP-13, it will now be necessary to decide what room utilization rate is to be used to convert visit hours to room hours. This may be done by using the existing visit hour to room hour ratio as has been done in the example above (see Table OP-10); or a decision will have to be made as to what a reasonable room utilization rate would be.

If visit hours have *not* been calculated, the existing number of room hours can be used as a planning base. As noted earlier, the room hours figure builds in the current utilization factor; if it can be assumed that this factor is satisfactory, the calculations indicated in the example can be abridged by dividing the number of room hours by the clinic utilization rate rather than by the combined utilization factor.

It will also be necessary to decide what clinic utilization rate may reasonably be applied. In the example the rate has been computed by comparing existing utilization to an assumed potential utilization. If there were sufficient knowledge about the existing clinic operation and sufficient certainty about how clinics would operate in the future, it would be possible to adjust the utilization rate. Any decision to do so would, however, have to come from the institution itself on the basis of its own experience and knowledge of the real constraints on efficient scheduling.

A further planning decision will have to be made with regard to the effect of peak loads. The data compiled in Table OP-2 showing the range of variation by day or month should be studied to determine if the utilization factors should be adjusted further to take care of uneven work loads, if the utilization factors provide sufficient flexibility without adjustment, or if peaks and valleys can be smoothed out by changes in scheduling and appointment systems.

Number of rooms

Procedure

Using the total annual visit hours developed in Table OP-13, calculate the number of exam rooms needed at the target date at the chosen utilization factors:

Table OP-14. Calculation of Exam Rooms Needed (1)

Clinic	Projected Visit Hours	Room Utilization Rate	Clinic Utilization Rate	Room Hours Needed	Rooms Needed (PCH = 1820)
Clinic A	30,100	60%	76%	66,009	36
Clinic B	—	—	—	—	—

Or, if the existing room utilization rate is to be retained, the average visit per room hour from Table OP-8 may be used as a planning base:

$$\frac{\text{projected visits}}{\text{average visits per room hour}} = \text{total room hours needed}$$

Compute the number of rooms needed by dividing the room hours by the clinic utilization rate and the total room hours needed by the potential clinic hours. Summarize as follows:

Table OP-15. Calculation of Exam Rooms Needed (2)

Clinic	Number of Visits	Visits per Room Hour	Room Hours	Clinic Utilization Rate	Total Room Hours Needed	Total Rooms Needed (PCH = 1820)
Clinic A	105,000	2.1	50,000	76%	65,789	36
Clinic B	—	—	—	—	—	—

Space requirements

Given the number of exam rooms needed, it is now necessary to determine the amount of space that will be needed *per exam room* for typical clinic space and the number and type of specialized facilities that will be needed in addition to this. One of two approaches may be used: If the present amount of space per clinic is generally satisfactory with regard to the ratio of total space to the number of exam rooms, the existing total clinic space may be divided by the number of exam rooms to arrive at a standard total clinic space per exam room figure, which can then be applied to the projected number of exam rooms. Data for this was summarized in Table OP-5.

Table OP-16.   Calculation of Space Requirements (1)

	Existing			Projected	
Clinic	Area	No. of Exam Rooms	Total Area per Exam Room	No. of Exam Rooms	Area per Clinic
Clinic A	6624	24	276	36	9936
Clinic B	—	—	—	—	—
Total	—	—	—	—	—

An alternative method is to develop a more or less arbitrary clinic module that will reflect the proposed organization of the clinics and to divide this module by the number of exam rooms included. For example, assume that a typical clinic module includes the following spaces:

Table OP-17   Determining Average Area per Exam Room of Standard Clinic Space

Type of space	No. of spaces	Area per space	Total space
Exam rooms	14	150	2100
Doctors offices	7	150	1050
Student offices	4	75	300
Nurses offices	2	120	240
Treatment Rooms	2	150	300
Seminar/conference	1	300	300
Reception/clerical	—	700	700
Specialized support	2	300	600
Utility rooms	2	120	240
Total			5830
	× 1.15 added for circulation		6700

Divide the 6700 net square feet by 14 (exam rooms) to arrive at a *total* area-per-exam-room figure of 480 net square feet. Multiply the number of exam rooms needed by this figure to estimate total clinic space. For example:

Table OP-18   Estimation of Standard Clinic Space Requirements

Clinic	No. of exam rooms needed	Area-per- exam-room	Clinic area needed
Clinic A	36	480	17,280
Clinic B	10	480	4,800
Clinic C	—	—	—
Total	46	—	22,080

The next step is to determine the number of specialized facilities that will be required to support the clinics as projected.

Procedure

With the information and calculations collected to this point, determine on the basis of discussion with the clinical staff the number and type of specialized spaces needed for each group of visits. Since the impact on efficiency of flexible, multi-purpose spaces is considerable, "uniqueness" of these facilities should be explored to determine whether or not joint use is possible. For example, a surgical clinic which meets once a week may need a minor operating room—it has to be available, however little it is used. If the operating room can, with minor changes in equipment, be used by other clinics meeting on other days the fact should be noted. As a practical matter it may be necessary to obtain a list of all special facilities required by each department or clinic and then attempt to match them by location requirements, size, and work-load. Any conclusions made in this regard will, of course, have to be reviewed by the clinical staff.

Special facilities and treatment rooms should be listed and described according to the expectations for their use, which should be expressed in terms of the visit-load as a whole: e.g., :(X) percent of surgical visits require treatment which cannot be given in the examining room. Such treatments take an average of (X) minutes." OR: "For the existing workload, a ratio of one treatment room to six examination rooms has proved satsifactory."

The utilization of such rooms could, of course, be studied in the same way as the utilization of exam rooms. However, since these rooms constitute a small proportion of total space, in most cases it will not be worthwhile to do so until detailed planning begins. A careful estimate should be sufficient. Summarize special facilities requirements and add to standard clinic space:

Table OP-19. Estimation of Additional Requirements

Clinic	Additional Facilities Area	Standard Clinic Area	Total Space Needed
Clinic A	1,400	12,600	14,000
Clinic B	350⎫		
Clinic C	120⎭	3,500	3,970
Total	—	—	17,970

Personnel

Procedure

Using data from Table OP-11 showing man-hours per visit, calculate the number of full-time equivalent personnel who will be required at the target date.

Table OP-20. Projected Personnel Requirements

Man-Hours per Visit	Visits	Total Man-Hours	Hours per FTE	Number of FTE Personnel
.67	240	160	8	20

3.4 SUPPORTING AND ANCILLARY SERVICES

Certain functions may be considered as being in exclusive support of an outpatient service—for example, reception, registration, accounting and billing, or even an outpatient snack bar. Others may be considered as central hospital services that provide support to the outpatient service as a part of their total function; a third category may be thought of as more or less autonomous satellite units of a larger hospital department. Whatever the relationships may be, it will normally be necessary to assess the activity in question as a whole and only then determine the locations and distributions of the parts that specifically support the outpatient services.

An outline of some of the kinds of functions that may be associated with an outpatient service, together with some of the primary questions that may be asked about them, is presented below. For the major functions, the planner is referred to the chapter or section of this book in which the function is discussed in detail. A format for summarizing requirement as they relate to outpatient services is suggested.

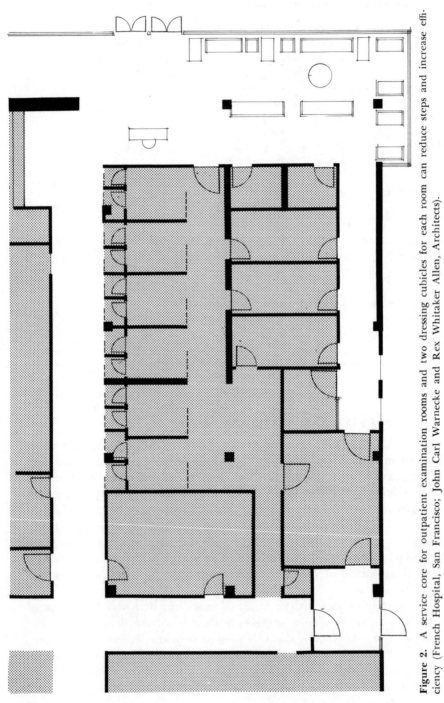

Figure 2. A service core for outpatient examination rooms and two dressing cubicles for each room can reduce steps and increase efficiency (French Hospital, San Francisco; John Carl Warnecke and Rex Whitaker Allen, Architects).

72

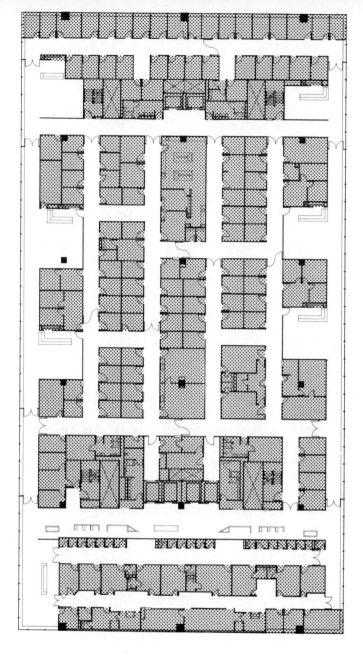

Figure 3. Decentralized and naturally lit waiting areas will create a less depressing environment for anxious patients. (Boston City Hospital, Boston; Hugh Stubbins/Rex Allen Partnership, Architects).

Beds

Will any provision be made for beds for outpatients? There are basically three categories of beds that should be considered with relation to ambulatory and emergency patients:

Observation or holding beds

These may be only day beds. They may be used for up to 24 hours for the observation of casualty patients from the emergency room; or for recovery and observation of patients who have undergone minor surgery or other therapeutic or diagnostic procedures that normally do not require admission but that the physician may wish to monitor because he wants to observe the effect of treatment or because he has some doubt about the patient's condition; or for holding and observation of drug-overdose, alcoholic, or psychiatric patients; or for holding of patients prior to transfer to other facilities. Unless there is need for a sufficiently large unit, staffing may be expensive.

Light care or self-care beds

Many patients are admitted to inpatient units who are merely under-going diagnostic procedures and who do not require nursing care or only a limited amount of care and perhaps special diet and instruction or counseling. A light care unit would reduce the cost of their stay con-siderably. It been estimated that from 10 to 30% of currently hos-pitalized patients do not need acute care and could be adequately cared for in other facilities. Ambulatory patients undergoing a series of diag-nostic tests can take advantage of such a facility on a short-term basis.

Hostel beds

Depending on local conditions and the availability of hotel and motel rooms in the area, the provision of hostel beds where ambulatory patients and their relatives could stay while the patients are undergoing diag-nostic or therapeutic procedures should be considered.

The following question should be asked with regard to short-stay beds of all types:

- What will be the criteria for admission?
- What will be the characteristics of the unit—level of staffing, length of stay, level of care, and so forth.
- What is the potential for shared use among several parts of the hospital?
- What will be the patient loading from each part of the hospital?
- What will be the effect of such a unit on inpatient admissions?

Outpatient Surgery

1. Which procedures currently performed on an inpatient basis can or will be done on an outpatient basis? What new procedures are anticipated? What is the average operating room time required for each type of procedure? What numbers of procedures are predicted for outpatient surgery by type of procedure? From the current inpatient load? From new patients? What types of anesthesia will be used?

2. Will outpatient procedures be done in special facilities designed for the purpose, or will they form part of the central operating room work load? If they form part of the central operating room work load, will they require separate induction and recovery facilities? Dressing rooms? Waiting rooms for relatives?

3. What will be the impact of outpatient surgery on work loads of the radiology, clinical laboratory, pathology, and service departments? What number of follow-up visits will be generated for scheduled clinics?

4. Will outpatient surgery be used for teaching, and if so, how?

Radiology

1. What volume of procedures of which types will the scheduled and unscheduled outpatient services generate? How can these procedures best be handled from the standpoint of (a) clinical excellence; (b) convenience of the service to patients and physicians; and (c) professional and administrative efficiency?

2. Will there be a radiology room for emergency patients within or adjacent to the emergency department itself? Will this be used by scheduled outpatient services?

3. Will nonemergency outpatients be handled in the same facility as inpatients, and if so, how will patient waiting and registration be separated? Or will there be a separate unit for outpatients?

Clinical Laboratories

1. What volume of tests will be generated per outpatient visit?

2. Will new procedures be introduced that will increase the work load as it relates to outpatients—massive screening programs, for example; or a multiphasic screening clinic?

3. Should there be a satellite laboratory to handle specific routine high-volume procedures for outpatients? Or merely a designated specimen collection and handling unit?

Medical Records

What systems of medical record keeping and retrieval are in effect or planned? Will there be a unit records system for all hospital patients? If the outpatient department is large, should the hospital medical record unit be located near it, since use of records by the outpatient department is heavier than by inpatient units? What technological changes in record entry, maintenance, and retrieval are in prospect?

Physicians' Offices

Will the outpatient department form a home base for certain physicians or groups of physicians? Permanently, or on rotation? What will be the contractural arrangement between these physicians and the hospital? Are there any legal or ethical questions that must be considered? If permanent offices are supplied to certain physicians, what would be their requirements as to space and supporting services? If offices are occupied temporarily, as part of the clinic operation only, how many must be supplied in relation to the number of exam rooms?

Reception, Registration, Information, Waiting, and Administrative and Book-Keeping Functions

What procedure will patients follow after they walk through the entrance? What procedure will be used for charging and billing? Where will patients wait? How many at average and peak periods? On the average, how many persons accompany each patient? What will be the scheduling and appointment system? How many employees will be involved at average and peak periods?

Social Services—Patient Advocate

What provision will be made for counseling patients directly, referring them for counseling, helping them find types of care offered by other institutions or services, arranging for home care or day care, guiding them through the hospital system or the health care system as a whole, and so forth? How many counseling professionals will be involved? What numbers and types of support personnel will be required? Where should the social services be located in relation to waiting or clinic areas?

Patient Education

Will any facilities be provided for individual or group instruction of patients in such subjects as nutrition, family planning, prenatal care, infant care, home care of sick, disabled, or aged relatives? What staff requirements would be associated with such activity? If individual instruction, what types of facilities would be required—for example, small offices or interview cubicles, conference room/library with media distribution? Standard classroom setting? Would patient education be a regularly scheduled function, or a drop-in area associated perhaps with the central waiting area?

Student Education

Will any form of clinical education or training occur in relation to outpatient activities? Will medical students, interns, nursing students, and paramedics be provided training, and if so, how and how many? Will they take over part of the examination process, and should they be provided office/exam room spaces in addition to those provided for physicians? Or will they participate with the physician in his examination? The latter will affect the time required per examination, increasing it perhaps by a third. The former method may or may not increase the time each physician spends per visit, but probably would not affect the time the patient spends in the main exam room. Will conference rooms be required, and if so, how many per clinic or group of clinic spaces? Will larger lecture facilities be required? Individual study spaces, perhaps with medi-equipped carrells? Library?

Nursery and Day Care

Will facilities be provided for patients, visitors, or staff? Such facilities may be especially desirable for psychiatric patients or physical rehabilitation patients undergoing long-term therapy. They may also help to attract staff in areas where shortages of qualified personnel exist.

Food Service Facilities

What provision must be made for staff if they cannot be accommodated in the central food service facilities? What meals will be served? How many staff will be on hand at noontime who will make use of the facilities, and what is the time-spread that they can make use of the facilities? Are full meals required for patients and visitors, or can their needs be met by a quick-service snack bar, or by vending machines. The volume of patients and visitors to be served will depend to a great extent on the efficiency of the appointment and scheduling system—if waiting times are long and a large number of patients accumulate, not only will the numbers available to use the facility be greater, but the need to relieve the boredom of waiting is likely to increase utilization of food services. How many patients and their relatives and friends will be on hand at noontime, and what proportion of them are likely to make use of the food services? How many times will seat occupancy turn over during the noon mealtime?

Table OP-21. Scheduled Outpatient Services—Summary of Supporting and Ancillary Services

Ancillary or Supporting Service	Planning Base	Planning Standards	Space Factor (NSF)	Estimated Space Requirements (NSF)
Outpatient surgery	40,000 surgery clinic visits	2 procedures per 100 visits, 400 procedures per room = 2 OR's	2000 NSF/OR	4,000
Observation beds	150,000 O.P. visits	65% occupany (days only) 1 bed/25,000 visits = 6 beds	250 NSF/bed	1,500
Light-care beds	150,000 O.P. visits	85% occupancy—AVLOS, 2 days — 1 bed/10,000 visits = 15 beds	250 NSF/bed	3,750

Radiology	150,000 O.P. visits	0.50 procedures per O.P. visits = 75,000 procedures 5000 average procedures per room/year = 15 rooms	1,100 NSF per procedure room.	16,500
Food services	Averages at noon: patients 150 visitors 70 staff 200 420	3 seatings at noon No. using facility: 40% = 60 70% = 79 60% = 120 Total 229 229 @ 3 seatings = 76 seats	30 NSF per seat for dining, preparation, serving	2,300
Clerical support services	150,000 O.P. visits	1 clerical worker for every 8000 annual visits = 19 FTE workers	120 NSF per FTE	2,280

Note: The planning standards and space factors shown are for purpose of example only.

Pharmacy

Will there be an outpatient dispensary—separate from the hospital pharmacy, or adjacent to it? Or will patients fill their prescriptions at community pharmacies? What number of prescriptions will be generated by the outpatient activities? Should the outpatient dispensary be located near the outpatient waiting areas? If outpatient dispensing is done as part of the central pharmacy function, are there suitable means of access by patients to the dispensing areas? How will patients be charged for their prescriptions?

Procedure

Once the basic workload for each of these supporting functions is worked out, the planning standards and assumptions should be summarized. The level of detail of explanation depends on the iminence of the project. In most preliminary planning efforts a shorthand summary such as that illustrated in Table OP-21 should be sufficient.

4

Nursing Services

4.1. BACKGROUND/DISCUSSION

Nursing services take place around the patient's bed, and patient beds are the key to the entire hospital plan: how many of them, what kind, how and how much they are used, how they are arranged, in what groups, for what patients. On the face of it, planning nursing units is perhaps the simplest part of hospital planning: The average area per bed is similar for most types of hospitals, and the sizes of nursing units— a question much discussed—is not an issue until design stages. However, so many issues surround the question of the number of beds that the matter is much more complex than it appears. In the context of this book it will only be possible to touch on some of the issues: The planner should be forewarned that a great deal of thought, analysis, and political ingenuity will be needed.

The number of beds planned for a particular hospital will depend on the total need for beds within the hospital's service area, the number of doctors on the staff, the number of beds that will be provided by other hospitals, the number and sizes of those hospitals, and the occupancy rate that can be anticipated given the range of sizes. There are a few basic facts that should be emphasized before the factors are examined separately.

- Health care planning is in its childhood, if not its infancy. Statistical health information that is routinely collected is crude, full of errors and inconsistencies, hard to interpret, and difficult to correlate.
- Governmental planning in the form of certificate of need legislation, professional review, and so forth is underdeveloped and is to a large degree functioning with inadequate information.

81

- It appears, but has not yet been proven to anyone's complete satisfaction, that hospital bed utilization drops when good preventive care is given. This is demonstrated by the lower use-rate for enrollees in health maintenance organizations such as the Kaiser Plan. On the other hand, it also appears that in areas where the use of outpatient services is higher the use of hospital beds increases. There appears to be no good standard means of calculating the hospitalization needs of particular populations that does not reflect practices already in effect and that must, therefore, be considered skewed in favor of things as they are.
- Anywhere between 10 and 30 percent of hospitalized patients may be in the wrong place. They could be in a nursing home, or receiving home care, but are hospitalized either because there is no alternative available or because the hospital is willing to keep them to help keep up the occupancy rate or because their insurance will cover them in the hospital but not elsewhere.
- The cost of hospitalization is so high that the pressure for change is enormous. But in what ways will changes occur?
- There is a dramatic mathematical increase in potential efficiency (occupancy rates) as hospitals increase in size—at least if there is good flexibility in the design of facilities. Where hospitalization is random (i.e., not elective) the daily census tends to be Poisson-distributed, and the number of beds needed to ensure an available bed for a selected ratio—say 99%—can be calculated. The proportion of extra beds needed decreases sharply as the total number of beds increases.* Thus most planning allows for differing occupancy rates for units of different sizes and encourages consolidation.
- Hospitals, communities, and doctors tend to be competitive, and the logical attempt to consolidate small and inefficient services may meet with opposition from many quarters.
- The number of beds needed at a particular hospital may seem to be a matter for rational exploration of population trends and travel distances, but in actual fact the patient loading may be based largely on the number of doctors on the staff and their level of success in attracting patients.

What, given all these uncertainties, are the steps that can be taken to proceed with planning?

The number of beds and the numbers of patients in those beds are the prime factors in predicting the work load of all other hospital inpatient

---

* "Dealing with Variability," *Hospital Industrial Engineering*, Ch. 18, Harold E. Smalley and John Freeman, Eds. 1966.

departments and services. The number of beds needed in a particular geographic area is determined by:

- The population density of the surrounding area.
- The age profile of the population.
- The geographic boundaries of the service area (travel times to the hospital).
- The availability of routine health care to the population.
- The availability of alternative modes of convalescent or terminal care.
- Policies of third-party insurers.

The proportion of total need that is met by a particular hospital will depend on its reputation, its geographic accessibility, the numbers of doctors it can attract to its staff, and the availability of public transportation.

The number of beds needed results from a calculation of how many people will require hospitalization; how long they will need to stay in the hospital; and a mathematical factor of extra beds that will ensure that a bed is available when needed. Hospitals keep records of the numbers of patients who are admitted and the number of days of care that are provided. The total days of care divided by the number of admissions gives an average length of stay figure which is frequently scrutinized for purposes of comparison among hospitals. The aim of health planners is to reduce the average length of stay, since this will reduce the total cost of health care. The length of stay is, on the average, shorter on the West than on the East Coast. Large hospitals tend to have a longer length of stay because they are usually the hospitals that take care of the most seriously ill patients. A large proportion of elderly patients will raise the average length of stay, and so many hospitals break their statistics down by age groups as well as by clinical division. The extra beds needed to ensure availability are the difference between the average daily census and the actual number of beds. Hospitals are constantly shifting beds, taking them in and out of service, closing wings and opening new ones, so that the number of beds available is frequently changing. The usual practice is to count up the total bed-days that have been available throughout the year, and to match this against the average daily census divide by 365 to arrive at an accurate occupancy rate.

As a key to most other hospital activities the number of patient days is probably the most accurate measure, since this represents actual work performed. There are, of course, costs and efforts associated with an empty bed, since the operation of an institution is not flexible enough to adjust to day-to-day differences. But radiological or laboratory services are performed for a patient, not for a bed, and thus the bed itself is not a good measure for such activities.

4.2. PROJECTIONS FOR INPATIENT CARE

Ever since the inception of the Hill-Burton Program, projections have been made defining the need for beds in various categories of care. Each year states have modified their policies in an attempt to reflect more accurately the real need.* Some states project future requirements directly from existing statistics and anticipated population changes. Such an approach obviously perpetuates existing patterns of care. Others take a more flexible approach combining statistical data with usage norms for basic services, comparing results with existing usage, and then determining if unusual circumstances, such as local patterns of usage, physician practice, or reimbursement mechanisms, would warrant variations from norms. In recent years there has been an increasing interest in making as full use as possible of existing facilities and in controlling construction of new facilities to keep capital investment costs to a minimum. It is suggested, therefore, that existing usage patterns be carefully examined, that consideration be given to population characteristics, such as age and social composition, and that there be full recognition of the effects of size of facility, type of accommodation, and other variables that would affect usage in individual institutions.

The establishment of regional health planning agencies and certificate of need legislation will obviously have a great effect on how individual institutions will develop. It is the intent of this manual to outline a method that will permit the injection of all pertinent data and thus provide a rational plan for development. Some factors to be considered are:

1. New, innovative, or other methods of providing or organizing the delivery of health care services that may not otherwise be available to the community.

2. Need for facilities to provide a specialized treatment or research program to serve a population in a broad regional base area that exceeds the boundaries of the health facility planning area in which the proposed facility is located (e.g., regional burn centers, cancer research center) and that is not being met by existing facilities.

---

* (1) *Policy and Procedures Manual—Determination of Need and Project Review,* Bureau of Facility Planning, Division of Health Facility Financing & Development, New York State Department of Health. (2) *California State Plan for Hospitals and Related Health Facilities,* Department of Health, Comprehensive Health Planning Program, July 1, 1972–June 30, 1974, pp. 70–72.

3.   Where patterns of medical practice are developed and introduced that require reassessment and redetermination of projecting anticipated utilization in an area.

4.   Where mergers or trade-offs between facilities make past utilization an invalid indicator of future use.

5.   Where it can be demonstrated that the programming of additional beds assigned to a specific facility will enable service components to achieve optimum size to effect economies in operation by increased efficiencies and improvement in the quality of care.

6.   Where beds and services may be needed to serve specific population groups that because of language differences are unable to receive adequate treatment in existing facilities.

A clear statement of an institution's goals, establishing its objectives and the categories of inpatient care it will provide, is the first step in determining how many beds are needed. For example, if an acute general hospital provides inpatient care for medical-surgical, post-partum maternity, and pediatric patients, these will normally be in distinct patient facilities. Except in emergencies, patients will not be admitted to a category of nursing unit other than the one that suits his or her status. The simplest process of determining a future need for beds in each of these categories is to examine current usage in patient days per thousand population in a rationally defined service area.* Existing adult medical-surgical patient days are related to an estimate of current population aged 15 and over, maternity patient days to current female population aged 15 to 44, and pediatric patient days to current population under 15 (see Table NS-1.). By comparing these rates to normal rates for each category, by considering whether or not there are any extenuating circumstances, such as local patterns of usage, physician practice, or reimbursement mechanisms that might increase or decrease usage, and by establishing a figure based on reasoned judgement, it then becomes a matter of simple arithmetic to determine the anticipated days for each category of care. Before translating this into average daily census and actual bed need, consideration should be given to the effects of size.

Effects of Size

The size of a distinct patient facility such as those listed above will influence its capacity. The smaller the distinct patient facility, the less likely it is that it can maintain a high occupancy rate—the effect of 1 patient in

* Feldstein, Paul J. and German, Jeremiah J., *Predicting Hospital Utilization: An Evaluation of Three Approaches*, p. 34.

Table NS-1. Determination of Projected Patient Days (for a Hypothetical Population of 500,000)

	(1)	(2)	(3)	(4)	(5)	(6)	(7)	(8)
Nursing Service	Age	Population (1000)	Patient Days	Pat. Days per 1000	Recommended Pat. Days/1000	Adjusted Patient Days/1000	Anticipated Population In 5 Yrs.	Projected Pat. Days
Med./Surg.	15 and over	350	220,000	629	600–1200	630	402.5	253,575
Post-Partum	Female 15–44	(100)	15,000	150	150–200	150	(117)	17,250
Pediatric	Under 15	150	15,000	100	100–200	100	172.5	17,250
	Totals	500	250,000	500	500–1000	501	575	288,075

a service with a capacity of 4 is 25%, whereas in a service for 40 it is only 2½%. Thus the fewer distinct patient facilities there are and the larger they are, the easier it is to maintain high occupancy rates. Alternatively, if a facility can be designed that will permit some degree of flexibility of assignment of patients between patient facilities, making them less distinct, it will have a greater likelihood of higher occupancy.

The optimum size of a distinct patient facility to meet a given need can best be determined by establishing the degree of risk involved at various capacity levels and deciding what is tolerable. The greater the capacity, the lower the risk of inadequate service, but the greater the cost; the greater the risk, the lower the cost. A decision on what is acceptable must be made by those responsible for providing care. Generally, if distinct facilities are filled to capacity 1/100 to 1/1000 of the days, or approximately from 4 days per year to 1 day every 3 years, they are adequate.

It has been observed that "the distribution of daily (midnight) census figures on a distinctive patient facility are generally Poisson distributed . . . The Poisson distribution is a form of skewed bell-shaped curve in which the entire shape of the curve may be predicted when only the average case load of the facility is known."[*] Or, in the case of projected need, when the need is used as the average census figure, a determination of number of beds for each distinct patient facility can be made by using Table NS-2. Also it is possible to determine the effect of establishing flexibility or swing beds between two distinct patient facilities or of subdividing a distinct patient facility into smaller components.

For example, if projections indicate an average daily census of 100 medical-surgical patients and if the beds are to be full no more than 1 day in 100, from Table NS-2, Column 3 there would be a need for 125 beds (an 80% occupancy rate) provided all beds are in a single facility where they are equally available to all patients. If, however, 10 of the patients are pediatric and 10 are maternity, each in separate distinct patient units, from Table NS-2, Column 3 there would be a need for 141 beds (19 + 19 + 103) dropping the average occupancy rate to 71%. If the adult medical-surgical beds were further divided, either into separate medical and surgical nursing units or equally by sex because all accommodations were in multibed rooms, the total beds needed to accommodate the same number of patients might increase to 150 (19 + 19 + 56 + 56).

[*] "Estimating Hospital Bed Needs from Average Census Data", Mark S. Blumberg, M.D., *The Modern Hospital,* December, 1961.

Table NS-2. **Bed Complements (C) for a Given Average Census (A) Which Result in a Completely Occupied Facility an Average of 1 Day in 10, 1 day in 100, and 1 day in 1000.**

	Number of Beds Completely Occupied			Percent Occupancy		
(1)	(2)	(3)	(4)	(5)	(6)	(7)
Average Daily Census	1 Day in 10 (p = 0.1)	1 Day in 100 (p = .01)	1 Day in 1000 (p = .001)	p = 0.1 (Col. 2)	p = .01 (Col. 3)	p = .001 (Col. 4)
1	3	5	6	33	20	17
2	5	7	9	40	29	22
3	6	9	11	50	33	27
4	7	10	12	57	40	33
5	9	12	14	56	42	36
6	10	13	16	60	46	38
7	11	15	17	64	47	41
8	13	16	19	62	50	42
9	14	18	21	64	50	43
10	15	19	22	67	53	45
11	16	20	24	69	55	46
12	18	22	25	67	55	48
13	19	23	26	68	57	50
14	20	24	28	70	58	50
15	21	26	29	71	58	52
20	27	32	36	74	62	56
25	33	38	43	76	66	58
30	38	44	49	79	68	61
35	44	50	56	80	70	63
40	49	56	62	82	71	65
45	55	62	68	82	73	66
50	60	68	74	83	74	68
55	66	74	80	83	74	69
60	71	80	86	85	75	70
65	76	85	92	86	76	71
70	82	91	98	85	77	71
75	87	97	104	86	77	72
80	93	103	110	86	78	73
85	98	108	115	87	79	74
90	103	114	122	87	79	74
95	109	119	127	87	80	75
100	114	125	133	88	80	75
120		147	156		82	77
140		168	179		83	78
160		191	201		84	80

Table NS-2 (continued)

(1) Average Daily Census	Number of Beds Completely Occupied			Percent Occupancy		
	(2) 1 Day in 10 (p = 0.1)	(3) 1 Day in 100 (p = .01)	(4) 1 Day in 1000 (p = .001)	(5) p = 0.1 (Col. 2)	(6) p = .01 (Col. 3)	(7) p = .001 (Col. 4)
180		213	223		85	81
200		235	245		85	82
250		288	301		87	83
300		344	357		87	84
400		448	465		89	86
500		552	572		90	87
600		658	679		91	89
700		763	786		92	89
800		867	890		92	90

Source: "Estimating Hospital Bed Needs from Average Census Data," Mark S. Blumberg, M.D., *The Modern Hospital*, December, 1961.

On the other hand, by making some of the beds swing beds, beds available to either of two distinct patient facilities, it is possible to accommodate the same number of patients with fewer beds. The optimum number of swing beds can be determined by calculating the difference between the total number of beds needed for two separate facilities and the number needed if they were combined. For example, if there is a projected average daily census of 10 pediatric patients and 80 adult medical-surgical patients, from Table NS-2, Column 3 there would be a need for 19 pediatric beds and 103 adult beds, a total of 122 beds. However, as a combined facility there would only be a need for 114 beds. Therefore, if 8 beds (122 − 114) could be assigned to either one unit or the other as needed, the chances are that neither of the distinct facilities would be fully occupied more than 1 day in 100. The configuration would be 11 beds (19 − 8) in pediatrics, 95 beds (103 − 8) in adult medical-surgical, and 8 that could be assigned individually to either unit on demand.

A similar analysis can be applied to determine the need for private rooms to permit separation of the sexes. In a medical-surgical facility with an average daily census of 80, assuming an even distribution of men and women, there would be a need for 112 beds (56 + 56) if men and women were accommodated in distinct patient facilities. With all private rooms and no discrimination, only 103 beds would be needed for the same average census; however, if there were no other reason to segregate

patients or assign them to private rooms, only 9 private rooms
(112 − ·103) would theoretically accomplish the same result. This also
assumes that the private rooms would be assigned only when no other
appropriate beds were available. Obviously this is not a usual method of
assignment.

To summarize, it is apparent that the greater number of distinct
patient facilities, the lower the occupancy rate. Also, the smaller the
distinct patient facility, the lower the occupancy rate, and the smaller
the institution, the greater the cost of providing distinct patient facilities.
On the other hand, if each bed were in a private room so that each might
be considered a distinct patient facility, there would be maximum flexibility to accomplish separation by age, diagnosis, level of care, and so
forth. If appropriate nursing care were equally available, this would
make the entire hospital a single distinct patient facility, and the increased occupancy rate might well offset any additional nursing and
capital improvement costs.

Sometimes it may be valuable to determine the number of days in a
year that beds in a distinct patient facility will be fully occupied. Table
NS-3 can be used for this purpose. It is also developed from a Poisson
distribution. In using the Poisson formula it should be borne in mind
that it assumes a random admission rate. Should there be epidemic,
severe overcrowding, seasonal variations, or a high percentage of elective
admissions, the Poisson distribution will probably not apply.

Determination of Bed Need

Using the hypothetical population and patient day figures in Table NS-1
as an example, it is possible to determine the projected average daily
census for each category of nursing service by dividing the patient days
per year by 365 (see Table NS-4). Thus 253,575 medical-surgical patient
days represent an average daily census (ADC) of 695, and 17,250 patient
days each for post-partum maternity and pediatrics represent an ADC of
47. In the hypothetical case illustrated in Table NS-4, there are presumed
to be 3 existing hospitals in the service area under study, a 341-bed
general hospital that includes a 36-bed maternity service but no pediatric
beds, a 150-bed hospital with only a medical-surgical service, and a 114-
bed children's hospital. Assuming that it is acceptable to have the beds
in each service filled to capacity 1 day out of 100, or between 3 and 4
days a year, the 305 medical-surgical beds in Hospital A could have an
ADC of 265. This is determined from Table NS-2 by calculating the
difference between 288 and 344 in Column 3 and interpolating between
250 and 300 in Column 1, thus:

$$250 + [(305 − 288) ÷ (344 − 288) × (300 − 250)] = 265$$

Table NS-3. Determining Bed Need from Occupancy and Census Figures

Number of days per year an administrator can expect to have an insufficient number of beds to meet needs

A \ B	1	2	3	4	5	6	7	8	9	10	11	12	13	14	15	20	25	30	35	40	45	50	55	60	65	70	75	80	85	90	95	100	120	140
1	97	30	7	2	a																													
2	217	119	53	20	7	2	a																											
3	293	211	129	64	31	13	5	2	a																									
4	332	279	207	136	79	41	19	8	3	2	a																							
5	351	320	269	205	141	87	49	25	12	5	2	1	a																					
6	359	343	310	261	203	144	94	56	31	16	8	4	2	1	a																			
7	363	355	336	302	256	201	147	99	62	36	20	10	5	2	a																			
8	364	360	350	329	296	251	200	149	104	67	41	24	13	7	4																			
9	b	363	358	345	323	290	247	199	151	108	72	46	27	15	9																			
10	b	364	362	355	341	318	285	244	198	153	111	77	50	31	18																			
11	b	b	363	360	352	337	313	281	241	198	154	114	80	54	34																			
12	b	b	b	363	358	349	333	320	281	239	197	155	117	84	57																			
13	b	b	b	364	362	356	346	333	305	274	237	196	156	119	87																			
14	b	b	b	b	363	360	354	343	326	301	271	235	193	157	121																			
15	b	b	b	b	364	363	359	352	340	322	298	268	233	196	158																			
20	b	b	b	b	b	b	b	b	364	362	358	351	341	327	308	161	41	5	a															
25	b	b	b	b	b	b	b	b	b	b	b	b	b	b	b	298	164	50	9	1	a													
30	b	b	b	b	b	b	b	b	b	b	b	b	b	b	b	353	298	165	58	12	2	a												
35	b	b	b	b	b	b	b	b	b	b	b	b	b	b	b	364	348	283	167	64	16	3	a											
40	b	b	b	b	b	b	b	b	b	b	b	b	b	b	b	b	363	343	277	168	70	20	4	a										
45	b	b	b	b	b	b	b	b	b	b	b	b	b	b	b	b	b	361	338	272	169	75	23	5	1									
50	b	b	b	b	b	b	b	b	b	b	b	b	b	b	b	b	b	b	360	334	268	169	79	27	7	2								
55	b	b	b	b	b	b	b	b	b	b	b	b	b	b	b	b	b	b	b	358	330	264	170	83	30	8	2							
60	b	b	b	b	b	b	b	b	b	b	b	b	b	b	b	b	b	b	b	364	356	326	261	170	86	33	10	3						
65	b	b	b	b	b	b	b	b	b	b	b	b	b	b	b	b	b	b	b	b	364	353	323	258	171	90	36	12	3					
70	b	b	b	b	b	b	b	b	b	b	b	b	b	b	b	b	b	b	b	b	b	363	352	320	256	171	92	38	13	4				
75	b	b	b	b	b	b	b	b	b	b	b	b	b	b	b	b	b	b	b	b	b	b	362	350	316	254	172	95	42	15	5	1		
80	b	b	b	b	b	b	b	b	b	b	b	b	b	b	b	b	b	b	b	b	b	b	b	361	348	313	251	172	97	45	17	5		
85	b	b	b	b	b	b	b	b	b	b	b	b	b	b	b	b	b	b	b	b	b	b	b	b	360	346	310	250	172	100	47	19		
90	b	b	b	b	b	b	b	b	b	b	b	b	b	b	b	b	b	b	b	b	b	b	b	b	364	359	344	308	248	173	102	50	1	
95	b	b	b	b	b	b	b	b	b	b	b	b	b	b	b	b	b	b	b	b	b	b	b	b	b	364	358	342	305	246	173	104	5	
100	b	b	b	b	b	b	b	b	b	b	b	b	b	b	b	b	b	b	b	b	b	b	b	b	b	b	364	357	340	303	245	173	19	3

Number of Beds in the Facility

Average Daily Census (Actual or Anticipated)

a Less than one-half day can be expected for all values to the right.
b 365 days can be expected for all values below.

Source: "Determining Bed Needs from Occupancy and Census Figures," by Vernon E. Weckworth, Ph.D., *Hospitals*, J.A.H.A., January 1, 1966, Vol. 40.

Table NS-4. Determination of Projected Bed Need

Nursing Service	(1) Projected Average Daily Census (ADC) Col. 8 of Table NS-1 ÷ 365	Existing Hospitals						(8) Projected ADC for New Beds Co. 1 less Cols. 3+5+7	(9) Projected New Bed Need p. = 0.01
		A		B		C			
		(2) Available Beds	(3) Optimum ADC p = 0.01	(4) Available Beds	(5) Optimum ADC p = 0.01	(6) Available Beds	(7) Optimum ADC p = 0.01		
Med./Surg.	695	305	265	150	123	—	—	307	347
Post-Partum	47	36	23	—	—	—	—	24	37
Pediatric	47	—	—	—	—	114	90	(−43)	—
Totals	789	341	288	150	123	114	90	331	384

Note: Columns 3, 5, 7, and 9 are derived from Table NS-2.

Note: If all these beds were in one facility, the service area would be equally well served with only 886 beds instead of the projected 1015 beds, provided the beds were divided into the same (no additional) distinct patient facilities.

By a similar process, the optimum ADC of the 36 post-partum maternity beds would be 23 and of the 150 medical-surgical beds in Hospital B 123. Deducting the 265 and 123 ADC from 695 leaves a need to accommodate an ADC of 307 and this, by a reverse process, using Table NS-2, results in a need for 347 medical-surgical beds. Deducting the 23 ADC from the 47 projected ADC for maternity indicates a need to accommodate an ADC of 24 or a need for 37 beds, a total of 384 beds in a new facility or in an addition to one of the existing institutions. No additional pediatric beds are needed as long as the existing hospital remains in service, as it could accommodate an ADC of 90 or accommodate its present ADC of 47 in 64 beds, a reduction of 50 beds from its present capacity of 114. Alternatives for the pediatric hospital, of course, would be for it to expand its service, perhaps to develop a maternity department or to merge with a general hospital.

It should also be noted that the actual patient days in the existing hospitals are not used because they might produce a distorted picture of the need if they are either overutilized or underutilized. It is the authors' experience that the Poisson distribution is amazingly accurate under

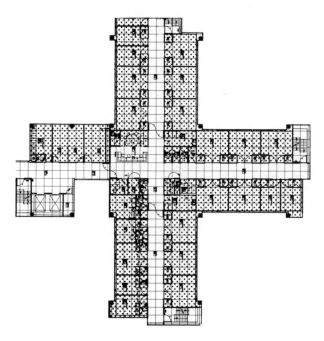

Figure 4. Walking distances in a potentially all private 36-bed nursing unit can be kept to a minimum by using a T-shape plan (St. Joseph Hospital, Clinton Township, Mich.; Hugh Stubbins/Rex Allen Partnership).

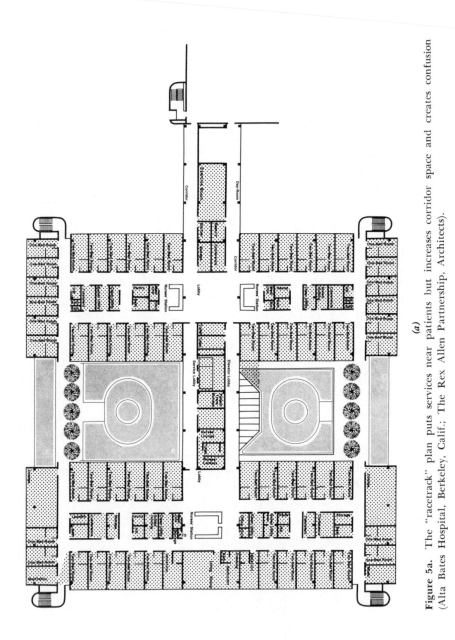

Figure 5a. The "racetrack" plan puts services near patients but increases corridor space and creates confusion (Alta Bates Hospital, Berkeley, Calif.; The Rex Allen Partnership, Architects).

(a)

normal circumstances and can be relied upon to give a dependable estimate of actual operating conditions. Also, the illustration is simplified. In practice, equal consideration using a similar approach should be given to nonacute nursing care and such other special services as intensive care, cardiac care, orthopedics, psychiatry, and other services that might require distinctive patient facilities.

4.3. DISTRIBUTION OF BEDS BY SERVICE AND LEVEL OF CARE

Policy Decisions Needed:

- Will nursing units be organized on the principle that the level of nursing care needed is the operative criterion for grouping of patients, or will beds be organized primarily by specialty/subspecialty?
- In either case, what exceptions will apply?
- What location requirements can be identified among nursing units and among nursing units and direct patient service functions?
- What proportion of beds should be in single rooms, double rooms, multiple bedrooms (if any)?
- How many intensive care beds should be provided, given the number of general care beds and the level of surgical and medical activity?
- Should medical and surgical intensive care beds be planned as a single unit? Will there be a separate pediatric intensive care unit? What will be the relationship between surgical intensive care and surgical recovery beds?
- Will there be special groupings, such as a cardiac surgery/cardiology unit or a unit combining neurological/neurosurgical patients?
- Will there be a unit of psychiatric beds, and what will be the criteria for admission and length of stay in such a unit?
- What proportion of patients currently under general care could be adequately handled in a self-care or light care unit? Is such a unit to be considered?

Planning Decisions Needed

For each distinct type of nursing unit, what special facilities, beyond the patient bedroom and the normal nursing station and clerical and utility space, are needed? For example, general care units may require a seminar/teaching/conference room. Units for ambulatory patients may require day rooms or dining rooms. A psychiatric unit will require a number of social areas, including lounge space, arts and education rooms, offices for conferences with social workers or physicians, and so forth. An

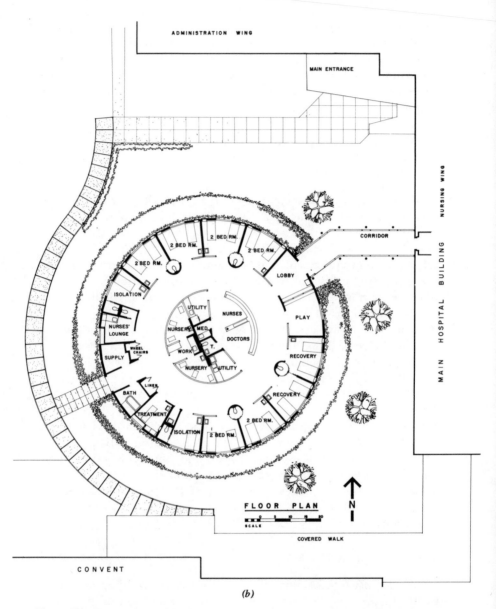

Figure 5b. For small specialized units not exceeding 24 beds the circular plan is efficient and provides excellent visibility; larger units have excessive interior space (Pediatric Pavillion, Mercy Hospital, Redding, CA.; Rex Whitaker Allen and Assoc., Architects).

obstetric unit will need a father's room as well as a number of supporting spaces not common to other units.

These special spaces may be developed by the planner from study of the literature and examples from other hospitals, but he should also attempt to elicit from the staff physicians and especially from the nurses ideas as to what additional facilities will serve to help the unit not only to function smoothly but to help the patient by providing an interesting and attractive environment for his convalescence.

The projection of beds as described in this chapter must be done in conjunction with the projection and planning of diagnostic and treatment services, as described in Chapter 5. The planning in these two major areas of hospital activity are inextricably interwoven and cannot be treated separately, nor is it easy to say which comes first. If the ability to predict the amount and distribution of illness were absolute, if there were only one hospital in a region, and if there were no impediments to access to hospital care, the particular clinical diagnostic and treatment services would be the prime factor, and beds would follow. In the world as it is, however, with the state of knowledge, economic and social conditions, and existing institutions in place as they are, the number of beds is often the key, with the services themselves following as they can or may.

Even for a standard nursing unit, where some proportion of the patients can be expected to be ambulatory for at least a part of their stay, it makes sense to consider places the patient can walk to, or can sit with visitors, outside the confines of his room. A full day room may not be needed, but if fire regulations are complied with, there could be places that could provide small groupings of seats, reading areas, or television viewing areas in circulation space.

The distribution of food must also be considered in planning for the nursing unit. Will there, with the development of the electronic oven, be a return to the ward kitchen—to the extent that frozen meals prepared in the central kitchen may be stored and heated on each floor, or in each nursing unit?

Size of the Nursing Unit

The term "nursing unit" seems to be used in two ways: as a definition of the number of beds a single nurse or team of nurses can manage and observe, (8-14 beds) and the beds supervisable by one head nurse. It may be helpful to keep in mind the fact that what may be a large nursing unit in total beds need not be a large one in the organization of nursing staff. A large nursing unit of 60 beds is too large for one nurse

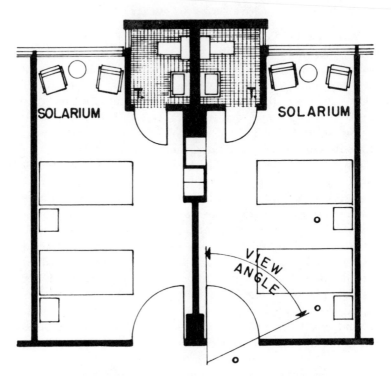

SOLARIUM SOLARIUM

VIEW ANGLE

(a)

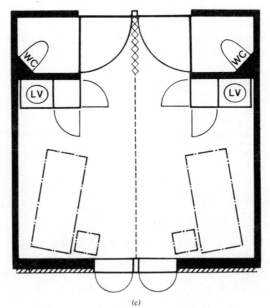

WC WC

LV LV

(c)

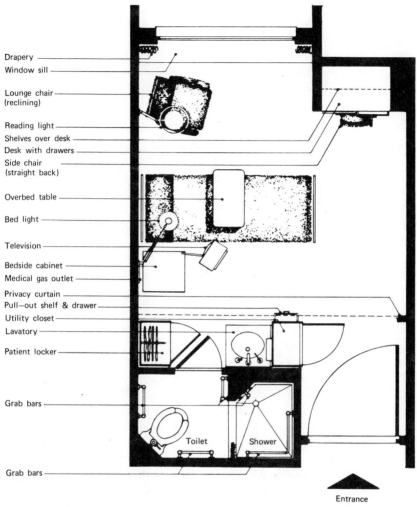

Drapery
Window sill
Lounge chair (reclining)
Reading light
Shelves over desk
Desk with drawers
Side chair (straight back)
Overbed table
Bed light
Television
Bedside cabinet
Medical gas outlet
Privacy curtain
Pull—out shelf & drawer
Utility closet
Lavatory
Patient locker
Grab bars
Grab bars

Toilet

Shower

Entrance

(b)

Figure 6a. Locating the toilet on the outside wall opposite the corridor door gives the nurse better visibility of the patient and provides a sitting alcove near the window (French Hospital, San Francisco; John Carl Warnecke & Rex Whitaker Allen, Assoc., Architects).

Figure 6b. The private room permits higher occupancy rates and, when the lavatory and supplies are located within arm's length of the nurse, greater efficiency (St. Francis Hospital, San Francisco; Rex Whitaker Allen and Assoc., Architects).

Figure 6c. Turning the bed perpendicular to the exterior wall and using folding partitions gives each bed its own window, door to the corridor, and toilet facility—potentially private accommodations in the space of a conventional two-bed room (St. Joseph Hospital, Mt. Clemens, Mich.; Hugh Stubbins/Rex Allen Partnership).

99

to monitor, but there may be more than one nurse. Such a unit may, however, be economical in terms of space because the requirements for supporting spaces—utility rooms, clerical space, and so on—may be not much more than they would be for a unit of half the size. Factors which enter into the decision as to the proper size of nursing units include:

- Federal or state regulation.
- The types of patients and the level of observation and care they require.
- The organization of nursing staffs and hospital administration.
- The organization of clinical departments and attending physicians.
- The layout of the unit; the distances to be traveled by the staff.
- The relationship to other nursing divisions.
- The type of accommodation; that is, single rooms will increase distances and reduce desirable number of beds.

Single, Double or Multiple-Bed Rooms

In the United States, but not in all developed countries, the trend in hospitals has been to provide increasingly greater proportions of single bedrooms and to eliminate the multiple bed room, or ward, entirely. A large proportion of single bedrooms has operational advantages, since it allows for a freer mix of patients and hence helps to increase occupancy in the hospital as a whole. The single room allows privacy for the patient and his visitors, lets the patient occupy himself as he wishes without disturbing a neighbor, and frees him from the disturbances a roommate may create. There are arguments for larger rooms, however, and they should be considered in allocating a distribution. Double and multiple rooms are somewhat more economical of space. Some patients are very uncomfortable alone and feel much more at ease with company, even if they have little choice about who the company is and even if the presence of others may be in some ways disturbing. For patients who do wish company, the double room may not be the best alternative, although it is the most common. Two patients in a room experience a kind of intimacy, quite different from the kind of human presence without intimacy that may be provided in a multiple bed room. The characteristics of the patient population, their economic, educational, and domestic status and life-styles should be considered before arbitrarily deciding that the single room is necessarily the optimum choice for everyone.

5

Diagnostic and Treatment Services

5.1. SURGERY

Background/Discussion

Surgical facilities and the staff required to use them are one of the most expensive single parts of the hospital. They also represent, of course, a central life-saving activity. Surgery is, by its nature, dramatic. It is expensive. Its successes and failures are highly visible. There has been a considerable amount of questioning about the numbers of surgeons in this country and the number of operations that are performed. It has been asked whether priorities are in order; is open heart surgery a luxury, when large segments of the population do not receive adequate routine medical care? The expense of maintaining operating rooms has led to many studies of how to improve utilization and efficiency. It is evident then that it will be necessary to justify both the level of activity and the utilization of facilities. On the other hand, it is unlikely that anyone would suggest that surgical facilities be scheduled so tightly that there would be a risk of patients being turned away or experiencing excessive waiting periods.

A basic assumption of this book—that as a planning guideline the numbers of beds alone is inadequate—is applicable here. Other commonly used standards—such as the numbers of operations per operating room per year—are likewise inadequate, taken alone. None of these methods takes into account the variations that are bound to occur among hospitals when it comes to such matters as differences in hospital organization, the types of doctors on the staff, the types of patients and the means of payment available to them, and so on. Clearly the number of 3-hour operations that can be performed in one operating room in a month is different from the number of 20-minute operations: nor is it

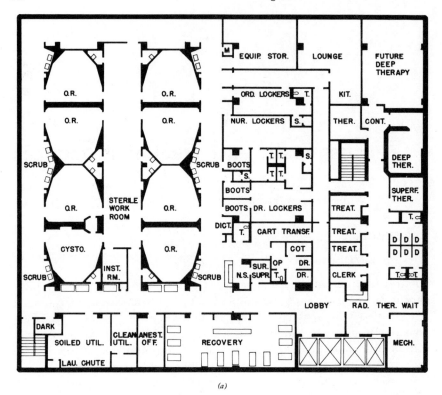

Figure 7a. The peripheral corridor ostensibly separates clean and soiled circulation—clean supplies and work area in the center; patients, scrub, and soiled utility on the outside (Alta Bates Hospital, Berkeley, CA.; The Rex Allen Partnership, Architects).

likely that the ratio of major to minor operations will be the same from one hospital to the next.

Some of the quantifiable factors which must be considered in greater or lesser detail include:

• The numbers and types of physicians and the numbers and types of patients.
• The number and nature of procedures.
• The numbers of beds available or needed.
• The average length of stay of surgical patients within each specialty.
• The average operating and preparation and clean-up time required in each specialty.
• The amount of time operating rooms can be staffed and available for use.

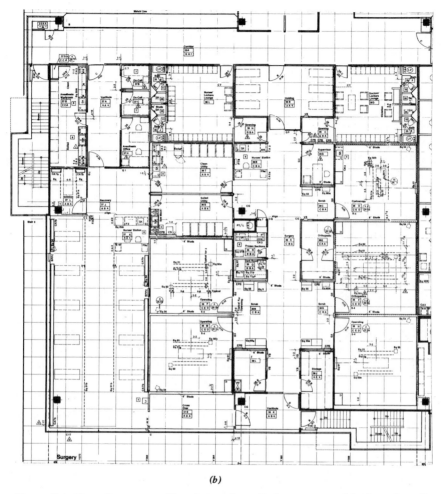

(b)

Figure 7b. Operating rooms with only one door eliminate any possible through traffic and force reliance on good techniques for sterility (St. Joseph Hospital, Clinton Township, Mich.; Hugh Stubbins/Rex Allen Partnership, Architects).

- The amount of operating room time that should be reserved for emergency procedures.
- The amount of idle time of operating rooms and staff that can be considered necessary or acceptable.

Equally important for planning but less subject to analysis and quantification are social, economic, and professional practice trends. At some stage in the planning—perhaps after an analysis of existing conditions has been made and before plans for the future are fully defined—it would

be well to ask questions such as those which are outlined below. It is unlikely that there will be answers to any of these questions, for the data
surrounding them are ambiguous and generally subject to varying interpretations, but the discussions may serve to slant interpretations of current activity and projections in a realistic direction.

- Can the major factors that control the number of operations be identified? Is it the number of physicians on the staff and the patient load
  generated by them? Is it the demand of a more or less defined population? Is it the hospital as an institution and the numbers of beds it can
  supply?
- Is there a trend towards shorter hospital stays, and will this result in
  an ability to meet a hidden demand for surgery by permitting a larger
  turnover of patients? If a good home care program were available,
  would this reduce the average length of stay of surgical patients? If the
  average stay in this hospital is longer than at either other hospitals in
  the area, or other hospitals of similar size and type in other areas, can
  the reasons be identified? If they can, can or should the situation be
  altered? How?
- Conversely, is there a trend towards older and sicker patients, and
  should one conclude that the average length of stay might increase
  rather than decrease? What changes would this imply for the types and
  numbers of surgical procedures and consequently for the utilization of
  surgical facilities?
- Are there changes in the character of the patient population, either
  observed or predicted, which may have an impact on the kinds of procedures that are performed, their number, and whether they are performed on an inpatient or outpatient basis?
- Could some of the procedures currently being done on an inpatient
  basis be performed on outpatients if suitable facilities were developed?
  What proportion of the total procedures?
- Are there educational programs on the horizon that may affect either
  the types of patients or methods of operation?
- Are there changes in the organization or delivery of professional services that may affect the level of activity? As mentioned earlier, there
  has been much discussion of the fact that there are great differences in
  the ratios of operations performed to apparently similar populations. In
  an article in the New England Medical Journal (Jan. 1, 1970), for
  example, Dr. John Bunker observes that while in England in 1967 there
  were 18 surgeons per 100,000 population, in the United States there
  were 39. He further comments that the rate of operations in the U.S.
  for persons covered by comprehensive prepaid plans was half that of

those covered by Blue Cross. In a 1969 article in the same journal, C. E. Lewis reported that within a single state (Kansas) the rates at which common elective procedures were performed varied three- to four-fold, depending, apparently, on the numbers of surgeons and hospital beds available in the region. While such statistics may not take full account of differences in the populations themselves or may suffer some degree of inaccuracy because of differences in definitions, the variations are sufficiently large to raise serious questions that it would be imprudent not to consider.

It should be obvious that such questions cannot be settled before planning begins, and perhaps a warning is in order not to allow discussion of such matters to stop the planning process in its tracks. It seems important, however, that such discussion occur. When it comes time for the community or a regulatory agency to review the planning, it would be awkward to explain that no serious discussion of these matters had taken place.

Utilization of Facilities

The efficient utilization of operating rooms involves the reasonable prediction of demand, effective scheduling methods, and a careful balancing between number of beds and operating room capacity.

Depending on where the constraints lie in a particular situation, planning can begin either with the number of beds available or with the number of operations anticipated. In most institutions a limited number of beds controls the number of operations that can be performed, and the operating rooms themselves have considerable excess capacity. Often the lack of a good match between numbers of beds and operating room capacity is the result of wide fluctuations in demand which, in many cases, could be smoothed out by an effective method of controlling admissions. Such a method is described by J. T. Stewart, management systems analyst for the Presbyterian Hospital in Dallas, in an article in *Hospitals* (Sept. 1, 1970). Application of the method resulted in increasing the numbers of operations from 750 to 900 per month, without any increase in operating room capacity or numbers of beds. The method involves analyzing the typical operating time for procedures by specialty and the average length of stay of patients by specialty, and determining the average monthly admissions also by specialty. With these data, it becomes possible to calculate to a considerable degree of accuracy both the operating room time that will be required and the average census generated. Conversely, it becomes possible to adjust the balance of admissions by specialty so as to smooth out fluctuations in occupancy. For both approaches, it is necessary to consider each of the specialties: In the figures which Mr. Stewart gives in his article, for example, the range in average operating room time varies from .95 hours per procedure for urologic surgery to 2.55 hours for neurosurgery. Similarly, the average length of stay varies from about 1½ days for oral surgery patients to a little over 11 days for neurosurgery patients. Mr. Stewart notes that this method is merely designed to predict and control average admissions and procedures and is not intended for day-to-day scheduling which cannot, of course, be based upon average figures.

A number of recent studies, including computer simulation studies, have dealt with operating room schedules. While it is not within the scope of this book to deal with these methods, it may be worthwhile to list some of the factors that may affect operating room time.

- Is this a teaching hospital?
- How complex is the procedure?
- What type of anesthesia is used?
- How and where is induction carried out?
- How much clean-up and preparation time are required?

In his book *Planning of Surgical Centers* (Lloyd-Luke, London, 1973) Ervin Putsep concludes on the basis of both American and European research that for general hospitals an average time for operations (including the necessary interval between operations for clean-up and preparation) a planning standard of 75 minutes would be satisfactory. He suggests that surgeries should not be in operation more than 6 hours a day, since procedures late in the day tend to cause both anxiety and discomfort to the patient. Assuming a 5-day week and 250 operating days per year, together with what he considers to be a reasonable efficiency rate of staff and facilities of 60%, he concludes that a normal number of operating hours per operating room per year would be 1500 at best. He points out, however, that if the room were in operation seven days a week, the capacity would be increased by about 40%.

Emergency Procedures

In a Scottish study, *Surgical Departments in Hospitals—The Surgeon's View* (Butterworths, London, 1972) Dr. Donald Macleod Douglas notes that an analysis of a year's surgical activity at the Dundee Royal Infirmary showed a considerable consistency throughout the year in the numbers of both emergency and elective procedures: Deviation was never over 15%. This and similar data suggest that while emergency procedures cannot be controlled in the same way as elective procedures, they may reasonably be predicted, and sufficient allowance made for them.

It is suggested that for preliminary planning purposes estimates be based on an average of the 2 or 3 months of highest activity in recent experience for elective cases. For emergency cases—if a separate facility is not a priori provided—it is recommended that the month of highest activity be used as a guide. The outlined calculations are presented in terms of monthly activity, but depending on the level of detail appropriate the project they can be developed in terms of weekly or annual activity.

Distribution of Facilities

It is generally agreed that central, multi-use operating suites are desirable not only because they ensure efficient use of staff and facilities but because they permit more effective professional supervision and hence produce a better quality of medical care. Such ideal arrangements may not always be possible, however. There may be reasons for exception, and alternatives should be explored. If there is a predictable and sufficient volume of work for a specialty such as ophthalmic surgery, for example, a separate facility may be able to function quite satisfactorily. Specific disease oriented institutes such as cancer or heart centers, whose aim is to approach a specific disease process or site on an interdisciplinary basis, may wish to maintain their own operating suites, supporting facilities, and highly specialized staff. There is a continuing conflict between the generalist and the specialist point of view; there are valid arguments on both sides. It should be pointed out that as far as utilization of facilities is concerned, the greater the pool of cases, the greater the potential for efficiency. Efficiency, however, is not the only criterion.

Another question that may arise is what operating facilities should be part of the emergency suite. If the main surgical suite is adjacent to emergency, it will be necessary to decide whether the emergency department should contain a discrete major operating room, or if not, what means of rapid access can be provided to the central facilities. In considering this question an external demand factor may enter the picture: Is there, or is there a prospect of, a formal regional emergency services plan with official designation of certain hospitals as trauma centers? Such a plan would make it unlikely that the emergency room of a hospital not designated as a trauma center would receive major surgery cases. Conversely, the designation of the hospital as a trauma center would draw to it an increased volume of such cases and might suggest the need for more elaborate facilities reserved for emergencies.

An increasing number of surgical procedures are being done on an outpatient basis, and this raises the question of whether these patients are to be brought into the central surgical system or into a separate system that is to be provided for them. The criteria for this decision are both medical and functional: Is it felt that the procedures contain sufficient risk that they should take place in an area immediately accessible to major operating rooms and related support facilities? Is the volume of such procedures sufficiently great and sufficiently predictable to allow a separate unit to function efficiently? If outpatient surgery takes place in a separate facility, what types of anesthesia will be used? What provision will be made for induction and recovery?

The relationship between delivery, obstetric surgery, and gynecologic surgery should be explored. In many older hospitals, facilities for these are grouped as a separate women's unit, and in such cases it will be necessary to determine which parts of such a system are to be retained and how they should relate to central facilities.

Ideally the surgeries and the diagnostic radiology facilities will be adjacent. If this is impossible, it will be necessary to determine what the best compromise may be. Will special radiology procedure rooms, such as heart catheterization facilities, form part of the surgical suite? Will mobile radiology units be sufficient, or are more sophisticated facilities needed in the surgical suite? For example, how will cystoscopy, bronchoscopy, and orthopedic work be handled? The question of what happens to the patient after he leaves the operating room must also be explored. Where does he go? How long does he stay? Where does he go next? How is he moved, and how often?

Existing Conditions

Purpose

To obtain a picture of current operations and trends for analysis and later projection by determining (a) the average numbers and ratio of emergency and elective procedures over a defined period, (b) the average number of procedures and patient days, grouped by type, over a defined period, and (c) the current utilization of staff and facilities.

Work load

Information needed

1. Monthly hospital statistics, preferably for a period of not less than 5 years, which show the number of operations by surgical specialty and the number of patients days by specialty. (Many hospitals use figures showing admissions and average patient census rather than total patient days.)

Table S-1. 5-Year Summary of Average Monthly Procedures by Type

Type	Year 1	Year 2	Year 3	Year 4	Year 5	Average Annual Percent Increase (Decrease)
Major	240	245	235	260	275	3.5%
Minor	590	610	595	650	675	3.4%
Spec. Proc.	10	15	17	20	25	25.77%
Emergency	40	45	39	47	50	5.77%
Totals	880	915	885	977	1025	3.9%

2.   Information that shows the number of emergency as opposed to elective procedures. The definition of emergency should be supplied by the person responsible for scheduling the operating rooms, as it may be used in different ways. The purpose of the distinction is to try to determine how much of the work load is controllable, and to what degree the noncontrollable portion is predictable. If records that would provide this information are not kept routinely, Table S-2 may be revised to give

Table S-2. 5-Year Monthly Summary of Emergency and Elective Surgery Procedures by Month

Months	Year 1		Year 2		Year 3		Year 4		Year 5	
	Elec.	Emer.	Elec.	Emer.	Elec.	Emer.	Elec.	Emer.	Elec.	Emer.
Jan										
Feb										
Mar										
Apr										
May										
June										
July										
August										
Sept										
Oct										
Nov										
Dec										
Totals										
Percent of Total										

merely the total operations per month. In that case it will be necessary to obtain an authoritative estimate of the ratio of emergency to elective procedures. It may also be possible to obtain an informed judgment as to the numbers' relative stability.

Utilization

From operating room records, determine for a typical month how many hours each operating room or group of operating rooms was *available* for use, and also for how many hours each was *actually* in use (including preparation and clean-up times). If appropriate to the situation, major, minor, or specialty operating rooms may be considered separately. Available for use is taken to mean either any time that staff is available or the normal operating hours of the facility. The fact should be noted if there are any circumstances that might be considered out of the ordinary, for example, if a room is not available for use because of staff shortages or if scheduled operating hours are longer than normal because of a lack of facilities. Tables S-3 and S-4 are examples.

Table S-3. Monthly Operating Room Hours Available

Room	Weekdays	All Nights	Sat & Sun	Total
Room A	140	—	—	—
Room B	140	—	—	—
Etc.	—	—	—	—
Subtotal, Elective	—	—	—	—
Emergency	—	—	—	—
Total	—	—	—	—

Table S-4. Monthly Operating Room Hours Used (or Scheduled)

Room	Weekdays	All Nights	Sat & Sun	Total
Room A	106	—	—	—
Room B	62	—	—	—
Etc.	—	—	—	—
Subtotal Elective	—			—
Emergency	4	12	10	26
Totals	—	—	—	—

Personnel

A list of personnel by category by work shift. Part-time personnel should be shown separately, with the percentage of full-time equivalency (FTE) indicated. The actual number of individuals who make up the part-time staff should be indicated in parentheses. Totals for both FTE and individuals should be shown.

Table S-5. Summary of Operating Room Personnel by Shift

Personnel Category	Weekdays		Nights		Weekends		Total FTE	Total Numbers
	F-T	P-T	F-T	P-T	F-T	P-T		
Anesthetists	2	1(2)	1	—	1	1(4)	6	10
Scrub Nurses	—	—	—	—	—	—	—	—
Floor Nurses	—	—	—	—	—	—	—	—
Etc.	—	—	—	—	—	—	—	—
Totals	—	(—)	—	(—)	—	(—)	11.3	17

Analysis and Summary

Purpose

To summarize data about existing conditions and to compare potential with actual utilization of facilities to arrive at the current efficiency rate. It is proposed that a three-way comparison be made, not only comparing operating room potential to actual utilization during a specific month, but also comparing the actual utilization with a hypothetical time requirement arrived at by using the actual numbers of procedures by specialty for the chosen month, and then multiplying them by the time estimated to be required per specialty, as described below and illustrated in Table S-6. Such a comparison will provide a rough empirical test of the accuracy of the estimates.

Planning assumptions needed

1. With the assistance of the supervisor of the operating rooms or the heads of the services, obtain data or estimates of the average time required per procedure within each specialty, either separately for major and minor procedures or in total (Table S-6, below). At the same time. determine what proportion of procedures within each discipline fall into the category of major. If there are plans to develop an outpatient surgery, determine what proportion of each specialty's cases might be dealt with in this way.

2. If available data is inadequate for a factual determination, obtain estimates from the heads of the specialties as to the average length of stay of patients for that specialty; again, if appropriate, separately for major and minor procedures.

Table S-6. Typical Operating Room Time per Procedure by Specialty

| | Operating Room Time (Minutes) | | | | | |
| | Major Procedures | | | Minor Procedures | | |
Specialty	Proc.	Prep/ Cleanup	Total	Proc.	Prep/ Cleanup	Total
General	62	28	90	24	21	45
Gynecol.	40	20	60	—	—	—
Neurosur.	105	35	140	—	—	—

While the questions above are being discussed with heads of the specialties, the following additional information may be collected from each:

• How much recovery room time do patients typically require?
• What proportion of patients will require intensive postoperative care, and for how long?

Procedure

Prepare a table summarizing the data collected earlier;

Table S-7. Characteristics of Work Load

Category	Average Monthly Procedures	Average Length of Stay	Average Monthly Patient Days	Percent Distribution of Procedures
Major	275	8	2200	26.8%
Minor	675	5	3375[a]	65.9%
Spec. Proc.	25	12	300	2.4%
Emergency	50	7	350	4.9%
Totals	1025	6.1	6225	100.0%

[a] For purposes of the example it is assumed that admissions are equal to procedures, however, see Table S-12

Using the data or estimates tabulated in Table S-6, calculate the total monthly operating room time needed for each specialty, separately for elective and emergency cases if this information is needed.

Table S-8. Estimated Operating Room Time for General Surgery for One Month

| Category | Total Procedures | Minor Procedures | | | Major Procedures | | | Total OR Hours |
		Minutes per Procedure	Monthly Procedures	Monthly OR Hours	Minutes per Procedure	Monthly Procedures	Monthly OR Hours	
Elective	950	45	675	506	90	275	412.5	918.5
Emergency	50	45	35	26	90	15	22.5	48.5
Totals	1000	—	710	532	—	290	435.0	967.0

Repeat for each specialty and summarize.

Purpose

To determine percentage utilization.

Procedure

Choosing a single month, compare the operating room utilization figures, separately for emergency and special operating rooms if data are available from Tables S-3, S-4, and the summary of calculations shown in Table S-8.

Table S-9. Comparison of Potential and Actual Operating Room Utilization— General Surgery

| Category of OR | Total Monthly Hours Available | Monthly Hours Used | |
		Number	% Utilization
Room A	140	106	76%
Room B	140	62	44%
Etc.	—	—	—
Totals	1225	918.5	75%
Emergency	720	48.5	7%

Purpose

To compare the number of personnel hours per month to the number of procedures.

Procedure

Multiply the figure in the last line of the "Total FTE" column of Table S-5 by the number of work hours in a month to arrive at total personnel hours. For more detailed analyses, the calculation may be made separately for each category of personnel. Prepare a table summarizing personnel hours per procedure:

Table S-10. Personnel Hours per Procedure

Full-Time Equivalent Personnel	Monthly Hours per FTE	Total Monthly Man-Hours	Monthly Procedures	Man-Hours per Procedure
11.3	173	1955	194	10

Surgery—Projections

Purpose

To determine for a target date the distribution, by specialty and by type of facility needed, of a projected number of procedures; to estimate the utilization rate applicable in each case; and to calculate the number of operating rooms needed. The projection of the surgical case load can be approached from two directions, depending on what the operative constraints appear to be in a particular situation: If the number of surgical beds available is controlling, it will be necessary to begin with the number of patient days and to develop from that the level of activity of the surgical specialties; conversely, if planning is to be based on the needs of a defined population for procedures or on the ability of the surgical staff to bring in patients, planning will have to begin with the number of procedures. In either case, it is unlikely that a detailed projection by specialty can be made initially. It is proposed that a general projection be made for total procedures or total beds and that this total projection then be distributed among the specialties according to the best judgment of the surgical staff and administration to provide a reasonable estimate of operating room time and patient days. Depending on the degree of refinement required in a particular planning project, adjustments and corrections may be more or less detailed. For a long-range planning project, where current decisions are not critical and can be refined in the future, a simple projection of averages and totals based on unadjusted current operations may be sufficient. The calculations outlined suggest a midlevel of detail. It will be obvious in the course of analyzing the data the points at which further refinements should be made. Several planning and policy decisions must be made before this part of the process can begin.

General planning decisions needed

1. How will the surgical case load be projected? On the basis of beds assigned? On the basis of physicians' anticipated work load? On the basis of procedures per thousand population? Such projections will presumably be based on both regional and hospital policy. The projections must be coordinated with other hospital projections as outlined in Chapters 2 and 3.

2. What trends observed in (a) the percentage distribution of cases (or patient days) by specialty, (b) changes in the average length of stay, and (c) ratio between simple and complex or emergency and elective procedures should be considered in adjusting current characteristics of the work load to project into the future.

3. What is the projection at the target date of total surgical procedures and of beds or patient days?

Information needed

1. Historical data summarized in Table S-1 and Table S-2.
2. Characteristics of the work load from Table S-7.

Specific planning decisions needed

1. Given the percentage distribution of procedures (or patient days) by specialty summarized in Table S-1, what adjustments, if any, should be made to reflect anticipated changes (for example, the development of a strong new department)?

2. Given the average length of stay by specialty indicated in Table S-7, are any adjustments required in light of observed trends or changes in policy?

3. Given the proportion of emergency procedures summarized in Tables S-2 and S-8, what adjustments are needed, if any, to reflect anticipated changes?

4. Are the estimates of average operating room time per procedure by specialty (Table S-6) a realistic basis for planning? Or does the data summarized in Table S-9 represent a more accurate or sufficiently realistic method of estimation?

5. What percentage occupancy should be projected for surgical beds?

Step One: Work load

Procedure

If beds are the controlling factor, assume a given number of beds and a chosen occupancy rate and calculate the number of patient days available:

$$\text{Monthly patient days} = \text{number of beds} \times 30 \text{ days} \\ \times \text{ percentage occupancy}$$

Correct the major planning factors (percentage distribution by specialty, average length of stay, operating room time per specialty) according to the decisions taken (outlined in "Specific Planning Decisions Needed"). Calculate the number of procedures that can be performed monthly, by specialty or in total. Summarize the calculations as shown in Table S-11.

If number of procedures is the controlling factor, assume that a total number of procedures is projected at the target date, correct the planning factors as outlined above, and calculate the number of patient days that will be generated. Convert these to numbers of beds needed at a chosen occupancy rate (for example, 85%):

$$\text{Number of beds needed} = \frac{\text{monthly patient days}}{30 \text{ days} \times \text{percentage occupancy}}$$

Table S-11.   Summary of Projected Monthly Activity—Based on Patient Days

Category	Percent of Distribution of Procedures	No. of Beds	Projected Patient Days	Average Length of Stay	No. of Procedures	Average Minutes per Procedure	Operating Room Hours Needed
Major	26.8	—	2650	8	332	90	498
Minor	65.9	—	4070	5	813	45	610
Spec. Proc.	2.4	—	360	12	30	140	70
Emergency	4.9	—	420	7	60	58	58
Totals	100.0	250	7500	6.1	1235	60	1236

Step Two: Distribution of the Work Load

Policy decisions needed

1.   Will separate facilities be provided for emergency or specialized surgery? If so, the numbers of procedures represented must be removed from the "Projected Number of Procedures" and "Operating Room Hours Needed" columns of Table S-11.

2.   Will any portion of the total projected procedures be performed on an outpatient basis? How many from each specialty? If this is planned,

the estimated number of patient days generated by these procedures must be removed from the total patient days and the estimate of beds revised accordingly.

3. Will outpatient surgery be performed in a discrete facility provided for this purpose? If so, the "Operating Room Hours" column should be adjusted by removing the hours attributable to this portion of the work load.

4. The number of procedures which is expected to occur *in addition* to procedures currently performed on an inpatient basis must be estimated.

Such adjustments might be displayed as follows:

Table S-12. Adjustment to Numbers of Procedures

Category	Total Projected Procedures	Percent Outpatient Procedures	No. of Outpatient Procedures	Added Outpatient Cases	Total Outpatient Procedures	Balance Inpatient Procedures
Major	331	—	—	—	—	331
Minor	814	20%	163	—	—	651
Spec. Proc.	30	—	—	—	—	30
Totals	1175	—	163	200	363	1012
Emergency	60	60%	36	—	—	24

Table S-13. Adjustment to Number of Patients Days and Operating Hours

Category	Number of Outpatient Procedures	Average Length of Stay	Total Patient Days to be Deducted	Average OR Time per Procedure	Total OR Hours to be Deducted
Minor	163	5	815	45	122
Emergency	36	7	252	—	—
Totals	199	—	1067	—	122

Planning decision needed

Determine how many outpatient surgical visits will occur in addition to those deducted from the present inpatient work load.

Procedure

Summarize the adjusted projections to show the work load, operating room time, and patient days associated with each category of operating room:

Table S-14. Summary of Procedures, Patient Days and Time

Operating Room Category	Number of Procedures	Patient Days Generated	Operating Room Hours Needed
Central OR	1012	6265[a]	1056[c]
Emergency OR	60	168[b]	58
Outpatient OR	363	None	272[d]
Totals	1435	6433	1386

[a] $2650 + 4070 + 360 - 815 = 6265$; [b] $420 - 252 = 168$; [c] $498 + 610 + 70 - 122 = 1056$; [d] $363 \times 45 \div 60 = 272$.

Step Three: Utilization

Information needed

Summary data from Table S-4 above, showing totals of procedures and operating room hours needed.

Planning assumptions needed

1. What percentage utilization of operating room time available is considered adequate (from the standpoint of efficiency) and acceptable (from the standpoint of necessary availability)? This assumption may be based on a straightforward projection of current utilization as developed in Table S-9 if the current rate appears reasonable. If this is not feasible, it will be necessary to decide how this rate is to be adjusted, with the reasons for doing so explained.

2. What changes, if any, may be anticipated in the numbers of hours during which operating rooms are available; for example, will there be a change to a 7-day week, or a longer or shorter day?

Procedure

Calculate the number of operating room hours that must be available at the chosen utilization rate in order to accommodate the projected work load, and determine the number of rooms that are needed at the chosen length of work day and work week.

It may be interesting to examine the effect of changing the number of hours during which the operating rooms are available. 140 hours a month represents a schedule of 5 days a week, 7 hours a day. A 7-day week of 6 hours a day would provide a total of approximately 180 hours a month

Table S-15.

Operating Room Category	Projected Operating Room Hours per Month	Percentage Utilization	Adjusted Operating Room Hours Needed	Available Hours per Operating Room per Month	Number of Rooms Needed
Central ORs	1056	65%	1625	140	12
Emergency ORs	58	10%	580	720	1
Outpatient ORs	272	75%	363	140	3
Totals	1386	—	2568	—	16

per room. In the example this would reduce the number of rooms required to 9 central OR's, and 2 outpatient OR's. Since a separate emergency surgery is shown as being available 24 hours a day, no change would take place in emergency surgery requirements.

Step Four: Personnel

Information needed

Data on current man-hours per procedure from Table S-10.

Planning decision needed

Does the current ratio of man-hours to procedures represent an acceptable planning standard? If not, what adjustments should be made?

Table S-16.   Projected OR Personnel

Projected Monthly Procedures	Man Hours per Procedure	Total Man-Hours	Monthly Hours per FTE	FTE Personnel Required
1012	10	10,120	180	55.2

Note: This projection is for *total* staff. For some purposes a *weekday only* estimate may be more useful.

5.2. OBSTETRICS AND RELATED FACILITIES

Background/Discussion

The number of beds, and consequently of facilities for delivery and neonatal care of infants, is of course dependent in a general way on the birth rate, but in the case of a specific hospital it is also dependent on the number of gynecologists and obstetricians on the staff and on the location of the hospital and its accessibility. Declining birth rates have created high vacancy rates in obstetric units of many hospitals, and concern for the quality of care that patients receive in an underutilized obstetric facility is one of the reasons for a series of guidelines issued in 1971 by the American College of Obstetricians and Gynecologists.* The guidelines deal with the organization and delivery of services and development of manpower and give recommendations specifically related to sizes of obstetric units.

Because a study initiated by the ACOG showed that a full range of hospital obstetric services could only be provided efficiently when annual deliveries exceeded 1500 per year, the recommendation was made that smaller obstetric services be consolidated in so far as possible. In sparsely populated areas a limited but adequate service could be expected when at least 500 deliveries occurred per year. An acknowledged constraint on consolidation is accessibility. The group recommended that a travel time of 1 hour could be considered acceptable. In some areas, travel might have to be by helicopter.

An attempt to predict obstetric service requirements by mathematical modeling, using the experience of 3 hospitals as a basis for comparison, shows that there is a dramatic reduction in the requirements not only for beds but for delivery and supporting facilities, when facilities are consolidated. A 1966 article by Fetter and Thompson† shows that efficiency of facilities decreases sharply when admissions are under 4000 a year, although from 4000 upward the rate of improvement is rather minimal. The authors compare the combined requirements for 3 separate hospitals, each having admissions of 1300-1400 per year, with a hypothetical hospital in which 3900-4200 admissions occur in a centralized facility. The results of the comparison clearly illustrate the smoothing effect of large numbers where events occur randomly:

* *National Needs in Obstetrics and Gynecology*, 1971. Issued by the ACOG, Chicago, Ill., March 1971, and approved by the Executive Committee of the ACOG as a guide for future action in the areas covered.
† *"Predicting Maternity Service Requirements"*, John D. Thompson and Robert B. Fetter in *Hospital Industrial Engineering* (p. 317-21). Harold E. Smalley, John Freeman, eds. 1966.

	Totals required for three hospitals @ 1300–1400 births per year each:	Required for a consolidated unit with 3900–4200 births/year:
Number of beds	90	75
Number of labor rooms	9	7
Recovery rooms	3	2
Caeserian section rooms	3	1
Delivery rooms	6	3

Health planning agencies generally acknowledge the difficulty of maintaining a high census in a specialized facility with a small number of beds and allow that in some cases a small unit may be necessary for geographic reasons. As a preliminary planning guideline, for example, the Massachusetts Comprehensive Health Planning Agency suggested that the following occupancy rates are realistic:

Size of Unit	Occupancy rate
10–15 beds	50–65%
15–20 beds	60–70%
20–50 beds	65–75%
50+ beds	75% +

From the preceding, it will be evident that neither the number of beds nor the number of delivery rooms, labor rooms, and supporting facilities of various kinds are subject to a straightforward rule of thumb. Because of its random nature, the obstetric patient load is particularly suitable for analysis by the Poisson distribution (see Chapter 4).

One authority suggests the following relationships among obstetric facilities:

> For every 16-18 beds—1 delivery room
> For every 8 beds—1 labor room
> For every 2-3 labor beds—1 recovery bed

These relationships can best be derived from an analysis of the time required for each stage of a woman's progress from admission to discharge. The modes in which obstetric care is given vary, depending on local customs and habits. The recent trend of introducing the father to the complete process of birth has implications for the way rooms are arranged, and it would be worthwhile in planning a new facility or adding to an existing one to examine the entire sequence of events afresh. Some of the questions that may be asked are:

- Where will a woman be examined upon admission? That is, in a labor room, an admission room, or will she be admitted to her post-partum room for the first stages of labor? Will the father be with her most of the time? How will they spend the time between admission and the next stage of labor? Will the first-stage labor room be the same room to which she will return after delivery, or will she go to a recovery room or the nursing unit? If to a recovery room, how long will she stay there? How will her progress be monitored?
- Will there be a second-stage labor room? Will this be a single room, and will the father still be along?
- If this is a high-risk patient, will her delivery be in a special room? If she is delivered by Caeserian section, will this be done in the delivery area or in a general surgery? During a normal delivery, will the father be present?
- What will be the arrangement for post-partum care? Will there be rooming in? Should there be a small nursery between clusters of rooms, or should the nursery be centralized? Should the rooms be multiple bed rooms with sitting and perhaps dining areas where patients and fathers can share meals and socialize? Or should rooms be private, perhaps with room for the fathers to stay, and assist in the care of the infant?
- What is the rate of high-risk births that will take place at this hospital?
- What provision is to be made for premature or ill newborn? Will there be an acute care nursery for them, and if so, will it be associated with the pediatric service or with the maternity service? Or will high-risk mothers and infants be transferred elsewhere, and if so by what means?

A question of some importance, as well as of some controversy, is whether an obstetric operating room can be used for clean gynecological cases. The trend seems to be to feel that it can, as long as appropriate precautions are taken. In fact, it is sometimes argued that there should not be an obstetric operating room at all and that obstetric operations should take place where the full range of operating room facilities are available.

Another issue that relates to obstetric facilities is whether or not abortions should be dealt with in the obstetric area and whether or not beds and facilities can be combined. Most early abortions are performed on an outpatient basis, but many physicians feel that the full range of hospital facilities should be available in case of trouble. A psychological question also enters into the decision: Should women who are giving up a child be located in an area where women are giving birth? The same question needs to be asked about gynecological patients, some of whom are often placed in the same nursing unit as new mothers. The physical design of a nursing unit can help here, by ensuring that any swing beds—beds that can be assigned to either unit—are in some manner separable from one of the neighboring units, if only by visual means.

In most hospitals having a fair volume of deliveries the volume of high risk patients will be somewhat higher than the average, since such patients are likely to be sent to a larger hospital where a fuller range of services is available. This suggests the need, in such hospitals, to plan for special facilities such as special on-call rooms for obstetricians, anesthesiologists, and pediatricians, anesthesia workroom, and special procedure laboratories providing equipment for patient monitoring.

Because births cannot be accurately scheduled, at least one room beyond the planned number of delivery rooms should be designed to be large enough and fitted out for emergency delivery.

Projecting Requirements for Obstetric Services

Because of the likelihood that facilities requirements will overlap, the planning of obstetrics services should be done in the context of planning for surgical services.

Information needed

- On the basis of hospital-wide and area-wide planning decisions, the numbers of obstetric beds that are planned.
- Status of current obstetric facilities as to occupancy, patterns of care, and so forth.

Planning decisions needed

- Given anticipated changes in length of stay, methods and styles of delivery, care of the post-partum patient, involvement of the father, and care of the infant, what will be the relationship between beds and facilities for: labor, normal delivery, Caeserian delivery, recovery, and nursery beds or bassinets? Infant intensive care?
- If an obstetric operating room is used for purposes other than delivery, what are the criteria for such use? If, conversely, obstetric surgery is performed in a general operating room, what special criteria will apply?

Summarize the projected work load and facility needs:

Table OB-1. Summary of Obstetric Facility Requirements

	Annual Number	Average Daily Census	Beds Needed	Delivery Rooms	Minor Procedure Rooms	Labor Beds	Recovery Beds	Bassinets
Normal births	—	—	—	—	—	—	—	—
High-risk births	—	—	—	—	—	—	—	—
Abortions	—	—	—	—	—	—	—	—
Other procedures	—	—	—	—	—	—	—	—

In addition, a brief verbal statement should be made as to the approach that will be taken to each type of patient and to infants and fathers. The relationship between obstetrics, gynecology, general surgery, and pediatrics should also be explored.

5.3. RADIATION MEDICINE

Background/Discussion

The relationships among diagnostic radiology, radiation therapy, and nuclear medicine vary considerably from one institution to another. A brief summary of the position of the Joint Expert Committee of the World Health Organization and the International Atomic Energy Commission will confirm that the problem of definition is universal. The committee concluded that at the time of their deliberations there were three principal branches of radiation medicine, described as follows:

- Diagnostic radiology has the object of providing information.
- Radiotherapy is the treatment of disease by ionizing radiation, making use of biological effects, particularly the selective destruction of tissue.
- Nuclear medicine partakes of characteristics of both. It consists of the application of unsealed radioactive materials for diagnostic and therapeutic purposes, making use of emissions of ionizing radiation from such materials and from their distribution within the body or *in vitro*. The committee noted that the exact definition of nuclear medicine is still a matter of study but that for purposes of its deliberation all medical uses of unsealed sources of radioactive materials were to be considered as part of nuclear medicine. The committee noted further, however, that in many instances the therapeutic uses of such materials is within the province of radiotherapy and also observed that some of the diagnostic procedures, which the committee had classified as nuclear medicine, might more properly be classified with diagnostic radiology.

The committee described the common features of the disciplines which justified their inclusion in an omnibus category of radiation medicine, namely: the use of various properties of ionizing radiation; the necessity for protection against hazards; the requirement for specially built facilities; a common need for the services of specially trained physicists and technicians; a common need for maintenance of complex high voltage and electronic equipment; and a common shortage of trained personnel.

Distribution of Facilities

It is evident that from the standpoint of the departments themselves the planning of facilities for radiation medicine must be considered together. Although it might seem that ideally the facilities of the three main disciplines should be located together, since there are overlapping requirements for support facilities and staff and since such an arrangement would assure that activities could flow from one area into another if one discipline grows as another shrinks, the categories of patients placing primary demand on the facilities vary, and this may cause constraints on location that are at variance with the concept of a centralized facility. On the average, outpatients may represent 90% of the work load of a therapy department, and the work load of a diagnostic department may be tipped heavily towards inpatients. It may be that the therapy department should be located so as to permit a multidisciplinary approach to cancer patients in a centralized facility including both inpatients and outpatients rather than maintaining its primary relation to diagnostic radiology.

For diagnostic radiology and nuclear medicine, access is required by wheelchair and stretcher patients coming from nursing units and the emergency room and by outpatients from clinics or on referral by private physicians. Some radiological procedures require a surgical or quasi-surgical setting, which may be at odds with other location criteria.

A diagnostic radiology department may have to be split a number of ways, perhaps owing to site constraints, to the need to maintain facilities already in place, or to a large and busy outpatient department that can sustain a satellite unit.

In order to approach the question of distribution of facilities it will be necessary to make a first-round rough estimate of space requirements for each type of facility and each group of patients. As projections are refined, a more detailed analysis can be done to explore the issues of centrality and adjacency. When decisions have been made as to the distribution of facilities it may be necessary to revise utilization and support facility estimates to reflect some necessary duplication of support spaces and possible lower efficiency of some units where decentralization turns out to be necessary or desirable.

Diagnostic Radiology

The growth of this discipline has been very rapid in the recent past and shows no signs of letting up. Although diagnostic radiology was originally used exclusively as an aid to clinical diagnosis, it is now used to follow the progress of a patient during and after treatment and to screen for diseases before symptoms develop. The shift in disease patterns away from infectious diseases has increased the use of diagnotic radiology as a tool, and the rapid development of increasingly complex and sophisticated procedures have added to the work load. Technologies such as thermography, xeroradiography, tomography, computerized scanners and ultrasonics, which are generally grouped with diagnostic radiology are new enough that considerable development can be expected. It is possible, therefore, that taken together these factors will contribute to maintaining the growth rate of procedures for some time into the future. However, it would be as unwise to *assume* the continuation of the recent growth as it would be to ignore it, and it is suggested that projections not be made explicit beyond a 5-year period. Clearly, though, all planning for diagnostic radiology facilities should include an escape route in the event that growth does continue. Since facilities are extremely expensive to move, under no circumstances should facilities be located so that they are locked in by other functions that cannot themselves be easily moved.

The basic questions to be asked about the radiology department include:

- What are the numbers and categories of patients who will make demands on the department?
- What are the types and numbers of procedures that will be required for each category of patient?
- How efficiently can (or will) the radiology procedure rooms be used?
- How can facilities be physically distributed for maximum efficiency of operation, quality of supervision, and convenience for patients and staff?

The work load of the department of radiology depends on the types of patients the hospital attracts. The number of radiographic procedures to be planned for is often predicated on the numbers of beds in the hospital. Projecting on the basis of numbers of beds alone appears to be too crude a method for any but the roughest preliminary estimate. A simple bed count does not take account of differences in occupancy rate or outpatient loads, and, furthermore, is too general to be checked and updated at later stages of planning. Discussing data that tabulate typical work

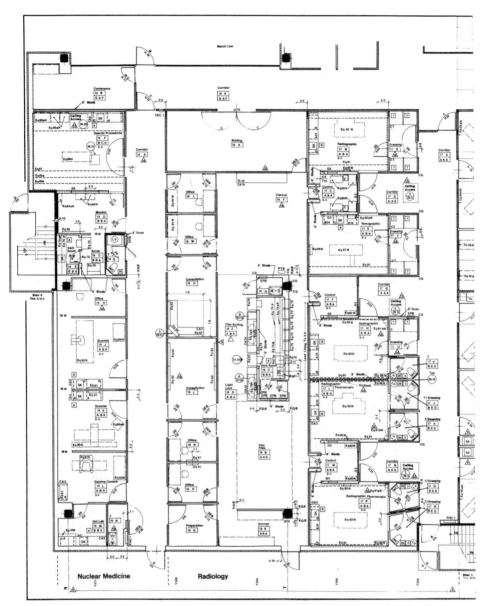

Figure 8. Radiology Suite: Alcoves for inpatient stretchers provide privacy and keep corridors free from obstructions (St. Joseph Hospital, Clinton Township, Mich.; Hugh Stubbins/Rex Allen Partnership, Architects).

loads and facilities, in terms of bed size of the hospitals, Drs. George
Cooper and Barton Young remark:

These statistics are interesting; they indicate trends. The averages and means
offer some planning guidance, but the very wide range behind the averages and
means lead to (our) . . . statement that in the final analysis *the estimate of
practice volume and nature of the radiological practice must be made on the
basis of local experience, and factors peculiar to the individual situation.*

Changes and advances in scientific medicine have added to the types
of procedures that generally fall under the heading of diagnostic radiology and have changed the distribution of procedures from the simplest
to the most complex. For planning purposes it is recommended that procedures be grouped and projected separately by level of complexity and
time required. The appropriate groupings will vary from one hospital to
the next, and the groupings illustrated in the following section should
not in any way be considered authoritative. It is recommended that procedures be grouped with the assistance of a radiologist or department
administrator who is familiar with the current operation and who can
decide on the basis of local conditions what a useful aggregation would
be.

Utilization

How to calculate room utilization or plan capacity is a troublesome issue
which, again, does not seem to be capable of resolution by reference to
norms. There is little agreement among authorities as to acceptable utilization standards. It seems on the face of it absurd to lump together procedures that may consume over 200 minutes of equipment or personnel
time with those that may consume at the most 7 or 8 minutes and to
average them together. For this reason we have chosen to combine procedures by the length of time they consume and to use averages for the
group as a whole. The proportion of the total work load represented by
the more complex and time consuming is thus a major factor in planning
capacity. Other factors that will vary considerably, depending on the type
of hospital, its geographic area, and its location, include the number of
trained professional and support personnel available, the numbers of
hours they are willing to work, the times at which patients present themselves or are presented by the hospital itself for its outpatient department,
and the internal organization of the radiology department. If detailed
data about patients—their source, the days and times they arrived, the
time they spent in the department, and so on—have been kept, it will be
possible to arrive at a useful profile of the work load of the department

and to explore some of the reasons for such factors as peak loads on certain days or certain hours of the day.

However, probably only a minority of departments keep full records and it may be desirable, in that case, to do a survey for the specific purpose of collecting planning data. Such a survey should include information about the patient and how he arrived at the department, about the procedure performed, and about the patient's total experience while in the department, including procedure time and waiting time. Additional operational information about the staff effort can be collected at the same time. Each procedure room can be monitored separately to determine the distribution of work in that room during the course of the day and the week.

One of the problems in discussing utilization is that it is often a touchy question. Most people are sensitive to any suggestion of inefficiency, and any analysis of efficiency, however discreetly approached, is likely to be met with a defensive reaction. It should be made clear immediately, therefore, that a daily room utilization rate of 50% is quite common and not a cause for criticism—although a rate higher than this should certainly be attempted. It is a good policy to ask the department itself for an evaluation of utilization and for suggestions as to the reasons for possible excessive loads at certain times of day or week or year, and for factors arising out of matters outside the control and jurisdiction of the department that might be changed. The primary tool for planning with the department, however, is a sequence of data and analysis that will allow the department itself to arrive at planning standards that are applicable to its particular situation. Although in the future the size of equipment may be reduced, the current rough planning guidelines for diagnostic radiology facilities, that is, a net area of 1100 to 1300 square feet per procedure room for total space (excluding research) is likely to remain applicable for some time.

Radiotherapy

The work load of a radiotherapy department is likely to be somewhat more predictable and subject to advance scheduling than is the case for diagnostic radiology. Because statistics on cancer have been maintained for some time, planning guidelines are fairly well established. The World Health Organization in 1964 quotes a figure of 3000 new cases per year per 1,000,000 population with an estimate that approximately one-half of all cases would receive radiation therapy during the course of the disease in areas of the world where programs were well developed. New York State currently proposes the following guidelines:

- One major radiotherapeutic center should be planned for every half million of population.
- To ensure an efficient operation, approximately 1000-3000 patients. At least 300 new patients per year are required for 1 supervoltage unit.
- 90% of all radiation therapy treatments are provided on an outpatient basis.
- 200 new patients per year is accepted as the maximum case load for a clinical radiation therapist under ideal conditions.
- Minimum staffing should include a full-time radiation therapist, a radiation physicist, plus clerical support. The services of a dosimetrist and a social worker should be available on a consulting basis.
- Provision must be made for the safe handling and storage of radioactive materials; for space and resources for planning treatments; for a standards laboratory for calibrating equipment, as well as office space for staff, additional laboratories for research, and receiving and holding areas for patients.

The radiation therapy department, much of whose work load comes from outpatients, should be located so as to take this into account. However, it must also be possible to bring bed patients to the facility. Particularly in a smaller unit, there are good arguments for placing the area adjacent to diagnostic radiology, except that construction and shielding requirements are considerably greater, suggesting a subgrade location. However, a close physical relationship can help to encourage the shared use of supporting staff, technicians, maintenance engineers, and so on. In a discipline where shortage of trained personnel is a perennial problem, this is particularly important. Because of the current multidisciplinary approach to cancer, serious consideration must also be given to a location for the radiotherapy unit that will facilitate such an approach. This may mean that diagnostic and treatment facilities and research areas may be organized into an interdisciplinary center. Again the problem of functional versus departmental planning arises. Such a facility, especially designed to deal with today's approaches to a particular problem, may quickly become obsolete.

Nuclear Medicine

Nuclear medicine combines diagnostic and therapeutic aspects, and as suggested by the WHO committee quoted earlier it is not yet clear where it belongs. Measurements of the movement and localization of radionucleides through the body are done by the introduction of low-level doses of radiopharmaceuticals which are then counted. High radiation doses can also be directed at specific tissues for therapeutic purposes. *In vitro* measurements are also made of body fluids, tissue, or excretions.

The WHO outlines a proposed distribution of services by category:

- Advanced nuclear medicine should take place only in major medical centers and should include a full range of services, including training and the development of new procedures. It is estimated that a major nuclear medicine department will require at a minimum about 7000 square feet, exclusive of beds, education, and research space.
- Smaller general units with simpler installations, but still capable of a range of diagnostic and therapeutic procedures, could be accommodated in an area of approximately 4500 square feet. Facilities can be provided in small local hospitals to perform simple diagnostic procedures, using radiopharmaceuticals supplied by major centers, and *in vitro* procedures that do not involve administration to the patient.

Planning for Radiation Medicine

In the planning outline which follows, procedures are described in terms of diagnostic radiology procedures. The same approach may be taken to deal with the needs of radiation therapy and nuclear medicine by revising the headings on the illustrative tables.

Most of the needed planning assumptions and decisions apply to the nuclear medicine and radiotherapy departments. An important added question arises in the case of a therapy department, however. High levels of public and government support for cancer research programs have, in some areas, led to a poor distribution of cancer treatment centers. For this discipline it is particularly important to determine the level of effort being planned by other institutions in the area and to avoid duplication of the more powerful and expensive equipment. This appears to be an area, similar to that of number of beds and occupancy rates, where governmental intervention may be anticipated.

Diagnostic Radiology—Current Operations

Purpose

To determine the number and distribution of procedures by type of procedure and patient category and to estimate current utilization of facilities.

Information needed

1. A list of procedures performed over the past full year, showing the types of procedures and the category of patient. The information may be tabulated thus:

Table R-1. Distribution of Procedures by Category of Patient, Year 19___

| | / | Patient Category | | | |
Procedure	Inpatients	Outpatients	Emergency Patients	Other	Totals
Type A	600	200	200	100	1100
Type B	1000	300	—	50	1350
Type C	400	—	—	—	400
Etc.	—	—	—	—	—
Totals	—	—	—	—	—

2. List of procedure rooms, showing which types of procedures are performed in which rooms. The department should note its impressions of which rooms appear to be functioning at, below, or beyond capacity.

3. Any logs which may indicate seasonal, weekly, or daily peak or slow periods.

4. From the hospital's statistics, the number of admissions (with breakdown by clinical department, if available) and the number of outpatient and emergency visits for the same period.

5. Optional: list of personnel by category, by work shift.

6. A list of the weekly hours during which each room is in operation (that is, the time during which the room can be staffed and available for use, whether it is in fact being used or not). The department should indicate whether rooms are being used in the evenings or on weekends because of functional necessity or desirability or because of a work load that is in excess of capacity. If rooms are available for shorter than normal hours, the department should likewise note the reasons such as lack of demand or shortage of staff.

Table R-2. Weekly Room Hours Available

| | Weekly Hours Available | | | |
Rooms	Weekdays	Nights	Weekends	Total
Room A	35	10	5	50
Room B	35	—	—	35
Etc.	—	—	—	—
Totals	—	—	—	—

Planning assumptions needed

1. The average procedure room time required for each type of procedure shown in the list described under Item 1 of *Information needed*.

2. Aggregation of these procedures into groups according to the type of procedure room or special equipment they require and the time they consume.

These planning assumptions must be developed with the assistance of a radiologist or possibly an administrator who is familiar with the procedures and equipment. A typical grouping might be as follows:

GROUP I   General Procedures: including chest, abdomen, skull, extremities, spine, and IVPs.

GROUP II   Routine Chest (as a separate category if the volume is very high and rapid).

GROUP III   Fluoroscopy (routine).

GROUP IV   Special Procedures: these may include urological procedures, cardiovascular and neurological procedures, tomography, ultrasound, and others; or, if the work load is sufficient they may be listed separately.

The purpose of grouping the procedures is to arrive at sets of procedures for which time requirements can be reasonably averaged, consistent with the types of rooms required.

A summary of these assumptions might look like this:

Table R-3. Summary of Procedures by Major Groups

Procedure Type	In-patients	Out-patients	Emer-gency	Other	Totals	Estimated Minutes per Procedure
Group I Procedures						20
Totals	18,355	7342	842	1129	27,668	Average
Type A	600	200	200	100	—	18
Type B	1000	300	—	50	—	9
Etc.	—	—	—	—	—	—
Group II Procedures						
Totals	—	—	—	—	—	—
Type X	—	—	—	—	—	—
Type Y	—	—	—	—	—	—
Etc.	—	—	—	—	—	—

Number of Procedures by Patient Category

Procedure

1. Prepare a table showing the average annual procedures for each group of procedures by patient category, and calculate the percent of total procedures each group represents, thus:

Table R-4. Average Annual Procedures by Patient Category—Year 19___

| | Procedures | | | | | | | | |
| | Group I | | Group II | | Group III | | Group IV | | Totals | |
Patient Category	No.	%	No.	%	No.	No.	No.	%	No.	%
No. of inpatient procedures	18,355	60	7342	24	3059	10	1835	06	30,591	100
Average procedures per admission (13,905 annual admissions)	1.32		.53		.22		.13		2.2	
No. of outpatient procedures	7,342	—	—	—	—	—	—	—	—	—
Average procedures per outpatient visit	—		—		—		—		—	
Etc.	—		—		—		—		—	

2.   Compute the average procedure time for each group of procedures as shown in Table R-3. For each patient category compute the total annual hours (number of procedures multiplied by the average minutes per procedure and divided by 60 minutes). Divide the total annual hours by 52 (weeks) to arrive at the computed average weekly room hours needed. Determine the potential number of room hours available for each group of procedures by multiplying the number of rooms available by the number of hours per week during which the rooms might be expected to be in operation (i.e., a 35-hour week or a 40-hour week). Compare the computed hours needed to the actual hours available to arrive at the percentage utilization thus:

Table R-5. Average Utilization of Procedure Rooms for Inpatient Procedures, Year 19___

Procedures	Annual Procedures	Average Minutes per Procedure	Total Annual Hours	Calculated Average Weekly Hours	No. of Rooms Available	Weekly Hours Available	Percent Utilization
Group I	18,355	20	6118	117.6	5	200[a]	58.8%
Group II	—	—	—	—	—	—	—
Etc.	—	—	—	—	—	—	—
Totals	—	—	—	—	—	—	—

[a] Assumes a 40-hour week.

3.   Optional: Compute total annual full-time equivalent (FTE) personnel hours and compare to total annual procedures:

Table R-6. Personnel Hours

Personnel	Total FTE Annual Hours	Total Procedures	Average Personnel Hours per Procedure
Radiologist	—	—	—
X-ray technician	—	—	—
Technical support	—	—	—
Total	—	—	—

Diagnostic Radiology—Projections

Purpose

To estimate the number of procedures that can be anticipated as occurring annually at a target date and the facilities and personnel required to accommodate them.

Information needed

1. Historical data showing admissions, outpatient visits, emergency vistis, and procedures performed for each of these categories of patients; with the rate of increase in procedures per patient indicated for a 5- to 10-year period.

Table R-7. Rate of Increase of Radiology Procedures

Year	Inpatients				Outpatients				Emergency
	Admissions	Procedures	Procedures per Admission	Percent Change	Visits	Procedures	Procedures per Visit	Percent Change	And so on
19—	—	—	—	—	—	—	—	—	—
19—	—	—	—	—	—	—	—	—	—
19—	—	—	—	—	—	—	—	—	—
Etc.	—	—	—	—	—	—	—	—	—

2. The information developed about the current operation, including data shown in Examples R-5, R-6, R-7, and R-8.

Planning decisions needed

1. Given the rate of increase in procedures *per patient* over the past x years, what rate of increase can be assumed for the next x years? Will

the rate of increase be the same for all patient categories? Will the rate be the same for each of the groups of procedures?

2.   Is the current utilization rate of facilities satisfactory? For all or some of the available procedure rooms? If not, can the causes be traced and corrected, and how? Is it safe to assume that the percent of total procedures represented by each group of procedures will remain relatively constant and likewise that the average time consumed will remain constant? (Typically, a small percentage of procedures may consume a much larger percentage of the total time. See Table R-10.)

Education

What kinds of training programs are planned? How many students of what types? Will basic science courses be taught within the department itself, or will these be provided by a nearby educational institution?

Research

How many persons will be engaged in research, and what provision will be made for them? (See Chapter 9)

Planning assumptions needed

These are questions which must be answered by the hospital administration for the hospital as a whole.

What projections have been made with regard to increases or decreases in the numbers of beds? What will be the distribution of characteristics of patients and of the clinical departments to which they are admitted? What projections have been made with regard to outpatient visits, and what will be the conditions of that population? Similar assumptions will have to be defined by the hospital administration with regard to emergency patients and private referrals or referrals from other institutions.

Procedure

1.   On the basis of planning decisions made with regard to the overall projected rate of increase of procedures per patient for each patient category and planning assumptions with regard to patient loads, calculate the numbers of radiology procedures anticipated at the target date:

Table R-8. Projected Average Annual Procedures for the Target Year—In-Patients

Patient Category	Projected Patient Load	Average Procedures per Patient	Projected Radiology Procedures
Inpatient Admissions	21,000	2.9	60,900
Outpatients	—	—	—
Emergency Patients	—	—	—
Others	—	—	—
Totals	—	—	—

2. Distribute the total projected annual procedures for each category of patients according to either the percentages applicable to the current year (see Table R-4) or adjusted according to planning decisions made with regard to anticipated changes in the ratios among the several groups of procedures:

Table R-9. Distribution of Procedures by Major Groups Projected for the Target Year

Patient Category	Total Procedures	Distribution							
		Group I		Group II		Group III		Group IV	
		%	No.	%	No.	%	No.	%	No.
Inpatients	60,900	60	36,540	24	14,616	10	6090	06	3654
Outpatients	—	—	—	—	—	—	—	—	—
Emergency	—	—	—	—	—	—	—	—	—
Other	—	—	—	—	—	—	—	—	—
Totals	—	—	—	—	—	—	—	—	—

3. Calculate the average annual room time required for each projected group of procedures at the target date either for the work load as a whole or by patient category:

Table R-10. Projected Average Weekly Room Hours Needed—Inpatients

Procedure Type	Projected Annual Procedures	Average Minutes per Procedure	Total Annual Hours	Average Weekly Hours
Group I	36,540	20	12,180	234.2
Group II	14,616	10	2,436	46.8
Group III	6,090	35	3,552	68.3
Group IV	3,654	120	7,308	140.5
Totals	—	—	—	489.8

4. On the basis of decisions taken with regard to: (*a*) acceptable room utilization rate and (*b*) available weekly hours per room (that is, the number of hours per week a room might normally be available for use) calculate the number of procedure rooms needed:

Table R-11. Calculation of the Projected Number of Rooms Needed—Inpatients

Procedure Type	Calculated Average Weekly Hours	Utilization Rate	Actual Weekly Room Hours Needed	Weekly Hours per Room	Number of Rooms Needed
Group I	234.2	.70	334.6	45	7.4
Group II	46.8	.60	78	35	2.2
Group III	68.3	.65	105	35	3
Group IV	140.5	.50	281	35	8
Totals	489.8	.61 avg.	798.6	—	20.6

5.4. SPECIAL PATIENT SERVICES

Into this general category fall the many diagnostic and treatment services not covered in the preceding sections. These services make modern medicine what it is—complex, sophisticated, subject to rapid scientific and technological change. The methodologies outlined in the preceding sections of this chapter can easily be adapted to deal with these services. The basic approach of examining existing conditions and determining the nature and source of the work load and the personnel and space required per unit of measure of the work load is the same. This section will, therefore, confine itself to a brief examination of some services and provide a checklist of others.

Some of the special services found in hospitals include:

• Audiology and ophthalmology testing and treatment facilities.
• Otorhinolaryngology.
• Minor procedure facilities for endoscopy, bronchoscopy, cystoscopy, dentistry.
• Respiratory therapy (inhalation therapy is sometimes included as a supply service).
• Hyperbaric laboratory.
• Cardiopulmonary laboratory.
• EKG and other measurements of cardiac activity.
• EEG EMG, biofeedback, and other measurements of neural activity.

- Renal services (acute or chronic)
- Rehabilitative services.
- Psychiatric and social services (primary or supporting).

Certain types of special services may be subject to independent demand —that is, they may be required for specific portions of the population's health care needs. Examples of this type of service are a hemodialysis unit, a psychiatric unit or a rehabilitation unit. Other services may be primarily in support of general patient care; facilities for cardiac, pulmonary, and neurological diagnosis, monitoring, and treatment are examples of functions that are essentially part of the working of the hospital as a whole. The distinctions are not always clear, however. A small physical rehabilitation unit might well be considered as being in the latter category rather than in the former, for example. A general sequence of analysis can be outlined which can be applied to any type of unit. The following questions should be asked about each:

- What determines the work load of the department? Demand based on population; size of a particular clinical division of the hospital; number of patients in intensive care.
- What official regulatory guidelines or constraints apply?
- Is there a maximum or minimum size at which such a unit is ineffective or inefficient?
- What are the characteristics of the unit in terms of staff and types of equipment, interaction with patients, and relationship to specific other hospital functions or to particular units of hospital beds?
- Is the function related to inpatient care, outpatient care, or both? If both, what proportion of services is provided to each group?
- What are the criteria for location?
- What social, economic, scientific, or technological changes are in prospect that may significantly affect either the nature, volume of work, or productivity of the unit?

Some examples of planning procedures for some of the more complex special services follow.

Renal Services

While chronic hemodialysis services may be provided within a hospital, they may also be provided in community health centers where there is a sufficient volume of demand to justify facilities, or they may be provided at home. Facilities for acute hemodialysis are provided only in the hospital setting. New York State guidelines* suggest the following predic-

---

* Policy & Procedures Manual, N.Y. Dept. of Health, 1971.

tion of demand for chronic dialysis, based on data provided by the New York State Kidney Disease Institute:

- That new cases for hemodialysis will occur at the rate of 60-65 per year per million population.
- That 15% of the total case load die per year.
- That of the 85% who survive, 25% can receive transplants, of which 60% will be successful. The balance or 40% of those receiving transplants will have to be returned to dialysis.
- That of the remaining case load, after the adjustments made above, 90% will require institutional dialysis, while 10% could be cared for at home. The 90% who require institutional dialysis will generate 125 procedures per case year—that is, each case will require a treatment approximately once every three days.
- Each dialysis unit (bed plus equipment) can handle 1½ cases a day, 6 days a week. Thus each unit could handle 9 procedures per week.

Assuming a population of 2,000,000, the figures work out as follows:

At the rate of 60 per million, there would be a 120 new cases per year of whom 18 would die, leaving 102 survivors of whom 25% or 26 would receive transplants. Sixteen of these transplants would be successful. Adding the balance of 10 whose transplants were not successful to the 76 who did not receive transplants, there remains a caseload for dialysis of 86. Of these, 10% can be treated at home, while the remaining 77 will require institutional treatment at the rate of 125 procedures each per year, for a total of 9625 treatments. Divided by 365 this suggests the need for 26 units at 100% occupancy—a figure that would have to be further adjusted to allow for emergency treatments.

The projected *use rate* indicated above corresponds fairly closely to those predicted by Australian authorities,* although the predicted number of patients per million of population is different. In Australia in 1968 the number of known patients was 20 per million, and the estimate was that the potential need was something over 30 per million—still half of the New York estimate.

A model organ transplant and renal unit described in the Australian paper consists of the following facilities: a minimum of 35 beds of which at least 40 percent should be in a low-pathogen environment, with at least 5 of these designed for full isolation. In addition, 8-10 beds should be provided for dialysis, as well as 600 square feet of routine laboratory space and 1000 feet of research laboratory space. Office, teaching, and outpatient areas would also be required.

* Report of the Ad Hoc Committee on the Rationalization of Facilities for Organ Transplantation. Medical Journal of Australia, Dec. 28, 1968.

Planning and policy decisions needed

The following planning and policy decisions will have to be made before more detailed planning can commence:

- Is a transplantation unit and acute dialysis unit to be considered? If so, is the predicted volume of patients sufficient to justify it? Are there other area hospitals that already have a unit, or are planning one? Should a joint unit be considered?
- Assuming a full range of transplant and acute and chronic dialysis services are planned, what will be the relationship between (a) acute dialysis and chronic dialysis and (b) between chronic dialysis and the outpatient services?
- Will the hospital provide its own tissue typing laboratory or have access to a central laboratory?
- A transplantation and dialysis unit will almost inevitably generate the need for research space. What will be the relationship of such research space to the unit and to the hospital as a whole?

Information needed

Given the level of services that have been identified above, what are the predicted number of patients per day?

- What proportion of these patients will be inpatients, and what proportion can be handled on an outpatient basis?
- How long will each procedure take? How even is the distribution of the patient load—that is, what factor must be added to allow for peak loads?

Procedure

Summarize the decisions and information to show the following:

CHRONIC DIALYSIS
    Population base: _____
    Annual case load: _____
    Daily number of
      procedures: _____
    Capacity of (bed) unit
      for procedures per day: _____

TRANSPLANT AND ACUTE DIALYSIS
    Annual predicted case load: _____
    Number of transplants: _____
    Required daily acute procedures: _____

Rehabilitation: Physical Medicine, Occupational Therapy, Recreation Therapy

Background/Discussion

Rehabilitation facilities may range from a single room for physical therapy to a wide range of facilities designed to handle a variety of physical, emotional, social, and occupational problems, including the management of the patient after his discharge from the hospital.

To some degree, almost any patient who has had an extended hospital stay or has been hospitalized for a serious illness is a candidate for rehabilitation. He must be encouraged to test himself during his convalescence and to engage gradually in normal activities, including personal care. This general need can be met by providing places for patient activity in nursing units and by the philosophy and attitude of the staff. But for patients who have suffered damage that requires relearning of basic functions and skills special facilities are needed. Candidates for rehabilitation include orthopedic patients, and patients suffering from a variety of disorders resulting in motor, emotional, or mental impairment, or blindness, or deafness, as well as victims of chronic disease, all of whom must be taught how to deal with their condition and helped to overcome or accept the limitations imposed on them.

The range of facilities may include facilities for physical rehabilitation such as hydrotherapy and exercise; facilities for occupational rehabilitation (which can be interpreted much more broadly than the traditional arts-and-crafts type of therapy and can include facilities for relearning household or occupational skills or learning new ones); facilities for the design, production, and fitting of assistive devices; and facilities for social workers and therapists as well as staff physicians. In addition, diagnostic facilities for testing hearing, vision, and other senses may be needed.

Rehabilitation services can be decentralized throughout a hospital, in both inpatient and outpatient areas. In some cases there may be a rehabilitation service, a subspecialty similar to any other specialized group of beds with supporting services. Alternatively, there may be a central grouping of rehabilitation services serving inpatients and outpatients and access to light care or motel beds for patients coming in for fitting for assistive devices.

Projecting requirements for rehabilitation facilities

Information needed

- How many patients of what types will be dealt with? What proportion of inpatients to outpatients?
- Will there be beds specifically reserved for rehabilitation patients?

Policy and planning assumptions needed

- What is the overall level of service that will be provided, and what are the criteria for patient services? How long will patients be associated with the service, and what affiliated organizations or institutions will be involved?
- Will the service be responsible for services to others beyond the inpatient and outpatients who come to the service—for instance to a neighboring chronic hospital or nearby housing for the elderly? What level of growth may be anticipated for the service over a defined period?

Planning decisions needed

- Given the level of demand suggested by the above, what facilities with what capacity will be needed?
- Given the anticipated level of inpatient and outpatient service, what are the requirements for access by inpatients and outpatients?
- Should the facilities be centralized, or can they be located in different areas? If the latter, what is the optimum location for each type of facility?

Procedure

Summarize the information and decisions made to show the work load and capacity for each type of facility, location, requirements, and necessary relationships among units.

Psychiatric Services

Background/Discussion

Generally, psychiatric services at general hospitals are limited to short-term admissions and outpatient services. The organization of psychiatric services everywhere is in a state of flux, and services may be provided in a variety of modalities and combinations.

The first step in projecting facility requirements for psychiatric services, then, is to clearly define the level of service, criteria for admission, and organizational and other aspects of the service, include patterns of affiliation with other components of the system and with other institutions.

Philosophy and orientation of the service

Some psychiatric departments function almost entirely apart from the other services in a hospital, except that they perhaps provide consulting services when medical, surgical, or pediatric patients show evidence of psychic disturbance. Others tend in the direction of integration and emphasize the physically based or chemical nature of mental illness and treatment. These differences in orientation may have implications for the location and design of facilities.

Patterns of care

Because treatment for psychiatric disorders tends to be long-term when compared to treatment for other types of illness and because a continuing relationship between therapist and patient is often required for the success of treatment, a psychiatric service will usually attempt to integrate its inpatient and outpatient services as much as possible and may want to use the same staff and facilities for both groups of patients. It may be helpful to summarize some of the ways in which psychiatric patients may receive their care.

A patient may start by visiting the outpatient clinics and may receive therapy there for some period of time. His illness may then become acute, and he may be admitted to a bed, possibly in isolation at first. As he improves, he will require a variety of activities, in addition to therapy, to keep him interested and occupied. These activities may go from simple arts and crafts to a full range of educational and recreational activities. As he improves even more he may be discharged to sleep at home, or at a so-called half-way house but spend his days at the hospital. Conversely, he may spend his days at work but remain in the hospital at night and on weekends. When he is finally discharged, he may return on a regular basis for outpatient therapy of various kinds. This therapy may be provided at the hospital or at community clinics.

It will be evident from the preceding that it is no simple matter of counting inpatient census and outpatient clinics to arrive at a typical population for the psychiatric facility. The course of treatment must be studied in some detail to determine how many patients of what types will be placing demand on facilities at a given time.

Types of facilities

Patient bed rooms for the psychiatric service can be assumed to be approximately the same size as any other patient room, although some details of design will differ. Some hospitals may feel that the configuration and grouping of rooms should be especially planned and that the typical hospital arrangement with central nursing stations and utility rooms is unsuitable and does not contribute to the patient's well-being. On the other hand, the construction of very specialized facilities is expensive and seriously limits the kind of flexibility that is so important to hospital design. Small clusters of rooms may not easily lend themselves to possible future conversion as general patient nursing units.

In addition to patient rooms, psychiatric facilities will require a considerable amount of space for activities such as individual and group psychiatric therapy, education, reading and study, games, arts and crafts, television monitoring and production, and physical recreation. It is safe to assume that without providing any major space-consuming facilities such as gymnasiums or assembly halls, the area per bed for psychiatric facilities may be at least double the area of other services, or to put it another way, that the supporting facilities may at least equal in area the amount of space normally required per bed for a nursing unit.

Projecting requirements for psychiatric facilities

It is assumed that the number of beds and the basic area per bed has been dealt with as described in Chapter 4, that is, the volumes of patients have been identified and the number of beds justified.

Information needed

- Projected distribution of patient by type of illness degree of illness, age, and sex.
- Projected number of beds and average census.
- Projected number of outpatient visits by age group.

Policy and planning assumptions needed

- A description of the orientation of the department and its relation to other departments of the hospital and to other institutions.
- A description of the patterns of patient care, with specific estimates of the distribution of patients as to type of category. The estimates must be made so that they show the typical demand on psychiatric central facilities during the day, separately for inpatients and outpatients if they are to be dealt with separately.

Planning decisions needed

What central supporting facilities are to be planned, given the volume of demand as identified above? What types of rooms, planned for occupancy by how many? Will special provisions need to be made in the emergency department to handle psychiatric patients?

Procedure

List the facilities that have been identified as being needed for inpatients and outpatients. If central facilities are treated seperately for inpatients, this space can be added up and divided by the number of beds to determine the amount of supporting space needed per bed. Be sure that outpatient areas identified here do not duplicate clinic facilities projected separately.

5.5. PATHOLOGY AND CLINICAL LABORATORIES

Background/Discussion

The work loads of hospital laboratories have been increasing at rates of between 8 and 25% a year. These increases are attributed to the increasing variety of tests available—the result of clinical application of recent basic research; trends towards more complex and time-consuming tests; increased reliance by younger physicians on clinical laboratory determinations in diagnosis; increasing liability problems; and larger numbers of screening programs. Factors that tend to indicate that recent growth will continue or even accelerate include trends towards a greater emphasis on preventive medicine, which will generate a heavy volume of screening activities involving laboratory work; application of computer technology to the interpretation and correlation of test results which, by making test data more useful, will tend to increase utilization; more sophisticated automated equipment which will increase the capacity of the laboratory to perform a wide range of determinations (with the corollary that the work load will tend to increase to fit capacity); and the fact that there is no indication that biomedical research has reached a plateau, so that it may be anticipated that such research will continue to generate clinical testing applications.

The growth rate for determinations per patient will vary from hospital to hospital, depending on the base from which the hospital is starting, the characteristics of its medical staff, and its geographic isolation or association with a major medical center. A hospital that has made a programatic commitment to preventive care would be likely to experience some increase in laboratory utilization as a result; but even a hospital without any such formal commitment might find that an increased awareness of the need for preventive care on the part of its staff may, in itself, generate increased use of the laboratory. Students and younger physicians in general tend to make more extensive use of laboratory services, partly perhaps as a result of their own uncertainties but perhaps also because medical education emphasizes scientific analysis.

Distribution of Facilities

Clinical laboratories represent an attractive investment for commercial entrepreneurs since an expanding market appears to be assured and since a high volume allows a commercial laboratory to provide services to hospitals at competitive prices while maintaining a good margin of profit. A commercial laboratory can, because of volume, provide tests that a single hospital would be unable to perform. The services of commercial laboratories must, therefore, be considered in planning the hospital's own service, and the extent to which commercial services will be used must be defined. In any case, a minimum laboratory for emergency procedures and for specimen collection will always be needed in-house. A central laboratory developed by a consortium of hospitals may provide services similar in scope to the commercial laboratory and with similar advantages and disadvantages. Whatever the nature of the external services available, it will be necessary to define the type of work that will be done in-house and the relationship that is to be developed with the external service. The decision about degree of utilization of external services should be based primarily on considerations of quality and secondly on questions of economy and convenience.

Some of the arguments for and against the use of central laboratories (including both commercial and shared nonprofit) are summarized below:

- A central laboratory can perform a wider range of complex tests because its larger volume makes automation and computerization feasible or economical. Quality may thereby be improved.
- A central laboratory may be able to perform routine tests faster and more economically by batching tests. It may be be able to operate around the clock, thus providing not only faster service but at lower cost because of more efficient utilization of equipment and facilities.
- As a separate organization (whether profit making or otherwise) it may be able to operate more effectively than would an in-hospital laboratory that might be subject to problems of organization and control.
- Laboratory facilities are expensive to build, equip, and maintain, and staff is expensive and difficult to find. It may be an advantage to the hospital to lay these responsibilities elsewhere.
- In some cases the hospital may not have the necessary resources for physical expansion and the use of external services then becomes a necessity.
- Savings that result from increased volume and efficiency may permit the use of sophisticated systems that serve to increase not only the quality of determinations but to improve the accessibility of results.

On the other hand:

- The absence of the more sophisticated laboratory resources within the hospital may discourage the type of research and educational activity that would otherwise attract a high quality staff at both professional and technician levels. It might also reduce the opportunities for physicians on the staff to become familiar with new procedures and developments in laboratory medicine in general.

- The hospital loses control of the quality of work.
- High volume may result in poor quality rather than improved quality.
- Distance may cause undesirable delays in the transmission of specimens and results.
- The laboratory may be one of the few units of the hospital that operate at a profit, and removing a large part of this operation might be economically undesirable. Further, the cost of collecting and handling specimens represents a large proportion of the total cost of routine tests, and the hospital would have to be responsible for this part of the work load in any case.

In addition to the question of in-house versus external laboratories, there is the question of how laboratories are to be organized and distributed within the hospital itself. A single flexible area allows the most efficient use of space, design of work flow, and supervision of staff, as well as maximum sharing of expensive and specialized equipment for any activity. This is particularly true of clinical laboratories, which require a heavy investment in special utilities distributed throughout the laboratory areas. Any function that depends on technology is especially subject to change as technical advances are made, and a single flexible area will permit a relatively easy shifting of functions as changes occur. A maximum consolidation of laboratory functions is thus indicated, although in specific instances it may not always be possible. Remodeling existing space for laboratory use can be considerably more expensive than building new space and should be considered only where there are no alternatives.

There are, however, a number of ways in which laboratories may be split up without major disruption of activities. Some alternatives that may be considered are:

- Distribution by type of laboratory: for example, Chemistry, Microbiology, Hematology.
- Distribution by service to patient type: for example, separate emergency laboratory, satellite laboratory for routine outpatient procedures.
- Distribution by handling method: for example, degree of automation used.

A number of areas associated with laboratory activity may be quite easily, and even desirably, separated. Examples of such areas are blood-drawing stations, which should be located where the patients will be; blood-donor area, which should be located so as to be easily accessible to the public; computer areas (although it is generally desirable to have data preparation areas near the sources of the data).

Utilization of Facilities—Productivity

Planning for physical facilities for laboratories is based on the numbers of people who require work space. Increases in the numbers of tests done may be partially offset by increases in productivity of technicians as the result of work simplification, increased mechanization, or automation. However, this may be reversed again by the increased complexity of tests, many of which are not subject to automation and continue to have to be done by hand. Extension of the work day or the work week will not increase the productivity of the technician but will reduce the amount of space required by allowing each work space to be occupied by a succession of workers. The figures used to estimate productivity per technician are based on standard work hours—approximately 1880 per year, if vacations, holidays, and sick days are included. If a two-shift system were used and productivity were measured by work space rather than by person, the number of tests done per space would, of course, be doubled. Where facilities and equipment are expensive, such an expansion of hours is worth considering, although a shortage of technical personnel may make recruitment difficult.

American Hospital Association studies show that, nationally, the productivity of technicians varies much less according to hospital size than, for example, do the numbers of tests performed per admission. Data from 1970 indicated that the number of tests per man-hour varies only from a low of 3.5 in the smallest hospitals to a high of a little over 4 in hospitals of middle size (200-300 beds) with the figure dropping down again slightly in the larger hospitals, presumably because of the increasing complexity of tests done in the larger hospitals. 1880 man-hours per year per technician with an average of 4 tests per man-hour would suggest a standard average of approximately 7500 tests per technician per year. If one assumes a substitute coverage for vacation, holidays, and sick days and thus assumes a 52-week, 40-hour standard of 2080-hours per year, the figure would increase to 8300. A 6-day work week would result in an additional 1700 annual tests per technician. At this rate, the figure correlates fairly closely with the standard suggested by the American College of Pathology of 10,180 tests per technician. It must be emphasized that these are average figures and do not take account of local differences in the balance of types of tests done, degree of training of technicians, degree of automation of the laboratory, and so on.

Increases in Productivity

This will, like productivity itself, vary according to local conditions and from year to year. In one large university medical center increases in productivity were calculated to average 7% a year over a 10-year period. However, the range per year was from 1 to 22%, with an actual decrease during one year. The introduction of automated equipment for high-volume procedures during a given year would tend to give a false picture when applied to the whole. One authority suggests that an increase in productivity of 20% over an 8- to 10-year period may be a reasonable estimate.

Summary of Planning Steps

- Determine the work that will be generated by each category of patient: What is the rate of increase of tests for each category of patient for each category of tests?
- Determine how many procedures of which types will be done in-house and which will be performed elsewhere. How many tests from outside will be performed in the hospital laboratory?
- For in-house tests, how many annual tests will be handled on the average by each technician?
- What will be the schedule of operating hours for the laboratories (how many technicians will occupy each work station?)
- How many support personnel are required per technician or per annual test load-unit?

Current Conditions

This section outlines the background information and analysis needed for the projection of future requirements. Prior to beginning his analysis, the planner should decide, on the basis of the particular situation and the availability of data, what the appropriate level of detail is. For a long-range plan where only broad blocks of space must be identified, it should not be necessary to deal with each type of laboratory separately. However, where laboratories may have to be fitted around existing facilities and fragmentation is inevitable, a more detailed approach will be necessary. Laboratories are used as the model, but other activities—such as autopsy, morgue, blood-banking, cytopathology, and anatomical pathology can be dealt with in the same way.

Work load

Purpose

To determine local trends in laboratory utilization over a chosen period, expressed as work per patient.

Information needed

1. Hospital statistics for the chosen period showing number of admissions (or patient days) and outpatient and emergency visits for each year.

2. Laboratory data showing the numbers of tests performed for inpatients and outpatients, either aggregated or separately for each type of determination (e.g., Chemistry, Hematology, etc.).

3. Laboratory data showing the numbers of tests sent out to other laboratories and the numbers of additional tests performed in the laboratory that are not attributable to hospital patients (e.g., referrals by private physicians or work done for other hospitals).

Procedure

Include the tests sent out, deduct the tests done for nonhospital patients, and calculate the number of tests generated by patients of each category. Calculate the percent change in tests per patient for each year of the chosen period. This may be done for all tests, aggregated without regard to type, or separately for each type.

Table CL-1. Current and Historical Pattern of Laboratory Work Loads

Year	Inpatients				Outpatients			
	Admissions	Tests	Tests per Admission	Percent Change	Visits	Tests	Tests per Visit	Percent Change
Year I	—	—	—	—	—	—	—	—
Year II	—	—	—	—	—	—	—	—
Year III	—	—	—	—	—	—	—	—
Year IV	—	—	—	—	—	—	—	—
Year VI	—	—	—	—	—	—	—	—
5-Year Increase	—	—	—	—	—	—	—	—

Productivity

Purpose

To determine changes in staffing and staff productivity. For long-range projects, this step may be omitted.

Information needed

1. Total tests performed in the hospital laboratories for all categories of patients (but excluding tests sent out) either aggregated or by laboratory type.

2. The number of full-time-equivalent laboratory technicians (defined as anyone who is occupying space at a laboratory bench, regardless of training or title) who were employed for each of the years in question. Full-time equivalency should be defined (total work-hours per year).

3. Information (such as acquisition of an autoanalyser) which may explain significant changes in productivity.

Procedure

Calculate the average number of tests per technician per year either in the aggregate or separately by laboratory type and the percent change per year:

Table CL-2. Changes in Tests per Technician, Years I-X—All Tests (or Chemistry, and so on)

Year	FTE Technicians	Annual Tests	Average Tests per Technician	Percent Change
Year I	—	—	—	—
Year II	—	—	—	—
Uear III	—	—	—	—
Year IV	—	—	—	—
Etc.	—	—	—	—
5-Year Increase				—

Personnel and space

Purpose

To determine the current ratio of support to technician personnel, and to calculate floor area of laboratories in relation to numbers of tests, and numbers of personnel.

Information needed

1. From data for the immediately preceding year, determine the number of full-time and part-time personnel in each category by work shift. This information may be summarized as follows:

Table CL-3. Summary of Personnel—All Laboratories

			Shift					
	Weekdays		Nights		Weekends		Total	Total
Personnel Category	F-T	P-T [a]	F-T	P-T	F-T	P-T	FTE	Individuals
Technicians	—	—( )	—	—( )	—	( )	—	—
Supports	—	—	—	—	—	—	—	—
Clerical	—	—	—	—	—	—	—	—
Administrative	—	—	—	—	—	—	—	—
Students	—	—	—	—	—	—	—	—
Totals	—	—( )	—	—( )	—	—( )	—	—

[a] Indicate the numbers of individuals represented by part-time FTE in parenthesis.

2. Net floor area of laboratory space, either total or by type of laboratory. Central shared space may be shown separately or prorated among the separate laboratories. Definition of net area appears in Chapter 2.

3. Data for the immediately preceding year showing numbers of tests performed in the hospital laboratories (i.e., excluding tests sent out) either in total or by type of laboratory.

Procedure

Calculate the number of tests per net square foot of floor area; and the number of net square feet per technician:

Table CL-4. Summary Table, Clinical Laboratories

Laboratory	Annual Tests	FTE Technicians	Net Area	Tests per Net Sq. Foot	Net Area per Technician	Net Area per Staff Member [a]
Chemistry	—	—	—	—	—	—
Hematology	—	—	—	—	—	—
Microbiology	—	—	—	—	—	—
Blood Bank	—	—	—	—	—	—
Subtotal	—	—	—	—	—	—
Shared	—	—	—	—	—	—
Total	—	—	—	—	—	—

[a] Total of technicians and support staff.

Summarize additional data: ratio of support personnel to technicians; percentage of total tests done which are sent out; percentage of total tests done which come from outside.

Clinical Laboratories—Projections

Space requirements for laboratories depend on the numbers of individuals who will be working in the laboratories at a given time. The numbers of persons who will be needed to do a projected level of work depends on their productivity, which, in turn, depends on their training, the amount of automated equipment available to them, and the overall efficiency of the laboratory layout and its management. In projecting future requirements, therefore, it is necessary to estimate not only the projected work load but to take into account productivity, operating schedule, and possible new developments both in the work load and in methods of dealing with it.

Projection of work load

Purpose

To determine the anticipated work load of the laboratories at a target date by category of patients or category of test. As mentioned earlier, the planner will have to decide the level of detail that is appropriate for a particular planning project.

Information needed

1. Historical data from Table CL-1 showing local trends in laboratory utilization.

2. Data indicating national or regional trends in laboratory utilization that may be reflected in the hospital laboratory.

3. General hospital projections with regard to projected patient loadings at the target date, including indications as to possible changes in characteristics of the patients.

Planning decisions needed

1. What rate of increase in tests per patient is to be used for projection?

2. What new programs (either from inside or from outside the hospital) such as preadmission testing, genetic screening programs, and multiphasic screening programs, should be considered in the planning?

3. What shifts are likely to occur in the balance of testing work among laboratories (e.g., increased work in immunology and virology)?

4. What rate of increase can be applied to work coming in from nonhospital sources, for example, a new doctor's office facility adjacent to the hospital or other hospitals.

Procedure

On the basis of historical data concerning laboratory activity, adjusted according to planning decisions taken, compute the work load of the

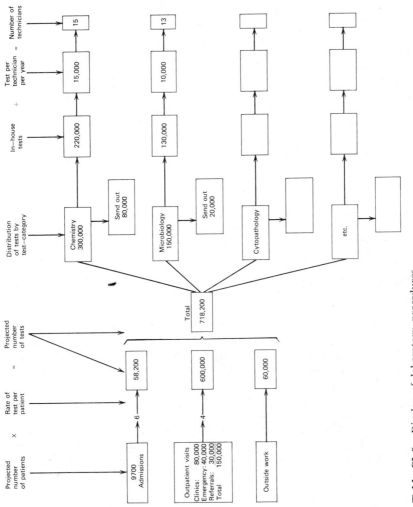

Table CL-5. Display of laboratory procedures.

clinical laboratories at the target date either in the aggregate or separately for each laboratory type:

Table CL-5. Projection of Laboratory Work Load, 19– All Laboratories (or Chemistry, and so on)

Patient Category	Current Tests per Admission or Visit	Annual Increase	Projected Tests per Admission or Visit	Projected Admissions and Visits	Projected Tests
Inpatients	—	—	—	—	—
Outpatients	—	—	—	—	—
Emergency	—	—	—	—	—
Subtotals	—	—	—	—	—
Plus tests from outside	—	—	—	—	—
Total	—	—	—		—

The above total represent *all* tests. For determining work within the hospital it will be necessary to deduct the number of tests that will be sent out.

Distribution of Work

Purpose

To determine policy with regard to the organization of laboratories, the amount of work that is to be done in-house, the amount that will be done on an emergency basis, relationships to central (nonprofit or commercial) laboratories.

Planning decisions needed

What are the minimal laboratory facilities that must be available within the hospital from a functional and quality-of-patient-care standpoint, by law or by regulation? What proportion of the work load will be done on an emergency basis?

Policy decisions needed

1. What level of teaching will occur in the laboratories (e.g., medical student rotation, house officer, pathologist, technician training).

2. Will there be programs of Ph.D. or postdoctoral training involving research?

3. What will be the professional levels of the laboratory director or supervisors of individual laboratories, and will they require research facilities?

The above questions should be considered before decisions are made with regard to the type and amount of work done within the hospital.

4. What proportion of the work load within each discipline or of the work load as a whole will be done in external laboratories? (See the list of pros and cons regarding the use of external laboratories in the introductory paragraphs of this section.)

5. What options are available for the consolidation of laboratory activities within the hospital? For consolidation of specialized laboratories among neighboring hospitals?

It is not possible to cover all the possible combinations of factors that may develop out of a particular group of circumstances. It is important that the kinds of questions indicated above be discussed, that conclusions, recommendations, and estimates of future developments be concisely summarized and documented where possible, and that for planning purposes some hard numbers be assigned—or at the very least that a range of possibilities be explicitly described.

Projection of Personnel and Space Needed

Purpose

To determine the probable productivity of staff at the target date and to estimate staff and space needed to perform the projected work load. In this method the number of technicians (here broadly defined as anyone performing work at a laboratory bench or operating a piece of laboratory equipment, regardless of professional status) is keyed to the work load, and support personnel are keyed to the numbers of technicians. The total numbers of personnel may also be used, but this provides less information and is, therefore, less useful in the long run.

Information needed

1. Data from Tables CL-2, CL-3, and CL-4 showing hospital trends in productivity of personnel, ratio of support personnel to technicians, and floor area per technician or tests per net square foot of the floor area.

2. Applicable data concerning national or regional trends or standards, as well as information as to laws or regulations that may have an impact on planning.

Planning and policy decisions needed

1. In light of current and past experience, technological develop ments, changes in types of tests, and so on, what average rate of increase in productivity (if any) can be predicted?

2. What proportion of tests should, for reasons of quality, or may, for reasons of volume, be automated? How will this affect staffing require- ments?

3. What level of computerization is in prospect, and what modalities will be used? Will this reduce the amount of clerical work done by technicians, thus increasing their technical productivity? Will it increase the numbers of support personnel inside the laboratory areas or in peripheral areas?

4. On the basis of policy decisions with respect to the distribution of work, what is the net volume of laboratory work to be performed in the hospital's laboratories?

5. What is the adequacy of current amount of space in relation to current numbers of technician and support personnel? For laboratory space itself? For supporting clerical, glasswashing, and supply areas? For patient blood-drawing and specimen collecting and handling areas?

Procedure—Method A: Annual tests per square foot

From Table CL-4, determine the average number of annual tests per net square foot per current practice. Adjust the figure as indicated to correct current inadequacies in space. For example, if currently 120,000 tests are being done in laboratories totalling 1800 net square feet, the rate of tests is 66.7 per net square foot. If the department estimates that there is 15% space deficiency, the figure can be corrected by dividing the annual tests by the optimal space (1800 × 1.15) of 2070 net square feet. The corrected figure is thus 58 tests per net square foot.

Using the total projected tests at the target date from Table CL-5, adjusted so as to omit tests that will not be done in the hospital, compute the floor area required for the net projected work load as a total or by laboratory type. The projections may be summarized as follows:

Table CL-6. Projected Hospital Tests and Floor Area (Method A)

	Current Tests per Net Square Foot	Adjusted Tests per Net Square Foot	Total Tests Projected In-house	Projected Net Floor Area
Chemistry	—	—	—	—
Hematology	—	—	—	—
Shared	—	—	—	—

Note: This method does not, as outlined, take account of factors such as hours of operation and changes in staff productivity. Obviously these factors could be plugged in, but the following method indicates the steps required more explicitly. For easier manipulation Method B can be converted to Method A after all relevant factors have been taken into account.

Procedure—Method B: Projection by staff

On the basis of decisions and estimates made with regard to the projected work load, adjusted so as to include only tests that will be done in the hospital's laboratories and planning decisions made with regard to the productivity of technicians, compute the numbers of technicians needed at the target date:

Table CL-7. Projected Technicians at Target Date

	Current Conditions			Projections		
	Annual Tests	FTE Tech-nicians	Tests per Tech-nician	Projected Tests	Projected Test per Tech-nician	Tech-nicians Needed
Chemistry	—	—	—	—	—	—
Hematology	—	—	—	—	—	—
Etc.	—	—	—	—	—	—
Totals	—	—	—	—	—	—

On the basis of the department's estimate of deficiencies in existing space, if any, adjust the net area per technician derived from current conditions (Table CL-4) on a percentage basis. Multiply the projected number of technicians by the adjusted net area per technician. Note: the area-per-technician figure does not represent actual work space per technician: It includes space for all activities, including space for all other employees.

Table CL-8. Projected Area per Technician

	Current Conditions			Projections	
	FTE Technicians	Area per Technician	Adjusted Area per Technician	FTE Technicians	Area per Technician
Chemistry	—	—	—	—	—
Hematology	—	—	—	—	—
Etc.	—	—	—	—	—
Totals	—	—	—	—	—

The two steps above may be performed for the laboratories as a whole or separately for each type. Further adjustments will be necessary if a significant change in operating hours is planned: This may be done by determining the average tests per man-hour and determining the number of technicians who will be needed per shift to handle the work load. It may also be necessary to determine the time of highest activity, since even if a lab operates on a 24-hour schedule it is unlikely that the work will be evenly distributed over the period.

6

Supply Services

6.1. BACKGROUND/DISCUSSION

In conjunction with the planning of circulation patterns for people, the planning of distribution paths for materials and equipment is a major factor in making a building or building complex function well. These paths or systems are difficult to modify once in place and difficult to insert where they do not exist. The planner may expect to spend a great deal of time with the architect and with consultant specialists in the study of alternative systems. Before such studies begin, it will be helpful to have completed a preliminary study of the basic organization of such services, the quantities of materials handled, and the functional relationships among supply and other hospital departments. Preliminary conclusions as to the best organization of services will undoubtedly be subject to revision as work proceeds. Constraints of space or access may require changes in a preferred system, or new technologies may suggest possible improvements. It is very important that these systems not be treated as an afterthought but be considered during the earliest steps in planning.

Some of the major questions that should be asked about each function that deals with supplies and the distribution of materials include:

- What determines the work load and volume of materials of each unit? For example, dietary services and laundry operations can safely be keyed to the number of patient days, with adjustments to reflect non-patient work.
- For each unit, how much material must be kept in ready storage, how much must be processed per day, and how much backup bulk storage is needed?
- For each function, how much material must or should be kept on hand at the point of use?

- For each unit, how much material is transported per day, how often, and where? Are there any special requirements for the handling of the material (e.g., must it be kept hot or cold)?
- Are there any critical environmental and location requirements? For example the sterilizing area should not be adjacent to the area where soiled linens or trash are handled. The receiving area must have access from an external loading dock.
- What grouping or centralization of internal functions would work to the advantage of each? To what degree is such centralization important?
- What services may be provided from outside either through a centralized service arranged among area institutions or by the purchase of contract services? Purchasing, bulk storage, hospital laundry, food services, and pharmaceutical manufacturing are examples of activities that may be undertaken jointly with other institutions.

What changes in materials, processing techniques, or external circumstances are likely to have a significant change on the operations or space requirements of each unit? An example of such change in the recent past has been the trend toward the use of disposable materials and instruments in a number of areas. This has generally meant a decrease in the areas required for processing and a concomitant increase in the amount of storage space. It is quite conceivable that this trend might reverse itself again as the costs of materials increases or as shortages of materials develop or as increased environmental regulation makes the disposal of these materials more difficult and costly.

The departments or work units that are here considered as supply departments include the pharmacy; sterile supplies; purchasing, receiving, and general stores; the laundry; and dietary services. These services are not the only ones that place a demand on the distribution system, of course. The definition of a supply department is necessarily rather arbitrary: The clinical laboratories and the pharmacy could both be considered as supply services, in so far as they store, collect, process, and distribute materials—and both could be considered to be part of the therapeutic/diagnostic system in that they directly serve the patient. Medical records place a heavy demand on the distribution system too. It is important, therefore, that the demands of all hospital functions be considered in planning for the distribution system: The supply departments do not exist *in fact* as a separate category of activity.

Communications and management systems are important elements of the supply and distribution system. If supplies are efficiently handled and if emergency requests are met promptly, the ordering departments will not feel the need to keep an excess of supplies on hand at the point of use.

In this chapter two units are dealt with in detail, the pharmacy and dietary services. The method illustrated for projecting pharmacy requirements is based on the characteristic of the work—that space depends on the number of people who are working and that the number of people who are working depends on both the amount of work they have to do and their productivity. If a similar analysis of sterile supply services or the laundry were needed the same approach could be taken. The dietary services are an example of an activity that involves a number of populations, not just patients, and here the key to an adequate projection of future needs lies in the projection of demand.

6.2. PHARMACY

Background/Discussion

Pharmacists in the United States have expressed considerable dissatisfaction with the state of their profession, particularly with regard to hospital pharmacy, pointing to lack of professional status, and inability or unwillingness of pharmacists to engage in research, professional training and teaching activities, development and evaluation of pharmaceutical products, and routine assay and control procedures. The Association of Hospital Pharmacists has recommended that their members make every effort to upgrade the profession by providing a wider range of services, not all of which are currently available even at larger medical centers. Particular emphasis is placed on developing facilities for assay and evaluation, because without these facilites it is not possible to control the quality of therapeutic and other agents or bulk chemicals; do research; or train professional pharmacists to a high level.

The organization, capability, scope of services, and facilities of hospital pharmacies vary widely. For example, the authors of "Mirror to Hospital Pharmacy"* report that a survey of short-term general and specialized hospitals of 200 to 299 beds showed a range of from 100 square feet to more than 5000 square feet assigned to pharmacy. Hospitals in other size ranges showed similar variations. Some of these differences are no doubt due to differences in definition of what constitutes pharmacy space: In some instances bulk storage might be included, for example, while other hospitals might include all bulk storage in a separate category. Nevertheless, it is clear that there are significant vari-

* Francke, D. E., et al., *Mirror to Hospital Pharmacy*. Washington: American Society of Hospital Pharmacists, 1964.

ations in the scale of operations. The first step in planning, therefore, will be to identify the activities of the pharmacy as it is currently constituted and to explore what developments are in prospect.

One of the key questions about pharmacy operations is the extent to which the pharmacy will engage in manufacture. Although the competition presented by industry makes it generally uneconomical to produce small quantities of pharmaceuticals, particularly the more complex ones that are likely to be under patent control, there are arguments in favor of at least small manufacturing capability. The preparation of solutions and dilution of concentrates may be classified as manufacturing, and this may be performed economically. The instrumentation necessary for manufacturing can provide a benefit, beyond the capacity of analysis and control, by enabling the pharmacist to become engaged in research himself or to assist in research by others. It will also provide a means of more sophisticated training of young pharmacists. But the primary advantage may be in enabling the physician to prescribe in forms that may not be available commercially. Since the pharmacist is responsible for the quality of drugs, it is recommended that he have facilities available for the analysis and testing of products. This will enable the medical staff to obtain informed assessments of specific pharmaceuticals.

If the pharmacy is to engage in manufacturing, it will be necessary to determine specifically the types of products that will be manufactured and to estimate the probable volume. This information will, in turn, provide information as to the amount and type of storage facilities that will be needed.

The system used to compound, package, and deliver pharmaceuticals to the user must also be explored. The pharmacy supplies inpatient prescriptions and other drug orders; it may also supply the outpatient clinics, emergency department, laboratories, surgery, and radiology. The types of products delivered to each of these should be identified, and estimates made of their volume.

Pharmacy—Existing Conditions

Purpose

To determine the current level of activity of the pharmacy as it relates to numbers of patients.

Information needed

1. Pharmacy data from the preceding year indicating the annual total number of prescriptions and other orders dispensed. Outpatient prescriptions should be listed separately.

2. Type and volume of items manufactured.

3. Hospital data for the same year showing number of inpatient days and number of outpatient visits.

Work load procedure

List and summarize the work load data by groups and categories suggested by the department itself. The basis for grouping items should be the type of laboratory or equipment required to produce or compound them. Divide the number of outpatient prescriptions by the number of outpatient visits. Divide all other activities by hundreds of patient days. (Patient days are a more accurate measure than admissions; numbers of drug and other orders per patient day are relatively constant regardless of hospital size.) The information may be summarized as follows:

Table PH-1. Volume of Activity

		Inpatients		Outpatients	
Work Category	Annual Volume	Patient Days	Volume per 100 Inpatient Days	Annual Visits	Volume per Visit
Outpatients* prescriptions	—			—	—
Inpatient prescriptions	—	—	—		
Other orders	—		—		—
Manufacturing:					
Bulk compound	—				
Solutions	—				
Reagents	—				
Etc.					
Totals	—	—	—	—	—

*Includes Emergency

Additional Workload

Purpose

To identify all activities and services of the department.

Procedure

Obtain from the pharmacy department a list of all activities, including committee meetings, consultations with physicians, drug information center, library, formulary, unit dose system, and so on. Time spent in these activities may not be quantifiable: The activities are included in the pharmacist hours shown in the following table. The purpose of listing all activities, however, is to be able to adjust the figures for projection to reflect increases in these kinds of activities.

Personnel

Purpose

To determine the number of full-time-equivalent pharmacists, support personnel, and the ratio between the two groups.

Information needed

1. The number of pharmacists employed and the annual hours of each.
2. The numbers of support personnel engaged in pharmacy activity and the annual hours of each. Do not include personnel such as messengers who may be assigned to the pharmacy as a part of other duties.

Procedure

Tabulate the data separately for full-time and part-time personnel, showing the numbers of part-timers who make up the full-time equivalency, and show total annual man-hours, thus:

Table PH-2. Summary of Pharmacy Personnel

Category	Full-Time	Full-Time Equivalents	Total FTE	Total Man-Hours
Pharmacists	1	1 (2)	2	4,000
Support Personnel	5	1.5 (3)	6.5	13,000
Pharm. Asst.	3	—	3	—
Technician	1	—	1	—
Clerical	1	1.5 (3)	2.5	—

The ratio of pharmacists to support personnel in the example is 2:6.5.

Productivity

Purpose

To determine the volume of work performed under the direction of each pharmacist. If more detail is desired, the analysis may be repeated using volume of work per all personnel.

Information needed

1. The annual volume of work by the chosen categories (Table PH-1).
2. The full-time-equivalent pharmacists (man-hours) (Table PH-2).

Procedure

Divide the volume of work per year by the number of pharmacists to obtain an average annual volume per man. Similarly, calculate the volume of work per pharmacist man-hour (in the example, full-time equivalency is figured at 2000 hours per year).

Table PH-3. Productivity of Pharmacists

Work Category	Annual Volume	Annual Volume per Pharmacist	Volume per Pharmacist Man-Hour
All prescriptions	—	—	—
All other orders	—	—	—
Manufactured items	—	—	—

Facilities

Purpose

To summarize net areas of the pharmacy in order to analyze space in terms of the number of pharmacists.

Information needed

1. Net areas of pharmacy spaces, including major storage area if specific to the pharmacy. If bulk storage is in a central storage area, the pharmacy portion should be estimated. Floor stock areas need not be included.
2. Full-time-equivalent pharmacists from Table PH-2.

Procedure

Calculate the net area in total or by category per FTE pharmacist.

Table PH-4. Pharmacy Areas per Pharmacist

Work Category	Net Area	FTE Pharmacists	Net Area per Pharmacist
Inpatient pharmacy:			
compounding and packing	600 NSF	2	300 NSF
Outpatient pharmacy:	200 NSF	2	100 NSF
Sterile lab	—	—	—
Narcotics and alcohol vault	—	—	—
Manufacturing	—	—	—
Control and assay	—	—	—
Bulk storage	—	—	—
Etc.	—	—	—
Total	—	—	400 NSF

Obtain from the department an estimate of the degree of deficiency, if any, of the space available to accommodate *current* activities.

Pharmacy—Projections

A reasonable method of projecting pharmacy requirements is to determine the estimated work load at the target date and to extrapolate from current ratios of pharmacists to work loads and space per pharmacist (adjusted as necessary to reflect changes in operation and scope of work and existing deficiencies) to develop estimates of future staff and space requirements.

Work load

Purpose

To determine the numbers of prescriptions, other orders, and manufactured items that are estimated for the target date.

Information needed

1.   Data from Table PH-1, showing volume of activity of the pharmacy at present related to inpatient and outpatient volume.
2.   Hospital projections with regard to numbers of outpatient visits and patient days at the target date. Estimates of increased activity in hospital departments that may affect the pharmacy and that is *not* keyed to increases in numbers of patient days or visits.

Planning decisions needed

1.   Is the current volume of prescriptions and other orders per patient valid as a planning standard? For purposes of discussion, it may be useful to compare the figure developed in the section of current conditions with the conclusions of the authors of "Mirror to Hospital Pharmacy" (1964) which indicated a range of from 0.6 to 1.1 prescriptions per inpatient day for short-term hospitals and an average of 0.5 for long-term hospitals. The range of ratios of prescriptions to other orders was between 1:1 and 3:1 or less, fluctuating according to size and type of hospital.
2.   Is the current volume of manufacturing per patient a valid basis for projection?
3.   Is there a disproportionate increase in the projected number of outpatient visits over the increase in inpatient days? Will this affect the volume of items manufactured? If so, adjust the volume of manufactured items by an appropriate percentage.

Procedure

On the basis of decisions made with regard to volume of work per patient, calculate the estimated work load at the target date:

Table PH-5. Projected Volume of Pharmacy Activity at the Target Date

Work Category	Volume per 100 Patient Days	Projected Patient Days	Annual Volume	Volume per O-P Visit	Projected Visits	Projected Annual Volume
Outpatient prescriptions				—	—	—
Inpatient prescriptions	—	—	—			
Other orders	—	—	—	—	—	—
Manufacturing	—	—	—			
Etc.						
Totals	—	—		—	—	

Productivity

Purpose

To determine the numbers of pharmacists and other personnel needed to perform the projected volume of work.

Information needed

1. Information from Table PH-2 and PH-3 showing the orders per pharmacist per year and the ratio of pharmacists to other personnel.
2. Total annual orders from Table PH-5 above.

Planning decisions needed

Is the current workload per person an acceptable basis for planning? What factors, if any, can be identified that might change practice? Would reduction of the pharmacists' paperwork by computerization of charging, billing, and patient drug profiles increase productivity of the pharmacist and possibly require added support staff? Will increases in the number and complexity of therapeutic and diagnostic agents result in an increase in pharmacists time spent in consultation with physicians and in educating patients? The U.S. Public Health Service found that in the late 1950's in hospitals of 100 to 500 beds there were between

100 and 150 prescriptions or orders filled per day per full-time pharmacist employed: How does this compare to current practice at this hospital? Are there changes in institutional or national policy with regard to pharmaceuticals that may affect work load or productivity?

Procedure

On the basis of decisions taken with regard to planning standards for productivity of personnel, adjust the figures for current practice and using the projected work load calculate the numbers of pharmacists and support personnel needed.

Table PH-6.   Projected Pharmacy Staff Requirements

Work Category	Projected Volume	Adjusted Volume per Pharm. per Year	Number of Pharmacists Needed	Pharmacist to Support Personnel Ratio	Number of Support Personnel Needed
Outpatient prescriptions	—	—	—	—	—
Inpatient prescriptions	—	—	—	—	—
Other orders	—	—	—	—	—
Manufacturing	—	—	—	—	—
Etc.	—	—	—	—	—
Totals			—		—

Facilities

Purpose

To estimate space requirements to accommodate the projected work load.

Information needed

Data from Table PH-4 showing current area per pharmacist.

Planning decisions needed

Is current space per person adequate, or should it be adjusted? Are there changes in organization planned that may increase space requirements per person, a separate outpatient pharmacy, for example, or more paperwork or a greater proportion of manufacturing?

Procedure

If the ratio of support personnel to pharmacists remains the same, the area per pharmacist guideline can probably be safely used. If it is felt that there will be a significant increase in support personnel, divide the total existing pharmacy area (adjusted to correct deficiencies) by the total FTE staff. The space estimate may be made on the basis of total area or separately by function. If the latter procedure is followed, it should be cautioned that this general method will not give a true picture of sizes of particular areas, since not all of these will increase at a constant rate. To avoid a false impression of specificity it is, therefore, suggested that the space projection be made for the pharmacy area as a whole. Possible exceptions are the outpatient pharmacy and bulk storage areas.

Table PH-7.   Projected Space Requirements

Projected Number of Pharmacists	Adjusted Area per Pharmacist	Net Area Needed	Projected Total Personnel	Adjusted Area per Person	Net Area Needed
—	—	—	—	—	—

Distribution of facilities

Purpose

To determine the optimal distribution of pharmacy facilities.

Policy decisions needed

1.   From the standpoint of volume, is it feasible to operate a satellite outpatient pharmacy if other required spatial relationships do not permit a unit adjacent to inpatient and manufacturing operations?

2.   What will be the relationship of the pharmacy to other supply departments? There may be some overlap in their functions—how will these be resolved?

3.   How will drugs be distributed to nursing floors?

4.   What provision will be made for night and emergency coverage of pharmacy activities?

5.   What physical or communications relationships are required among pharmacy activities and units? This may perhaps best be described in a diagram showing the path of materials and indicating the daily volume.

6.3. CENTRAL STERILE SUPPLY

Background/Discussion

In most modern hospitals the sterile supply department, which used to form a part of the surgical suite, has been relocated so that it can more readily serve sterilizing functions for all hospital departments. It is also generally charged with issuing sterile disposables and is, therefore, closely related to other supply functions. After articles have been cleaned, they are packaged and sterilized; after they are sterilized, they can be stored in the sterile supply storage area, together with prepackaged sterile supplies or disposables. In some hospitals all supply, processing and distribution functions are consolidated into a single department and single responsibility.

Existing Conditions

Purpose

To examine existing operation as it relates to number of patients.

Information needed

1. Average work load by type of activity (preparation and sterilization of packs, cleansing and sterilization of utensils, etc.) and by user (i.e., inpatient, outpatient, emergency, surgery, obstetrics, etc.) for the preceding year.

2. Hospital data for the same year (inpatient days, outpatient visits, emergency procedures, surgical procedures, obstetric deliveries, etc.).

Procedure

List and summarize the work load data by user and by categories of activity suggested by the department itself. The basis for grouping should be the type of equipment and supplies needed for processing. Data may be documented by shift and multiplied by number of shifts per year. The information may be displayed as follows:

Table CSS-1. Volume of work

	Units per Year						
Category	Nurs. Units	O.P.D.	Emerg.	Surgery	Obstetrics	Other	Total
Packs:							
Major Surgery	—	—	—	—	—	—	—
Minor Surgery	—	—	—	—	—	—	—
Etc.	—	—	—	—	—	—	—
Utensils	—	—	—	—	—	—	—
Flasks	—	—	—	—	—	—	—
Instruments	—	—	—	—	—	—	—

Potential Changes

Purpose

To determine the extent of use of disposables and the effect of changing requirements and methods analysis on the sterile processing department.

Information needed

1. Inventory of usage of current disposables.
2. Evaluation of environmental effects of disposing of disposables.
3. Estimate of the effect of new techniques on need for sterile supplies.
4. Analysis of methods used to produce sterile supplies.

Procedure

List disposables by category and state method of disposal including nature and environmental impact of waste products. Evaluate impact of new techniques as outlined by other departments (see Chapters 3, 4, & 5). Examine each step in processing reusable supplies to determine whether or not it is being done in the most logical and efficient manner; this should be done periodically, perhaps once every six months, as it is almost inevitable that existing work patterns will be used for new tasks without adequate consideration of suitability. All proposed changes should be included in a methods analysis report.

Economics of Disposables

Purpose

To compare cost of disposable with reusable items.

Information needed

1. Unit cost of disposable items.
2. Unit cost of reusable items.
3. Average number of possible reuses of reusable items.
4. Unit processing cost of each reusable item.

Procedure

Determine average cost per use of reusable items by dividing unit purchase price by average number of uses; add estimated unit labor cost for washing, inspection, sorting, packaging, and sterilizing reusables; add estimated unit cost of utilities and supplies used in processing; add amortization, installation, and maintenance cost of equipment per unit. Compare with unit cost of disposable item (including cost of disposal). Result may be displayed as follows:

Table CSS-2. Comparison of Unit Costs

Item	Reusable							Disposable		
	Cost	No Uses	Cost/Use	Labor	Util. and Sup.	Equip.	Total	Cost	Disposal	Total
Gloves	0.56	8	0.070	0.042	0.021	0.013	0.146	0.312	0.001	0.313
Syringe	—	—	—	—	—	—	—	—	—	—
Solutions	—	—	—	—	—	—	—	—	—	—
And so on	—	—	—	—	—	—	—	—	—	—

Distribution System

Purpose

To examine the existing or proposed distribution system to determine its suitability to the size and nature of the supply and processing operation.

Information needed

1. Method of controlling inventory (i.e., user requisition, fixed inventory, or exchange system).
2. Type and number of carts and conveyors used for distribution of supplies.
3. How supplies are stored at point of use—on carts, in cabinets, or on open shelves.
4. Available space for cart shortage both at points of distribution and use.

Procedure

Consider alternatives to current methods and weigh advantages of on-cart storage and daily cart rotation with cost of increased inventory and cart storage space. Compare pros and cons of automated distribution systems with hand delivery and messenger service. Maintenance cost as well as first cost should be given careful consideration. Systems to be evaluated include:

- Elevators.
- Automatic Unloading Cart Dumbwaiters.
- Dumbwaiters.
- Conveyors—horizontal, vertical, and combination.
- Monorails.
- Powered Carts and Cart Trains.

- Pneumatic Chutes.
- Pneumatic Tubes.

Personnel

Purpose

To determine the number of full-time-equivalent personnel on each shift.

Information needed

1.   Number of supervisory and support personnel by shift and by task employed in the central sterile supply department.
2.   Number of work stations for each task.

Procedure

List the number of full-time-equivalent personnel per shift and existing floor area and calculate units per FTE by dividing total units per year (Table CSS-1) by present employees and tabulate results as follows:

Table CSS-3.   Personnel

Category	Present Employees (FTE)	Existing Floor Area (NSF)	Area per FTE	Units per FTE
Administration	1	150	150	—
Sorting and cleaning	2	900	450	—
Processing:				
Packs	2	400	200	—
Utensils	0.5	200	200	—
Flasks	0.5	150	150	—
Instruments	1	200	200	—
Etc.	—	—	—	—
Totals	—	—	—	—

Projections

Purpose

To estimate the volume of work and number of employees for a given target date.

Information needed

1. Data from Table CSS-1 showing volume of work at present.
2. Data from Table CSS-3 showing number of employees and existing floor areas.
3. Estimate of change in work load in response to methods analysis report and changing demands of departments served.

Planning decisions needed

Will the use of disposables increase or decrease? Will the change in work load affect the number of employees needed?

Procedure

From Chapters 3, 4, and 5 determine percentage increase (decrease) in patient days, outpatient visits, emergency procedures, operating room procedures, OB deliveries, and other pertinent changes and calculate effect on volume of work.

Table CSS-4. Work Load Projection

Category	Units per Year						
	N.U.	O.P.D.	Emerg.	Surg.	OB	Other	Total
Percent Change	+15	+25	+20	+5	−10	+10	—
Packs:							
Major Surgery	—	—	—	—	—	—	—
Minor Surgery	—	—	—	—	—	—	—
Etc.	—	—	—	—	—	—	—
Utensils	—	—	—	—	—	—	—
Instruments	—	—	—	—	—	—	—
Etc.	—	—	—	—	—	—	—

Planning decisions needed

Does the methods analysis report recommend changes in procedure that will increase production?

Procedure

Estimate effect if any of changes on productivity of employees. Adjust units per FTE to reflect such changes and calculate number of full-time employees required for each task.

Table CSS-5. Work Load Projections per Task

Category	Units per Year Total (Table CSS-4)	Units per FTE (Table CSS-3)	FTE Required per Task
Packs	—	—	—
Utensils	—	—	—
Flasks	—	—	—
Instruments	—	—	—
Etc.	—	—	—

Facilities

Purpose

To estimate space requirements to accommodate the projected work load.

Information needed

1. Data from tables CSS-3, CSS-4, and CSS-5.
2. Methods Analysis Report.

Planning decisions needed

Will there be changes in the delivery system that will affect space requirements? How many shifts will be operated? Is current space per person adequate? Will the use of disposables be increased or decreased?

Procedure

List area per full-time-equivalent (FTE) employee from Table CSS-3 and number of FTE needed for each task assuming only one shift from Table CSS-5. Determine number of FTE for two or more shifts (note that total number of FTE with more than one shift may be higher due to need for supervisory personnel).

After reaching a decision on the number of shifts, add to the total areas in Table CSS-6 the following percentages for:

Receiving	5%
Sterilizers	12%
Unsterile Storage	25%
Sterile Storage	25%
Total	67%

more NSF than is required, for administration, cleaning, and processing areas.

Table CSS-6. Personnel and Area Requirements

| Category | Area NSF per FTE (from CSS-3) | One Shift | | | Two Shifts | | |
		Total FTE (from CSS-5)	Area Needed NSF	Max FTE per Shift	Area Needed NSF	Total FTE
Administra-tion	150	1	150	1	150	2
Sorting and Cleaning	450	3	1350	2	900	3
Processing:						
Packs	200	4	800	2	400	4
Utensils	150	1	150	0.5	150	1
Flasks	—	—	—	—	—	—
Instruments	—	—	—	—	—	—
And so on	—	—	—	—	—	—
Totals	—	—	—	—	—	—

Work Flow

The centralization of supply functions makes it possible to apply production techniques to the department. To realize full benefit from such techniques it is essential that careful consideration be given to work flow. Generally, it is desirable to consider the department as a whole, to produce as efficient a circulation pattern as possible, and then to study separate areas within the basic organizational framework. Figure CSS-A is a typical work flow diagram. For best control it is also desirable to locate receiving and issuing close to each other; this will produce a horseshoe circulation pattern.

6.4. GENERAL STORES AND PURCHASING

Purchasing, Receiving and General Stores

Under this category should be included bulk storage of supplies and materials, storage of nonsterile equipment and instruments and general storage of all types, including the storage of volatile materials that will require special handling, used equipment, or furniture that may be awaiting disposal or repair, and temporary storage for items that have been received but are awaiting checking prior to installation. With the increasing amount of highly technical equipment that is used in hos-

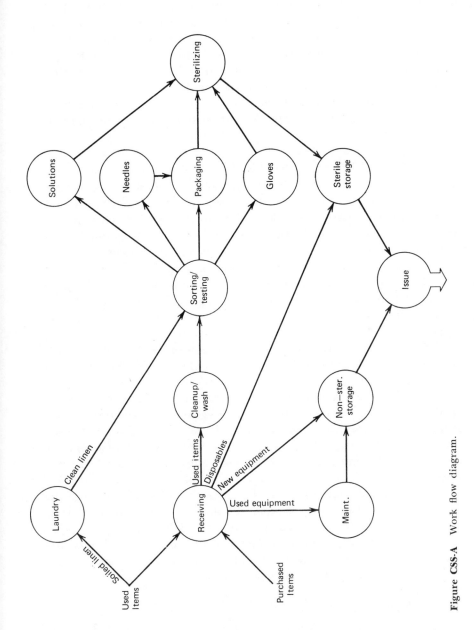

Figure CSS-A Work flow diagram.

pitals, the processing of purchasing and receiving goods becomes a highly professional matter and may well include the evaluation of complex types of equipment and the testing and calibration of such equipment prior to its acceptance and installation. The interrelationship of types of equipment and medical instrumentation and the question of shock hazard suggest the need for establishing overall responsibility for co-ordinating types of equipment purchased and ensuring that they are properly used and maintained and that all necessary warnings and instructions are observed. This responsibility may be placed with the purchasing department.

Projecting Requirements—General Stores

It will be necessary to establish the type and level of activity that is to be included and to define how functions are to be distributed. For example, what proportion of total stores are to be kept centrally and what proportion are to be distributed throughout the hospital? The more the stores are centralized, the better will be the inventory process—and this can significantly affect costs. The ability to keep a minimum of essential items scattered throughout the hospital depends a great deal on the effectiveness of the communication and ordering system and, hence, the confidence that departments can have that their needs will be met quickly.

The best way to describe the activity and requirements of this unit will be to draw a diagram which shows how items will be handled from initial acquisition through disposal or reuse.

There is no rule of thumb for an activity where so many levels of operation are possible. It may be possible to generalize that storage space should not fall below approximately 5% of total building area, but even this is not a very safe guideline. It should be said, however, that very few institutions ever have enough storage space—especially not the older ones where storage is often converted to more productive uses. Bulk storage, however, may not need to be in the central facility. It can easily be located across a street or even some distance away as long as there is adequate contiguous area for frequently used and emergency items. In addition, space requirements must be identified for such activities as unpacking and uncrating, checking, labeling, and inventorying and for the administrative functions of the department.

6 5. LAUNDRY

The demands on laundries have decreased as the use of disposables has increased, but this trend may be reversed. A hospital laundry may be an off-site activity and may be shared with other hospitals. In such a case, there will still be a requirement for the pick-up and handling of soiled items and for a place for receiving, storing and distributing of clean linens.

Projecting Requirements—Laundry

The work load for the laundry, whether it is an internal or external operation can be keyed to the number of pounds of laundry produced per patient day. This will vary, depending on general hospital policy as to the frequency of linen changes and the method of distribution. The amount of work and machine space needed can be calculated by determining the capacity of the required machines and the number of persons needed to do the manual work of sorting, bagging, folding, and so forth. How the linens are to be distributed should be identified, as this will affect the overall distribution system as well as the inventory.

6 6. DIETARY SERVICES

Oddly enough, one of the most basic activities of man—feeding himself— is subject to almost as much technological change and development as some of the most sophisticated diagnostic activities. Or at least that is the eternal hope of food service planners and designers. Technology will probably continue to have a great impact on food handling and processing; the planning of food services is thus not the simple matter it might appear to be. As with any area of change, it is advisable to employ the services of a specialist early in the planning process.

A hospital typically provides food for several different populations, including patients, most of whom will receive tray service, but some of whom may be served family-style meals. In addition, most hospitals provide a cafeteria for their own staff, and many provide services to visitors and outpatients. Some hospitals, perhaps inadvertently, provide meals to the general public. These differing populations may or may not have different hours of peak demand, but almost universally it is the noon meal that creates the heaviest volume. It is thus this meal which must serve as the basis for planning.

The questions to be asked about food services include:

- Who will be fed, in what groups, how often, and at what times?
- Where will raw and processed food come from, how much will be stored, and where?
- By what means, or by what combination of means, will the food be prepared for consumption?

- How and where will it be served?
- What types of trays and tableware will be used, and how will it be handled before and after use?
- How will food and patient trays be transported throughout the hospital?

Distribution of Facilities

Although centralization of food service facilities is generally desirable from a standpoint of efficiency, it may be worth considering some degree of decentralization where volume warrants or when the configuration of the hospital and the location of existing facilities suggest it. In almost all cases, however, it is advisable to consolidate receiving, rough processing, and storage areas as much as possible. Depending on local conditions, it may be feasible for the hospital to buy service from a commercial concern or to join with other institutions in a centralized food service system that would take out of the hospital the most space-consuming activities.

Current Conditions

Purpose

To summarize and evaluate the current type and level of services provided.

Information needed

1. Food services statistics showing the typical daily number of meals served—by meal and by category of service.

2. Hospital data showing the number of patients, staff employees, students, visitors, and others who are present during the day at the noon meal.

3. A list of food services net areas, including: cafeteria (seating areas and number of seats); cafeteria (line, check-out, and serving area); kitchen areas (cooking, warming, mixing, etc.); tray assemblage and loading areas; food preparation; refrigerated storage; dry foods storage; bulk storage; dishes, utensils (washing and storage areas).

4. Food service personnel by shift.

Procedure

1. Determine the proportion of the daily hospital population who take their meals in the hospital by comparing the total hospital popula-

tion with the number of meals served at noon. If there are different dining areas to serve different groups, the ratios can be derived for each category separately. (It is safe to assume that the number of patient-meals will equal the daily census.)

Table FS-1.   Utilization of Hospital Food Services

Hospital Populations	Number	Meals Served at Noon	% Utilization
Physicians, Hospital Personnel	600	400	67%
Outpatients and companions, Visitors, Students, Others	250	100	40%
Totals	850	500	59%

2.   Turnover rate—Determine the average turnover of seats at the noon meal by dividing the number of meals served (in each area) by the number of seats. The turnover rate is affected by factors such as personnel policies and shift schedules, the presence or absence of alternative lounge spaces, the overall pleasantness of the facility, and the degree of crowding. A typical turnover rate in a cafeteria might be between $2\frac{1}{2}$ and 3 times per meal, while in a table-service dining room the rate would be lower—perhaps 2 or $2\frac{1}{2}$ times. If a cafeteria has 200 seats, and 600 meals are served at noon, the turnover rate would be 3; that is, each seat is used, on the average, 3 times during the meal period.

Table FS-2.   Summary of Turnover Rates

Category	Meals Served	Seats	Turnover Rate
Physicians	32	12	2.7

3.   Summarize current food service space by main categories and break it down by area per seat for each category of general use space. Areas used exclusively for inpatient meals—such as floor pantries, if they are used, and tray assembly of special diet preparation areas should be listed separately.

Table FS-3. Summary and Analysis of Food Services Areas

Space/Type	Total Area	Number of Seats	Area per Seat	Daily Trays	Area per Tray
Seating Areas	3600		12		
Prep/Serve	3600	300	12		
Storage	1800		6		
Tray Prep	300			675	1.0
Floor Pantries	375				

4. Summarize food services personnel by category and shift.

Food Services—Projections

General planning decisions needed

- What will be the sizes of the several different hospital populations at the target date?
- What external factors may affect the utilization of hospital food services in the foreseeable future? For example, is the area near the hospital developing commercially in a way that might provide competing services?

Specific planning decisions needed

- What factors may change within the hospital that would affect the pattern of food services utilization? For example, some hospitals have experimented with a variable patient mealtime, which not only spreads the work more evenly over the day but enables the scheduling of patients' other necessary activities to be done more flexibly. A change in personnel practices might spread the employee work load more evenly over the noon meal period.
- What technological changes in processing and serving of food are in prospect, and how would they affect the operation and design of food services?
- Are affiliations with other institutions or contract arrangements with commercial concerns in prospect?

Procedure

Summarize the total projected population (except inpatients) expected to be in the hospital at the noon hour at the target date. Using current experience and whatever informed judgments may be made as to prospects for the future, assign to each group a utilization rate. For each group estimate the turnover rate that can be expected. Divide the percentage of the total population who will be using hospital food services by the suggested turnover rate to determine the number of seats required.

Table FS-4. Projected Food Services Utilization and Seats

Category	Numbers on Hand	Percent Using Food Services	Turnover Rate	Seats Needed
Physicians	80	40%	2.7	12
Employees	500	75%	3.4	110
Visitors	100	20%	2.5	8
Etc.	—	—	—	—
Total	680			130

Space Requirements

As suggested earlier, the variety of food handling methods and the number of changes on the horizon make it difficult to generalize about space requirements. Guidelines such as one square foot per daily meal for tray make-up may have a certain validity. For the rest, if current types of service are projected, the best method is simply to extrapolate from current experience. For a new facility the advice of a food services expert who can evaluate economic and quality tradeoffs should be sought as early as possible.

Procedure

Multiply the number of seats needed at the target date by the areas per seat or per tray from Table FS-2, adjusted to correct current deficits. It may be that not all areas require equivalent increases in space—for example, a kitchen may have excess capacity, but storage and seating areas might be short. The projection may be summarized as follows:

Table FS-4. Summary of Food Services Space Requirements—Target Date

Space/Type	Area per Seat	No. of Seats	Area Needed	Area per Tray	No. of Trays	Area Needed
Dining	15		1950			
Prep/Serve	14	130	1820			
Storage	8		1040			
Tray Prep				1.0	900	900
Floor Pantry				—	—	—
Totals		130	4810		900	900

Locations Requirements

Determine where food services will be needed, and how they should be distributed. A variety of types of food service may be offered, from vending machine rooms to snack bars. A general guideline of food service planners is that a facility serving under 500 meals is likely to be costly in terms of staff time and space. However, there may be good reasons for providing a variety of smaller eating areas: This is essentially a matter of policy and must be decided by the hospital administration. The architect, however, should be responsible for determining the optimum location for food services, since this is largely dependent on general circulation patterns, and must be developed in the context of the total hospital distribution system.

7

Administrative and General Services

7.1. BACKGROUND/DISCUSSION

As the level of interaction of hospitals with government, with social agencies and organizations, and with the general public grows, the supporting services and administrative activities of the hospital will also expand. Developments in private and public health insurance have led to a higher level of accountability to outside agencies, which increases the amount of documentation that is needed, which increases the amount of paperwork. As medicine has become more complex and expensive there has been an increased need for nonmedical specialists to administer and manage the hospital's activities.

Similarly, supporting social services for patients and services and amenities for employees continue to expand. It appears likely that such activities and services will proliferate, either within the hospital itself or nearby.

Projecting Requirements for Administrative and General Services

It may be sufficient at an early stage of planning simply to add up the numbers of people associated with all of the services in this category, to determine the total amount of space they occupy, and to project future space requirements on an estimated percentage increase. Location criteria for most of these functions are not as critical as they are for the highly interdependent clinical activities. Nevertheless, a smoothly running operation may depend to a considerable degree on good communication patterns among administrative work units, and this may, therefore, be considered sufficiently important that the hospital will want to go into a fairly detailed level of planning early in the process.

7.2. ADMINISTRATIVE AND BUSINESS FUNCTION

Included would be general administration, billing and accounts, statistics, nursing and other administrative units, data processing, and possibly computer operations, personnel office, and so on. Purchasing could be considered part of administration or part of supply services. Large hospitals may also have a legal officer and public relations and publications departments.

A quick and reasonably accurate means of estimating space requirements for office personnel is to estimate the projected total of people in all categories who will be working during the typical day and to multiply by 150-200 net square feet. Averaged out over a reasonably large staff, this allows for office support areas such as machine rooms, reception and waiting space, larger offices for executives, and clerical stations. Not included would be conference or meeting rooms, the need for which should be calculated separately.

A more detailed analysis can be done if the administrative and management structure is known. The question then is how the organization chart will look and what the management policies of the hospital are. One common controversy is whether the heads of administrative departments or functions should be located together to facilitate and encourage their daily communication or whether the head of each activity should be located so as to maintain maximum contact with his subordinates.

The planner should list all functions that are considered to be related to business administration and personnel, and he should identify the number of personnel by category. A summary might look like this:

	Persons or Stations		Planning Allowance	
Personnel Category	Current Number	Projected Number	NSF Per Station	Total NSF
Director	1	1	200	200
Assistant	—	1	150	150
Secretary	1	2	150	300
Waiting	3	6	30	180
Clerical	6	20	80	1600
Machine Room	—	—	—	150
Conference	—	15	20	300

7.3. ADMITTING

The admitting activity is largely clerical but may include clinical aspects such as preliminary diagnostic testing and history taking and social service. The space requirements for admissions will depend on the average number of daily admissions, the policy and practice of the hospital with regard to preadmission, and the level of service that is provided to both patients and relatives.

An important question that should be explored early in the planning process is whether or not there should be a single patient entrance to the hospital, combining elective inpatient admissions, outpatient clinics, and emergency visits. The arguments for a unified entrance and registration/ admissions system is that it serves to centralize activities that are similar, ensures good communications, and simplifies life for the patient who may otherwise be faced with a confusing choice of entrances, information desks, and offices. The ambulance entrance should always, of course, be separate.

The main argument against a combined entrance with admission/outpatient or emergency registration in the same area is that the volume of patients in the outpatient and emergency areas is large and creates confusion. This can probably be solved by good design of spaces, clear graphics, and a sufficient amount of space.

Projecting Requirements

Specific questions that must be asked are:

- Will inpatient admissions be combined with outpatient registration?
- How many visits and admissions will be handled on the average day? How many patient and clerical or other stations must be available at any one time? Waiting space for how many?
- What are the location requirements of admissions and registration activities relative to other units, such as medical records, nursing administration, bookkeeping, patient accounts, insurance, and credit offices? What social services will be provided in this area?

7.4. PATIENT AND PUBLIC SERVICES

This category can include such general services as the activities often operated by the hospital's auxiliary, such as flower and gift shops, hairdresser, lending library, and snack bar; services directed towards the spiritual and social well-being of patients and relatives, such as chaplain services and chapel, social services and counseling; and public information or the new position of patient advocate—an advisor, often a volunteer, charged with the responsibility of guiding the patient and his family through the health care maze.

As the hospital becomes more complex, and medical practice more difficult for the layman to understand, personal attention and careful explanations become essential. The small quasicommercial services offered by the auxiliary provide a needed relief to the anxious and harassed relative faced with unfamiliar surroundings and can help to make the hospital atmosphere less threatening. An area of public service that seems to be gaining importance is the area of education both for patients and their relatives. It is not ureasonable to think of a part of the hospital lobby being devoted to a classroom or to automated individual audiovisual carrels where relatives could be instructed in a specific disease process, its diagnosis and treatment, and in home care procedures.

A hospital might also provide day care or nursery services for the benefit of visiting relatives, especially if it is felt that such visits are important to the patient's recovery. Such a service would probably gain heaviest use in the outpatient clinics; it might be combined with a day care service for employee's children.

Projecting Requirements for Patient and Public Services

A list of such services should be drawn up with input from all segments of the hospital population—including patients and their relatives and friends. The size of the hospital may limit the numbers and kinds of services that can be provided, but there is no reason why a "blue sky" list should not be made initially. Some quantification will be needed in order to judge the relative demands on space. Then priorities can be established and choices made. Some of these services can be not only self-supporting but income-producing and should not, therefore, be considered merely as luxuries. Conceivably the income produced by one group of activities might serve to offset the costs of others. In fact, it may be in the hospital's self-interest to provide the kinds of services mentioned, if merely to mitigate community resentment of hospital costs.

For each service, estimates should be made of the volume of activity of daily number of users. Most of these kinds of activities require a location near the entrance or waiting areas of the hospital, ideally as part of the lobby.

7.5. SOCIAL SERVICES

Mention of social services is made throughout the description of clinical and general services. However, since facilities for the less visible services are sometimes forgotten, it may be a good idea to summarize the requirements for social services and their distribution throughout the hospital. A central administrative office will be needed where records can be centralized, liaison with outside social service agencies maintained, and meetings of the staff held. A meeting room combined with a library may be desirable. In addition to the centralized office, office/counseling facilities may be needed in a number of areas of the hospital, including admissions, outpatient clinics, emergency, and patient care areas.

The level of social services will be a matter of hospital policy—but the trend is to increase the level of such services, particularly in city hospitals where a large proportion of patients are both indigent and inexperienced in dealing with large institutions. Some hospitals may also want to give house room to outside social service organizations or agencies.

7.6. EMPLOYEE FACILITIES AND SERVICES

The kinds of facilities that are needed (or that may be desired) for hospital personnel include such necessities as: lounge, dressing and locker space; food services (covered in the preceding chapter); parking (covered in Chapter 10); and health services; not to mention the personnel function itself. The shortage of well-trained personnel, the typically low pay scales of hospitals, and the high demand on hospital personnel in terms of personal commitment and dedication will make it well worth the hospital's while to provide an adequate level of amenity for employees. The investment in space should return high dividends in employee satisfaction and reduce turnover rates. A day care center for children, provided free or at low cost, will enable the hospital to attract employees who would otherwise be unavailable. Attractive lounges, and even recreational facilities, may be provided.

Not long ago a major university medical center was considering including in its building program an employee social and recreation center, to include lockers, lounges, food services, shops, daycare and nursery, a library, and exercise facilities, including a multipurpose gymnasium and swimming pool. The difficulty that was encountered in planning such a facility was an old one: The doctors would not mix with the nurses, the registered nurses did not want to mix with the aides, the aides did not want to mix with the orderlies, the technicians did not want to mix with the craftsmen, and craftsmen especially did not want to mix with the maintenance men. This difficulty relates to a number of employee functions—status distinctions must either be broken or accepted, and this will involve a difficult policy decision that the hospital will have to make. Complicating the issue further may be union requirements. The stronger unions may be in a position to demand certain kinds of separate facilities for their own groups.

Projecting Requirements for Personnel Services

The best procedure for calculating personnel services may be to develop a list of desirable facilities and services, to make a rough estimate of space requirements for each, and then, in the light of operative priorities and constraints, to select those that are either essential or seem to provide the best value.

The space requirements for such facilities as day care, lounge facilities, and recreation can be developed from the needs of the full-time-equivalent day-shift population. Lockers, if they are to be provided to every employee, would have to be based on the total headcount and could represent a large amount of space.

Distribution of Facilities

The hospital will also have to decide, as a policy as well as a practical question, whether employee facilities should be provided centrally or small units of, for example, locker and lounge space should be provided in each major work unit. There are good arguments for providing facilities for employees near their places of work. Employee health services could readily be integrated into the outpatient clinic area or could form part of a central employee service area.

7.7. MEDICAL ILLUSTRATION AND PHOTOGRAPHY/AUDIOVISUAL SERVICES

These functions are really quite different—one dealing largely with clinical applications, the other having primarily an educational or communications character, but for practical reasons (at least in the smaller hospitals)—they are sometimes operated together. Medical illustration provides documentary services to the clinical departments and pathology: a studio where patients can be brought and photographed may be needed as well as a work area. The same personnel may also provide graphics services for medical education and may be responsible for audiovisual materials.

An audiovisual service may be merely a center for the maintenance and issuing of equipment such as projectors or television monitors, but it may also be responsible for production of materials and the collection and distribution of these materials.

Projecting Requirements for Medical Illustration and Audiovisual Services

A full definition of the departments responsibilities and activities should be obtained, along with necessary speculation as to future directions. It is hardly possible to generalize about space requirements except to point out that they may range from a few hundred square feet for a photographic studio and work area to several thousand where the design, production and distribution of audiovisual materials, services, and equipment is considered. In many cases, production is the responsibility of one unit, the cataloging and maintenance of materials that of another (often the library) and the maintenance and distribution of equipment for the use of materials that of yet a third.

7.8.   MEDICAL RECORDS

Background/Discussion

The medical record—the case history that describes the symptoms, diagnoses, course of treatment, and progress of a patient during his hospital visit as an inpatient or outpatient—requires information from a variety of sources and provides information for a variety of purposes. The medical record represents not only a resource to the physician but to the hospital in analyzing its services; in assessing how well it meets the needs of the population and the amount and quality of care that that population is receiving; as a source of epidemological data; and as a resource for retrospective research.

With the increased awareness of health professionals and planners that health care can and should be a comprehensive system rather than a series of isolated episodes, it has become evident that no matter how sophisticated a hospital's record-keeping system may be and no matter how well-integrated internally, it is still merely a recording of one hospital's activity with regard to that patient. It is not a record of his whole health history and gives only a fragmented image. With our mobile population it seems probable that in the not too distant future a person's entire health and illness record should travel with him wherever he goes and be available to any physician or institution he may encounter. Such records would also facilitate research into hereditary disease.

How such a comprehensive medical record system may be achieved is less a technical problem than a philosophical, social, and legal one. How to provide wide access to information without violating privacy or laws of confidentiality is a matter of concern in many fields. The thought of a central data bank for health information raises alarm, and justifiably. All the same, without a universal unique numbering system and a central repository of data and without administrative and management data linked to the patient record, comprehensive health planning and management will necessarily fall far short of what could be achieved.

The Special Problems of Medical Records

In addition to the complexities that surround any data-gathering activity and record-keeping, medical records provide some special difficulties. For example, it must be possible to retrieve a record at any time during the day or night, and quickly. The record's path must be accurately tracked once it leaves the record room. But probably the greatest problem of the record lies in its substance and format. It is essential that records be legible and that important information can be quickly located in it. If physicians' entries are made by hand they are likely to be hard, and sometimes impossible to read. This means that the history simply cannot be read by a physician in the time available to him, even in a nonemergency. If entries are transcribed, either from oral or handwritten notes, they may be subject to gross inaccuracies and errors—and the physician may be hard pressed to find the time to carefully proofread the typescript.

Initial computer recording of data may be an answer in the future, as diagnostic and monitoring instruments increasingly become tied to computer recording and analysis systems. The computer allows for concise and correlated presentations of data of a general nature, but the differences in language used by different specialties and subspecialties create a problem in extending their use to information generated by the physician himself. One might guess that it would be some time before physicians were routinely trained in a computer language suitable for use not only in their own specialties but in those of other disciplines. However, since computer scientists are increasingly turning their attention to the development of language and software there is, perhaps, hope of development in this area as well.

The basic questions that must be asked about medical records include:

What information is to be recorded, by whom, and how?

- What are the statutory requirements with regard to medical records?
- Who records the information initially and by what means?
- Who enters the information on the permanent record and how?
- What information is abstracted or summarized, how, and by whom?
- How is the record reviewed for accuracy?
- Where is the record stored, for how long, and how is access achieved?

How is the information used and by whom?

- Inpatient admissions, outpatient service?
- Physician and nursing staff, day-to-day?

- For professional review?
- For hospital statistics?
- For health planning and analysis? For example, morbidity, diagnostic studies, professional activity, and medical audit programs?
- For epidiomological statistics?
- For retrospective research? Clinical research? Historical research?

How long will records be retained and in what form?

- What are applicable statutory requirements for the retention of records?
- For how long are records to be considered current?
- For how long must the record be kept in its entirety, or how long is desirable to do so?
- Should *certain* records be kept in their entirety because of statutory requirements or a particular need (e.g., pediatric records, records of patients with malignancy, neurological or psychiatric illness) and may others be weeded, summarized, or abstracted?
- Can the discharge summary and pathology reports serve as an adequate record summary, with most other data discarded after a certain period?
- Should records be kept in their entirety in a form different from the original, such as microfilm or microfiche, videotape, or computer tape? Should abstracts or summaries be kept in one of these forms?
- At what point can records be disposed of in their entirety, if ever?
- Where can noncurrent records be stored?

Work Load and Personnel

Purpose

To give an approximate measure of the work load generated by the current volume of patients. The work load consists of information entered and abstracted from records, transcribing, coding, filing, pulling files, and the distribution and collection of records within the hospital. A detailed analysis of the activities should not be necessary at the level of planning to which this book addresses itself: it should be sufficient to make a general estimate that ties together the patient load, the amount of work generated, and the numbers of personnel in the medical records department.

Information needed

- Hospital data on average census and average number of outpatient visits.

- A list of personnel involved in medical records work, excluding messengers.
- An estimate from the medical records librarian of the daily volume of work, expressed in some constant unit of measure, such as average number of pages entered in records during a typical day or the number of records handled.
- A brief verbal description or diagram of the records system: How the records are handled and what path they follow from initiation to archiving or disposal.

Procedure

1. Calculate the ratio between units of work (here called entries for reasons of brevity) and the average daily census and number of out-patient visits.

2. List the categories of personnel, and show the full-time-equivalent staff members for each category. Divide the number of entries per day by the total staff in the medical records area to obtain a measure of the number of entries handled per day per person on the average.

The results of these calculations might be shown thus:

Table MR-1. Medical Records Workload

Personnel Categories	Daily Entries per Inpatient	Entries per Outpatient	Total Entries	FTE Staff Members	Entries per Person
—	—	—	—	—	—

Records Storage

Information needed

- Number of records on hand (considered current).
- Number of record volumes added per year.
- Number of records withdrawn from active use and put in archives.
- Method of storing records (e.g., on open shelves, in a mechanical storage and retrieval file).
- Method of filing (e.g., terminal digit filing will permit withdrawal of inactive records without requiring relocation of all remaining records).

Procedure

Using the number of records on hand as a base, calculate the actual net accession rate by subtracting the number of records annually withdrawn and adding the number of records annually added.

Space

Information needed

- The net areas of medical records work space, including such areas as dictating and transcribing rooms (wherever they may be located throughout the hospital) indexing, reference, and administrative areas, coding, keypunch, and machine rooms, and research.
- Separately, the net floor area of records storage space, including the space occupied by shelving, aisles, and work/study tables immediately associated with the records.

Procedure

Calculate separately the amount of space, per full-time-equivalent medical records employee for the first category of space, called, in the example below, work space, and the number of records that are stored per net square foot of floor area in the second category, thus:

Table MR-2.   Medical Records Space Analysis

Number of MR Personnel	Total MR Work Space	Work Space per Person	Total MR Rec. Volumes	Total MR Floor Area (NSF)	MR Volumes per NSF Floor Area
—	—	—	—	—	—

Medical Records—Projections

Space and location requirements for medical records will depend on the methods used to collect, process, transmit, and store information and on the ways in which medical records information is integrated with other parts of the hospital information system. Since the medical record is not only crucial to patient care but also is a source of information necessary to the general administration and management of the hospital, it is advisable that the entire information system be studied, and its needs projected, at one and the same time. Such a study should be taken early in the planning process; while all recommendations may not be capable of implementation immediately, at least the planner can be assured that future possibilities are taken into account. In so far as one can speculate about such a complex subject, it might be possible to predict that developments in the field will tend to decentralize the system rather than to continue placing demands on centrally located hospital space. However, the increasing need to know what has happened to the patient in the hospital and to link that information to hospital administrative data for cost analyses, demographic and patient-origin analyses, and so on may put the medical record into more active use by a larger number of interests.

General planning decisions needed

- What is the target date for which the medical records facility should be planned?
- What are general hospital planning projections with regard to daily volume of patients?

Workload and Personnel

Information needed

Data and estimates from preceding section.

Specific planning decisions needed

What changes can be predicted for (a) the volume of records work per patient and (b) the volume of work that can be done per person. If changes are in prospect, how would they affect the figures for current operations on a percentage basis?

Procedure

1. Calculate the number of entries that will result from multiplying the projected daily number of patients by the current average entries per patient from Table MR-1 (adjusted to reflect decisions made above).

2. Using the current rate of work from Table MR-1 (adjusted to reflected changes in productivity, if necessary) divide by projected total number of entries per person to determine the number of persons who will be required to handle the projected work load.

The projections can be displayed thus:

Table MR-3. Projected Work Load and Personnel at Target Date

Projected Patients Daily	Estimated Entries per Patient	Total Entries	Estimated Entries per Person	Number of Staff Needed
—	—	—	—	—

Record Storage

Information needed

Information from the preceding section, showing current patterns of record inventory, accession and disposal.

Planning decisions needed

What changes are in prospect with regard to patterns of retention and disposal of records?

Procedure

Calculate the number of records that will have to be accommodated at the target date separately for active records and records that may be archived. Note: If a steady increase in the number of patients were anticipated, the rate of accession would be correspondingly more rapid than the rate of archiving, and the arithmetic would get somewhat more complicated than in the example below.

Example

Assume that a hospital has 60,000 records currently in its active section and an accumulation of 120,000 in its archives. New records are added at the rate of 6000 a year, and records are put into the archives at the rate of 3000 volumes a year. In 10 years the active records would have grown to 90,000, and the archive (assuming that none are disposed of) would have grown to 150,000.

Space Requirements

Purpose

To calculate the area required for medical records separately for work area and storage area(s).

Information needed

- Projected number of personnel and projected number of records from the preceding paragraphs.
- Current net square feet per person and number of records per net square foot from Table MR-2.

Planning decisions needed

1. What changes in method of handling records or storing them are in prospect that should be taken into account when projecting future needs: For example, if by statute records must currently be kept for, say, 10 years, would it be legally and practically possible to transfer the records to microfilm after 3 years, at which age utilization of the record

usually drops significantly? What would the effect of this be on storage requirements?

2.   Does the current figure of space per person (employee) and number of records per net square foot of floor area represent workable allowances, or should adjustments be made?

Procedures

1.   For work areas, multiply the projected number of personnel by the current (or adjusted) figure of space per person.

2.   For record storage, divide the projected number of records by the current (or adjusted) figure of volumes per net square foot of floor space.

Table MR-4.   Projected Space Requirements—Target Date

Projected Personnel	Work Area per Person	Work Area Needed (NSF)	Projected Med. Records	Volumes per NSF	Storage Area Needed (NSF)
—	—	—	—	—	—

Note: If a more accurate method of calculating record storage space is needed, the following procedure may be followed:

1.   Count the average number of record volumes per linear foot of shelf space.

2.   Using a typical double-faced shelving unit of 5 shelves, calculate how many record volumes it will hold.

3.   Measure the floor space the unit itself takes up, and calculate the amount of aisle space that should be assigned to each such unit. Into this area, divide the number of records that will thus be accommodated to arrive at a figure of volumes per square foot of floor space area that accurately reflects specific conditions.

4.   Consider the effect of changing the type of storage shelf.

5.   Consider structural requirements to support weight of records to be stored.

7.9. MEDICAL LIBRARIES

The elements to be considered in library planning fall into three main groups:

• Numbers of volumes.
• Numbers of reader stations.
• Technical processing and administration.

Numbers of volumes can be interpreted to include all forms of information that can be stored and used by a reader or viewer, such as audio or video tapes, slides, photographs, film records, and a variety of microforms.

Reader stations includes seats at tables or carrels, small study rooms, group study rooms, computer terminals, microfilm readers, lounge seating, and so forth.

Technical processing includes all the work areas associated with selecting, ordering, receiving, cataloguing, and shelving of acquisitions.

The determinant of staff needs and technical processing space is the rate of acquisition, and this, therefore, becomes an important piece of information. The acquisition rate will also, of course, determine the rate at which new space will be needed for volumes. The net number of volumes added per year may be less than the annual acquisition rate if old books are weeded out as new ones are added.

Distribution of Libraries

A community hospital may have only one small library for reference material and major journals. A large teaching hospital may have a more extensive central library and in addition may have decentralized departmental libraries. The problem with departmental libraries is that they are usually too small to be able to maintain a librarian and thus quickly become disordered. An alternative is to install major reference works and current journals in a combined reading room/staff lounge or conference room.

As a rough planning guideline, the area required for books can be computed at 8-10 volumes per net square foot of floor area for the large reference works that are found in a typical medical library. This figure allows sufficient free shelf space so that a few books can be added to a shelf without moving every book in the library. Shelving that displays current periodicals with preceding issues stacked below will allow for about 5 periodical volumes per net square foot. Other forms must be calculated separately, as sizes and types of shelving required vary widely.

In a university setting, it is traditional to plan on a number of reader stations equivalent to one-fourth to one-third of the student population. In the case of a medical school this standard would probably apply. In the case of a hospital, an estimate of the required number of reader stations would have to be based on the local situation. It may be worth cautioning that where there is a shortage of general lounge space the library often becomes the only alternative place to go and sit. This may artificially inflate estimates of numbers of readers if they are made on the basis of current conditions where alternative seating space for general use is absent. Planning allowances for seating may range from 25 to 50 square feet per station, depending on the type of station that is needed. As a general guide, technical processing and catalog areas can be computed at 15-20% of the total of reader and book space.

Projecting Needs for Medical Libraries

Planning and policy decisions needed

- Should there be a central library or departmental libraries or a combination of these?
- If there are decentralized libraries, who will maintain them?
- What is the base collection of the central or departmental library?
- What is the anticipated annual rate of accession of all types of material? What are the implications for library staff?
- At what rate are items weeded?
- What is the defined target date at which the library (ies) will be full?
- What plans can be made for expansion beyond this point?
- What level of reader services is proposed? What are the implications for library staff?
- What number of reader stations of what types are planned for what hospital populations?

Procedure

Summarize the assumptions and calculate the implication for space.

Table L-1. Library Space Requirements

Volumes	Current Number	Added per Year	Number at Target Date	NSF Needed
Reference	—	—	—	—
Circulation	—	—	—	—
Periodicals (volume-equivalent)	—	—	—	—
Audiovisual Materials	—	—	—	—
Microforms	—	—	—	—

Readers	Number	Type of Station	NSF per Station	NSF Needed
Students	—		—	—
Faculty	—		—	—
Physicians	—		—	—
Nurses	—		—	—
Paramedical	—		—	—
Others	—		—	—
Totals	—		—	—

Compute the total area requirements and add 15-20% to allow for circulation desk and technical processing space.

8

Housekeeping, Maintenance, Engineering Service, and Systems

8.1. HOUSEKEEPING

Housekeeping is as essential to the operation of the hospital as any other department. In some institutions the housekeeping department is responsible for laundry and linen supply. However, in this book the housekeeping department is limited to janitorial services. Generally, hospitals use more equipment for cleaning than other institutions of comparable size. It is essential, therefore, that adequate space be provided. Each department should have a janitor's closet at least 4 by 6 feet. If carpets are used, additional space will be needed for shampooing equipment and supplies. There should also be a central storage room for janitorial supplies.

8.2. MAINTENANCE

Maintenance and operation costs are seldom given much attention during programming and design phases, but conventional emphasis on first cost with the problems of financing and resultant desire to obtain the lowest bid often causes the use of materials and methods that adversely affect the life cost of the building. Unfortunately, there is no dependable body of cost information on the intricate problems of operation and maintenance of hospital buildings. It is estimated that such costs have exceeded 5% per year and are continuing to rise due to the increasing amount of remodeling being done.

Hospital buildings are subject to extremely heavy demands upon both building fabric and mechanical systems and, therefore, require high standards of durability. Small savings in annual operation and maintenance costs will have a significant effect on life costs. Yet this does not mean that no effort should be made to analyze and justify the quality selection of materials and subsystems. On the contrary, an attempt should be made to estimate the life expectancy of each element of the building and to choose accordingly. The activities housed and the highly specialized equipment, the range of utilities, the need to create exceptional sterile environments in certain areas, the effect of chemicals on materials, and yet the need to deinstitutionalize insofar as possible create conflicting demands that defy simple solutions and present unique problems of operation and maintenance.

Certain utilities present their own specialized problems of supply and quality; cases in point are distilled water and vacuum installations, repeatedly the objects of criticism. Fumes and spillage of a highly noxious or corrosive nature place very special demands upon the materials employed in mechanical systems, building construction, interior finishes, and equipment. All these specialized requirements are in addition to the normal problems of operation and maintenance such as cleaning, wear and tear on materials, repair and replacement of mechanical parts, which occur in any building. Another factor that should not be overlooked in estimating maintenance costs is downtime required. Preventive maintenance done on a regularly scheduled basis can greatly reduce maintenance cost because downtime can be anticipated and planned for. And finally, the extent of provisions for change, the adaptability of the design, can further reduce maintenance cost.* Perhaps a first approach to analysis of material selection consistent with life expectancy would be to prepare an adjunct to a preliminary finishing schedule as shown in Table SYS-1:

Table SYS-1.   Estimated Life Expectancy

Room No.	Description	Estimated Life Expectancy (Years)					
			Finishes				
		Room	Floor-Base	Walls	Clg.	Equipment	Comments
101	General Laboratory	10	G / 10	B / 4	R / 10	5	
—	Etc.	—	—	—	—	—	—

Legend: [X / 0]   Finish Designation/ Life Expectancy of Finish

* Paraphrased from *Academic Building Systems*, A Joint Effort of Indiana University and the University of California, July, 1971.

8 3. ENGINEERING SERVICES AND SYSTEMS

The rapidly increasing complexity and extent of mechanical and electrical services have significantly affected the design of hospitals. Mechanical and electrical systems now comprise approximately half the total construction cost. In addition, changes in space requirements for new technologies and equipment suggest that greater consideration be given the ability to adapt mechanical and electrical services to meet the changing needs. The design of these support services should become an integral part of the architectural and structural design. Each system while remaining independent should work well with all other systems so that conflicts during construction, and later when changes may be required, are minimized. Further, systems should be designed insofar as possible for multiple use of spaces served. For example, although it would not be practical to design all floors to support the weight of x-ray film storage files, the heaviest normal loads should be anticipated and perhaps consideration should be given to a structural system that could be easily strengthened in limited areas if required. Or, an airconditioning system should be considered that can be easily modified to anticipate reasonable changes in occupancy of the spaces it serves, and such a system should work well with the structure and lighting requirements.

Another consideration should be the advantages of fabricating elements of structural, mechanical, and electrical systems off-site. The greater the standardization of such elements, the more likely it is that economies can be realized. Standardization will also tend to prevent over-specialized design, thus increasing flexibility and substantially shortening construction time.

A concept that is gaining increasing acceptance is the provision of a separate accessible floor, known as an interstitial floor or systems space, for the mechanical and electrical distribution systems. Such a floor is normally provided above all ancillary departments and below a nursing tower if it is on top of the ancillary departments. It may also be advantageously placed like a sandwich between every two nursing floors if there is a good chance that such floors may be converted to other uses. (See Table SYS-1). The reason for, and advantages of, the separate systems floor are:

- As the awareness grows that the true costs of a building are its life costs, a design that simplifies maintenance and facilitates repairs and remodeling becomes the more economical and desirable design.
- Time can be saved during the design process since the structural, mechanical, and electrical systems are designed to accommodate the maximum internal environment demands, thus permitting decisions on basic systems to be made much earlier in the design process.

- For the above reasons it is possible to consider the start of construction on foundations and strucural frame while departmental planning is finalized. Potentially, this offers tremendous economies in time and dollars.
- The shorter construction time reduces the costs added by inflation during an extended construction period and places the facility in operation sooner.
- A structural system that uses large preassembled members simplifies delivery scheduling as they can be lifted directly into place without the need for large staging areas for storage and sorting.
- The ability readily to remodel the spaces above and below with minimum disturbance of the used spaces will bring about savings in future construction costs.
- Maintenance personnel can easily inspect, maintain, replace, or revise the supporting systems serving a hospital floor without disrupting the operation of that floor.
- Much of the noise and possible contamination from the passage of mechanics and inspectors will be eliminated from patient areas.
- Floor-to-floor height need not be set by spaces which require exceptionally high ceilings since these areas can be accommodated by occasional infringement on the interstitial space.

It has been the experience of the authors that a systems floor can be provided at no increase in cost if contractors are aware of the significant savings in time that result from the fact that mechanical and finishing trades can work simultaneously. The successful planning of a systems floor requires a synthesis of the following systems:

1. Structural System.
2. Utility and Piping Distribution System.
3. Air Handling System.
4. Electrical System.
5. Material Handling System (if automated)

Maximum economies in time and money will be achieved when the design of all systems is coordinated and their influences on each other is properly understood.

To best meet the structural problem of long spans and to maximize the potential for unrestricted horizontal mechanical distribution, a system is recommended that makes efficient use of the depth of the required mechanical spaces for moment-resisting efficiency while providing as much free area as possible through the web for passage of mechanical and

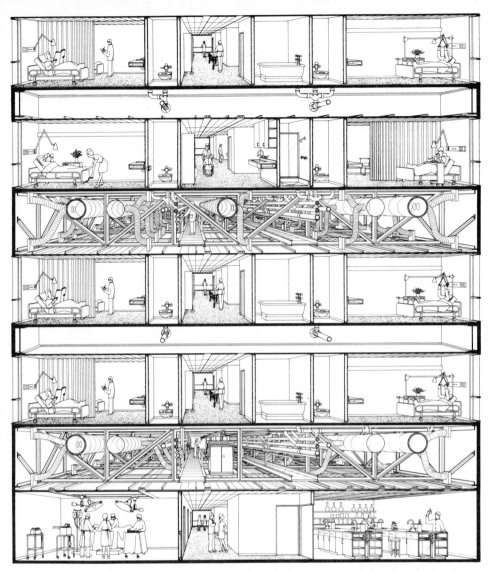

Figure 9. Increasingly complex mechanical systems combine with the desirability of eliminating fixed elements which inhibit change to suggest long span trusses whose depths can be used as a systems floor (The Rex Allen Partnership, Architects).

materials-handling systems as well as personnel. The structural form that best meets the criteria is a truss.

Whether such a truss is steel or concrete is a matter for detailed analysis. Generally, steel has proven more economical and will be less bulky. Consideration should also be given to the form of truss. Obviously a Vierendeel truss that has no diagonal members will interfere least with duct work. However, since it is generally the most expensive type of truss, justification must come from savings in a well-integrated mechanical system.

Contrary to what might be expected, the volume of a building is *not* significantly increased by the systems floor design. The reasons for this are:

1. The mechanical space requirements in a modern hospital are high and particularly so in core service areas. Therefore, even conventional hospitals have large floor-to-floor dimensions.

2. Only 20% or less of the structural space normally allowed is actually occupied by structural elements. The remaining 80% of the space is *not* utilized.

3. The systems floor, by contrast, utilizes a combined mechanical and structural space to achieve complete utilization of available space and at the same time provide increased structural depth for efficient spans. The conventional design approach of assigning an exclusive structural layer over an equally exclusive mechanical layer, sized for the worst crossover condition is surely not an efficient use of space.

In conclusion, the systems floor permits a design which reduces to a minimum the number of fixed vertical elements, such as columns and mechanical shafts, which limit adaptability of usable space. It is therefore suggested that a careful analysis be made of its advantages at an early stage of design.

9

The Effect of Education on the Hospital

This chapter briefly explores some of the broad effects of education on the medical center and hospital and outlines in a general way the added factors that must be considered in a program for the development of physical plans.

The clinical training of young doctors and nurses will add to the demands on space within the hospital itself, since an added component of teaching and study space will be required in almost every unit of the hospital. The greatest demand for space, however, will come from the fact that a large proportion of the teachers of the young physicians will be engaged in research—and it is research that presents the greatest problem to the planner. Research is expensive, space consuming, demanding of staff time, and, worst of all, unpredictable.

The greatest effect of education will be felt by the major medical center, where the training of medical students takes place. But nurses, pharmacists, hospital administrators, technicians, paramedical personnel, and most other hospital employees also receive some portion of their training in the hospital setting, and inevitably there is an effect on space.

Putting aside for the moment the training of doctors and nurses, let us consider the other people who will require training. The hospital may, as an institution, be involved in a variety of training programs in collaboration with a number of other organizations and institutions, including professional schools such as schools of dentistry, pharmacy, allied health sciences, and medical technology. Usually on an ad hoc basis, the hospital may be involved in the training of community groups or groups from public service or charitable organizations.

The hospital will, of necessity, be required to offer some training for its own employees. In a large hospital the annual hours spent in orientation and training, or retraining of employees and volunteers may run to the thousands, representing a large investment in staff time. A survey at one medium-sized university medical center suggested that a third of the time spent in training employees could be saved by a coordinated program in which most of the didactic instruction required for every training program was presented jointly. Most hospitals do not have adequate teaching space for employee instruction unless they are part of a medical center and can use conference/classrooms that have been provided for medical and nursing students, and most feel the lack.

There are two other groups who may be involved in education in the hospital setting: practicing physicians, who are continuing their education, and patients, their relatives, and the population at large to whom the hospital is in a position to provide instruction on health care in general and on specific types of care associated with particular conditions.

To take the latter group first: Responsibility for patient and public education on health related matters appears to fall largely to the hospital either as a direct service or with the hospital in the role of initiator and coordinator. The education of patients and their friends and relatives is receiving increased attention, particularly in the areas of nutrition, maternal health, and rehabilitation; the care and treatment of patients suffering from diabetes, cancer, and heart conditions; and the dying patient.

The vast and rapid accumulation of new knowledge in the clinical disciplines has suggested that physicians should be recertified at regular intervals and that to do this programs of continuing education for the medical profession must be widely available. It has been proposed that, in effect, every community hospital should be a teaching hospital, drawing in not only its own staff for seminars and conferences but all area physicians.

There are then six major groups for whom the hospital will, in one sense or another, be an educational setting: physicians and nurses in training; allied health professionals; administrative, technical, and support personnel of the hospital itself; patients and the public; and medical practicioners. It should be obvious that a considerable amount of space can be saved if these several types of programs can share facilities to some degree—and there is no reason why they should not. Although some types of facilities for teaching must be highly specialized, much of any type of teaching takes place in a classroom/seminar/conference room—which is merely a fairly large room equipped with tables and chairs or tablet armchairs and certain equipment for visual presentation.

Another fact that should be self-evident, but is often forgotten, may be repeated here: Space and time are inextricably related in the planning of facilities. The effective amount of space available for an activity depends upon the flexibility with which its use can be scheduled.

9.1. THE RELATIONSHIP BETWEEN HOSPITAL AND MEDICAL SCHOOL

There are a number of very fundamental issues that surround the education of future doctors and the relationship between their needs and those of the patients who serve as teaching material. Perhaps the most fundamental issue, and the one that is potentially most emotionally charged, is the question: Does the patient primarily serve the educational process, or is his care the first concern? The posing of the question should not imply that the interests of the participants in the process are necessarily at odds. Studies of teaching versus nonteaching hospitals tend to show that the quality of care a patient receives is generally higher at a teaching hospital than at a community hospital—logical enough, if one considers the enormous resources of professional and technical expertise available at a teaching hospital and the number of physicians who are on hand at any given time, compared to the staff and technical resources available at most community hospitals.

Nevertheless, the opposition of interests exists and is heightened, in the eyes of patients at least, by the common and insensitive use of such terms as "teaching material" to refer to ill human beings. Historically, it has been the poor who have provided the teaching material, with an occasional private patient with a particularly interesting condition added if the patient himself was willing. Patients were classed as resident staff patients if they were available for teaching purposes and as private patients if they were admitted by the clinical teaching staff or attending staff with admitting privileges.

To some extent these distinctions still exist, but they are fading. For one thing, the need to train physicians is so great that the pool of underprivileged patients is simply not large enough to provide the necessary experience for expanded classes of medical students. Private patients must, therefore, be used. Expansion of third-party coverage hospitalization has also vastly increased the number of patients who are able to pay for their care and reduced the charity patient to a small group. Persons covered by government programs are still somewhat at a disadvantage, since their care is paid for at a predetermined and contracted rate which is often below actual costs—but in theory, at least, they are equally provided for.

In addition to the potential conflict between the interest of the student and his teacher and between the interest of the patient and his insurer, there is another area of possible controversy. This is the conflict between the need of the teaching hospital to select its patients so as to represent a broad range of specialties and subspecialties and the need of the community to have available to it care for all patients, whether their condition is clinically interesting or not. Most health planning agencies and organizations agree on the need for certain hospitals to be designated as centers of specialization, but the immediate community may have a different opinion. Most large university medical centers are located in central city areas, in neighborhoods that have deteriorated and whose populations are often poor, overcrowded, underemployed, and that include a large proportion of old people. It is hard for these people to understand that the medical center's higher duty is the training of physicians and not the care of all the sick.

Another basic question is: How many patients are needed to provide adequate training for medical students? There seems to be little agreement on this question; estimates range from 2 to 4 or 5 beds per student. The question is complicated by the number of variations that can occur in teaching methods, patterns of affiliation with other hospitals where some undergraduate training may be provided, and differences in opinion as to how much hands-on experience is really necessary. Other factors affect the answer: A trend toward introducing medical students to patients earlier in their training; a trend toward compressing the clinical education of the medical student into a shorter period of time; and a trend toward making more use of outpatients in the training of students.

9.2. INTEGRATION OF HOSPITAL AND MEDICAL SCHOOL ACTIVITIES

The degree of integration of clinical, research, and teaching activities is another important issue, and one that is critical for the organization of space in the hospital. Fundamentally, the issue is one of functional flexibility versus territoriality. The hospital, seen as an intricate machine designed to care for patients in as smooth and efficient manner as possible, works best when like spaces and like functions are grouped together. This kind of physical organization allows for a relatively easy expansion and contraction of functions and activities as technology and demand change. From the standpoint of a clinical teaching department, however, a territorial arrangement is preferable—one in which all of a department's space, including patient care units, diagnostic and research laboratories, offices, seminar/conference rooms, and in certain instances outpatient clinics, are all grouped together in one area. Such an arrangement enhances communication among the faculty, students, and scientists associated with the department and saves a good deal of time that might otherwise be spent in moving back and forth between patients scattered throughout different floors or wings of the hospital or between patient care areas and research laboratories.

Centralization of Laboratories

This question of functional flexibility versus territorialty extends into specific areas of activity. Of particular concern are laboratories, both research and hospital laboratories. The configuration and utility systems required for laboratories are not very different from one type of laboratory to another. Differences exist in the configuration of equipment and the height of benches, but these are relatively superficial matters. In a sophisticated medical center, the line between what is a research and what is a patient care laboratory may be hard to draw. If a particular diagnostic procedure is successful in research, it will eventually become a routine part of hospital diagnostic activity. This argues that all laboratories, whatever their described purpose and whoever has jurisdiction over them, should be planned as a single unit. This argument is reinforced by the fact that research is often a creature of fashion and that government and private support for particular types of research may fluctuate rather unpredictably. If laboratories are planned together, a lost contract or a departed expert will merely mean that some remodeling may be needed to put the laboratory to other uses, providing expansion for a successful program perhaps or for the hospital's own clinical labs. If the laboratories are scattered among departments, this becomes extremely awkward.

Another example of this issue that relates particularly to research is the question of centralized versus decentralized animal research facilities. Most researchers will prefer to have their own animal facilities—it makes it easier to have the things you are using around you. However, it is impossible to maintain the kinds of conditions that should obtain in much animal experimentation except in a central, especially designed facility where absolute environmental control can be maintained. It is estimated that only between 10-20% of all animal experimentation requires frequent direct observation by the investigator himself and that the rest can quite readily take place in a central laboratory without real inconvenience. Animal research is not only becoming increasingly expensive but is coming under more careful government regulation and scrutiny. It is not only a question of humane treatment of animals, but more and more a question of the quality of research: Grants and contracts will not go to investigators who are not able to guarantee the quality of the animals themselves and the environmental conditions under which they are used. And these conditions are specialized and expensive to provide.

These then are some of the basic issues underlying the relationships among teaching, research, and staff training in hospitals:
• The potential conflict between patient care and physician training.
• The potential conflict between the needs of the medical school and the needs of the community, focused on the hospital and the patient.
• The question of which patients should be used as teaching material.
• The number and distribution of types of patients needed for a medical education.
• The issues of functional flexibility versus territoriality.

This list is by no means exhaustive, but it does suggest the areas that the planner may find to be most troublesome, emotionally charged, and important to explore. It is unlikely that all such issues can be resolved, and clear directions established all at once; but facing them will help to clear the air for the future. The only question for which it is absolutely necessary to get a clear answer before any physical planning is done is that of territoriality.

Research

At any but the smallest hospital there is likely to be some sort of research in progress. At a community hospital it may be limited to work being done by those physicians who by the nature of their specialty are hospital bound—the anethesiologists, radiologists, and pathologists. At a major medical center research may occupy more space than any other single type of activity.

For planning purposes it is useful to make a distinction between two types of research: clinical research and laboratory research. In medical parlance the term "clinical research" refers to the intent of the research rather than to its means, and much of it may, in fact, be done in a laboratory. For physical planning, however, a different kind of distinction is needed. Here, therefore, clinical research will refer only to work *that requires the physical presence of the patient* and that, therefore, requires a location proximate to patient care areas. The term "laboratory research" will be used for any type of work that may be done in a more remote location *and without the presence of patients.* In a medical school, basic science research is done by the faculty who teach the medical students during the early years and who may also have graduate and postdoctoral students in addition to the research which is done by the clinical faculty.

The largest problem of planning for research, as suggested in the introductory section of this chapter, lies in its unpredictable nature. The fact is that most institutions are not in a position to exercise very much control over the type, quality, and amount of research that is done under their auspices. The funds for research usually come from outside, the research itself enhances the image of the institution, and research facilities have to be provided if an institution wants to attract a distinguished faculty. The demands for research facilities spiral, as the distinguished faculty attracts others and as the reputation of the institution itself attracts further grants and contracts. For all of this, it is necessary to make an attempt at rational planning for this area, as for any other.

For a medical school the key to research facilities requirements is the number of faculty (both clinical and basic science faculty) who will be engaged in research work. Some of these faculty may require no more than their normal office space or a small individual laboratory—others may be chief investigators for a major project involving a number of research associates, fellows, graduate students, and technicians.

The first step therefore, is to determine what percentage of each group of faculty will be engaged in research and at what level. The second step is to draw the distinction between clinical research, which must be located close to patient areas, and laboratory research, which need not be.

An analysis of existing research facilities, their type, and location can be helpful in drawing a picture of current activities and space allotments. A problem here is that in the clinical areas it may be very difficult to draw a line between hospital-supported patient care facilities and research space. Very often this may have been done for fiscal purposes by prorating space used for a joint activity, and this data will give an acceptable measure of the level of clinical research.

Information about faculty and their research might be summarized thus:

Table ED-1. Summary of Research Faculty

| Departments | Number of Faculty | | | | |
| | Total | Engaged in Clinical Research | | Engaged in Laboratory Research | |
		No.	%	No.	%
Clinical Depts.	—	—	—	—	—
Basic Science Depts.	—	—	—	—	—
Totals	—	—	—	—	—

Information about the number of supporting staff (including research fellows and other graduate students) their ratio to faculty, and space assigned to research might be summarized thus:

Table ED-2. Summary of Research Staff and Space

Type of Research	No. of Faculty	No. of Support	Ratio	Total NSF Research	Area per Faculty
Clinical Research	—	—	—	—	—
Basic Science Research	—	—	—	—	—
Totals	—	—	—	—	—

In order to make projections for the future, it will be necessary to make a great many assumptions. The following planning decisions will be needed:

1. Will the total number of faculty increase, and if so by how much?
2. Will the percentage of total faculty engaged in research change?
3. Will there be a change in the balance between clinical and laboratory research?
4. Will the total amount of research or the balance among types of research change for reasons other than increases or decreases in the number of faculty?
5. Is the current ratio of supporting personnel to faculty likely to remain the same?
6. Is the current amount of space available per faculty member adequate *on the average?*

Using the same format as the tables above, future requirements as suggested by answers to these questions can be summarized.

Planning for Teaching Space

Teaching space can be divided into two main types—specialized or laboratory types space and multipurpose or classroom type space. Two kinds of use of the space can be considered—scheduled and unscheduled use. The planning of classroom type spaces is easiest, because, except for size, classrooms are essentially interchangeable and may be used by anyone. Space requirements per seat do not vary a great deal, although a bit more space will be needed per seat for seminar rooms than for lecture halls with fixed seating.

Laboratories, because they contain fixed furnishing and equipment and because their use may be limited to one discipline, require more careful planning. A laboratory station will vary in size, depending on its function, and will also require a larger area than a classroom. In addition, space must be allowed for supporting rooms that do not contain student stations at all, such as balance and instrument rooms. A teaching laboratory may be scheduled for a certain number of hours a week, but students taking a laboratory course may also require unscheduled access to the laboratory for class preparations. Thus the utilization of teaching laboratories must generally be considerably lower than is the case for classrooms.

Scheduled Space

The amount and type of space needed depends on the following factors: numbers of students, the teaching schedule, the sizes of classes, the subjects taught, and the way they are taught. An examination of teaching schedules is needed to ensure that the utilization of space is as efficient as possible—that is, that every student station is reused as often as possible, given the necessary constraints. Some definitions and an example may be helpful in discussing teaching space:

Example

Assume that 100 students take a course in gross anatomy. The course consists of 6 hours of laboratory work per week, during which time the students are divided into 4 sections of 25 students each. In addition, the course requires 1 hour a week in lecture, which all students take simultaneously; plus another 2 hours in seminars where the students again break up into groups of 25. Each student thus takes 9 weekly hours of instruction in this course.

Definitions

Weekly Student Contact Hours (WSCH).   The hours that all students spend in a class. In the example, there are 900 Weekly Student Contact Hours, broken down by space type as follows: WSCH in laboratory, 600; WSCH in lecture, 100; WSCH in Seminar, 200.

Weekly Section Hours (WSH).   The hours during which each *section* is in contact with an instructor. This gives a measure of instructors' time needed for the course. In the example there are 24 section hours in laboratories (6 hours × 4 sections); 8 section hours in seminar, and 1 section hour in lecture. To meet the requirements of the course as described in the example, a total of 33 hours of instructors' time is required per week. If the number of class sections could be reduced by increasing the sizes of sections, the demand on instructor's time would also be reduced, at least in so far as direct teaching time is concerned.

Student Station. The space required to accommodate a student, whatever the type of station may be. A station can be a place at a laboratory bench, a seat in a lecture hall, a tablet armchair in a classroom, or a chair and a portion of a table in a seminar/conference room.

In the example, the lecture hall would require a minimum of 100 student stations. The laboratory sections each require a minimum of 25 stations. The number of stations needed does not in itself define the size of the space. There could be a single large laboratory in which 4 instructors were teaching simultaneously. Or there could be only 1 laboratory for 25 students, with sections being taught successively during the week. This would be the most economical arrangement in terms of efficient utilization of facilities, since the single 25-student laboratory would be in use 24 hours a week. (However, the constraints of scheduling might be such that this arrangement would be impossible.)

Average Room Hours. The number of hours per week a room can be scheduled. This varies according to factors such as the amount of unscheduled time that must be available in that room; the constraints of faculty and student schedules (which may limit the time a particular course can be taught); and the pool of similar rooms. The average number of hours during which a room can be scheduled is generally low for specialized facilities and higher for general purpose rooms such as 30-station classrooms.

Average Station Occupancy. The percentage of stations that will be occupied during the time that the room is scheduled for use. This is considered in order to provide excess capacity to allow for the fact that enrollments in particular class sections will vary from time to time.

It is not possible to plan the amount of teaching space that will be needed without a relatively detailed study of teaching programs and schedules. Too many factors can vary from institution to institution and between one program and another. The following format for collecting data about all types of teaching programs may help to clarify the factors and the effects of different teaching modalities. In addition to the numerical data, the planner should also collect descriptions of program sequences, prerequisites, and other factors that will place constraints on scheduling.

The following type of tabulation should be done for each course that is to be taught. Care must be taken that what is counted is actually weekly *hours,* and not credits, which have a variable value. The concern here is only with time. The duration of a course and the time of year during which it is (or must be) offered should be noted.

Space Type	Enroll-ment	Section Size	No. of Sections	Weekly Course Hours	Weekly Section Hours	Weekly Student Contact Hours
Laboratory	⎫	25	4	6	24	600
Lecture Hall	⎬ 100	100	1	1	1	100
Classroom or						
seminar	⎭	25	4	2	8	200
Totals	100	—	—	9	33	900

These course tabulations may be summarized by space type, grouping together only those course sections that can share facilities.

The number of student stations needed for each category of space can now be calculated. Assumptions must be made with regard to average room hours and station utilization, defined earlier. General planning standards for colleges and universities suggest that there may be common utilization rates for laboratories and classrooms, and they are used in the examples which follow. However, teaching at a hospital or in a medical school follows unique patterns, and it is not safe to assume that such general guidelines apply. The utilization rates can only be tailored to the institution by studying the curriculum and teaching patterns individually.

The formula used for general planning of teaching space is as follows:

1. average room hours $\times$ percentage station occupancy = utilization rate.
2. $\dfrac{\text{total weekly students contact hours per space type}}{\text{utilization rate}}$ = number of stations needed.
3. number of stations needed $\times$ planning allowance per station = area needed.

Example

Assume that in addition to the gross anatomy course used earlier as an example, physiology and pharmacology can be taught in the same type of laboratory. Assume that an average station utilization rate of 80% is judged to be reasonable and that a reasonable expectation for average room hours is 18 per week; that is, out of a possible 40 hours it will be possible to schedule the laboratories for 45% of the time and during that time the expectation is that 80% of the stations will be used.

Anatomy generates a total of 600 weekly student contact hours. Assume that the other two courses each require an equivalent amount of laboratory time. The total weekly student contact hours is thus 1800. Following the formula, the arithmetic works like this:

1. 18 weekly room hours $\times$ .80 station occupancy = 14.4 utilization rate.

2. $\dfrac{1800 \text{ weekly student contact hours}}{14.4 \text{ utilization rate}} = 125$ laboratory stations needed.

3. 125 laboratory stations @ 80 net square feet per station (services included) = 10,000 net square feet.

Note that the validity of this method is entirely dependent on the ability to schedule flexibly. If each of these courses required a separate type of laboratory and no shared use were possible, the space requirements would triple, thus:

1. 6 weekly room hours × .80 station occupancy rate = 4.8 utilization rate.
2. $\dfrac{1800 \text{ weekly student contact hours}}{4.8} = 375$ stations needed.
3. 375 student stations @ 80 net square feet = 30,000 net square feet.

This clearly illustrates the danger of generalizing planning guidelines of this kind. The guidelines can serve as a shortcut but should only be used when the constraints of a particular situation are known.

Classroom and lecture space can be dealt with in the same way as laboratory space—with a good deal more confidence, since the pool of similar facilities will be much greater, which helps to level out peaks and valleys in the utilization curve.

Unscheduled teaching space

Class and seminar rooms in the clinical areas should usually be considered as unscheduled space. Their scheduled use is likely to be sporadic and may only be partially predictable. An approach to quantifying requirements for this kind of space is as follows:

Collect data on all potential uses of classroom/seminar space in the hospital, including irregularly scheduled training sessions, regular rounds, conferences, and classes of all types. A format similar to that used to collect data on scheduled courses can be used. Basically what needs to be discovered is the demand for teaching space over a typical week, but to do this it will be necessary to find out what occurs throughout the year. Data should include:

- A description of the groups, including numbers of participants and the nature of their activity.
- The time of day (morning, noon, evening) at which they must or prefer to meet.
- The length of the typical session.
- The frequency of meeting.
- Location criteria.

The meetings can be divided into groups according to size—those requiring conference space for 10 to 15, those requiring classrooms of up to 30, and lecture-sized groups. Within these groups, the number of weekly hours can be added up separately by time of day. This will provide a factual base from which a reasonable estimate of requirements can be built in discussion with interested departments and groups.

The educational component of hospital activities, whether the hospital is directly connected to a medical or nursing school or not, will require a number of supporting facilities beyond research and teaching space.

Even if there is a main library, some departments may require their own libraries and study facilities; or the hospital may contain one or more satellite libraries for reference works. Residents, interns, medical and nursing students, as well as certain others, will require offices or study cubicles. Media equipped carrels for self-instruction may be needed either in a central location or in locations scattered throughout the hospital. Offices will be needed for administrators and faculty and their supporting staff. Students may require housing, union, and recreational facilities: They will certainly add to the volume of cafeteria meals served.

The process of education and training adds immeasurably to the complexity of a hospital's operation. We have hardly skimmed the surface here—to do more would require a book in itself. We can only warn the planner that the educational component should be considered in exploring every hospital function and activity.

10

Planning Guidelines

10.1. GENERAL PRINCIPLES

It has been the intention of the authors of this book to avoid philosophizing about hospital design. However, this last chapter will indulge in stating some general principles of planning that apply to any complex building and particularly to medical facilities. It is hoped that these principles may at least provide some guidance to architects inexperienced in hospital design and to others who have responsibility for judging the effectiveness of a design solution.

Perhaps the most important current principle is to anticipate change. Yet providing for change becomes increasingly difficult because of the demand for specialized design to suit specific unique occupancies and the multiplication of mechanical services. Such demands suggest consideration of new solutions. When the cost of mechanical and electrical systems becomes a large proportion of the total building cost, it is not difficult to justify greater consideration of space requirements for such systems in order to simplify the problems of installation, maintenance, and alteration. In addition, since most functions in buildings take place on horizontal planes, if flexibility of usage is desired, it is reasonable to eliminate as many fixed vertical elements as possible. An analogy might be removing trees to cultivate land. In a building this would mean reducing the number of columns, consolidating mechanical shafts, and keeping elevator shafts, stairs, and other vertical circulation from dividing floor space into small compartments. All of these elements once built are practically impossible to move and, therefore, inhibit change.

The second principle, which relates to the first, is to provide for growth without destruction of established values. The most desirable way to do this is to plan each department with a corridor leading to an outside wall so that it can be extended when necessary. Care should be taken

222

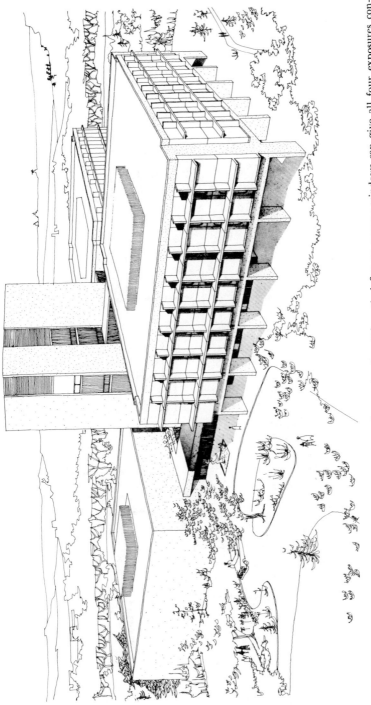

Figure 10. Turning a building 45° to the compass points and using 45° vertical fins on narrow windows can give all four exposures controlled energy-saving north-south light (Woodland Community Hospital, Woodland, CA.; The Rex Allen Partnership, Architects).

223

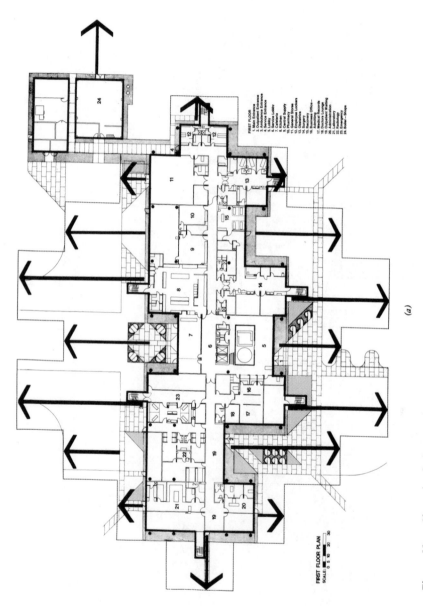

Figure 11a. Clear circulation arteries and departments extending to outside walls permit easy expansion without disruption of service (Madera Community Hospital, Madera, CA.; The Rex Allen Partnership, Architects).

(a)

FIRST FLOOR PLAN
SCALE IN FEET
0 5 10 20 30

FIRST FLOOR
1. Main Entrance
2. Outpatient Entrance
3. Ambulance Entrance
4. Service Entrance
5. Lobby
6. Service Lobby
7. Cafeteria
8. Kitchen
9. Central Supply
10. Pharmacy
11. General Stores
12. Employee Lockers
13. Obstetrics
14. Surgery
15. Recovery
16. Business Office—
17. Medical Records
18. Doctors Lounge
19. Outpatient Waiting
20. Administration
21. Laboratory
22. Radiology
23. Emergency
24. Boiler—Shops

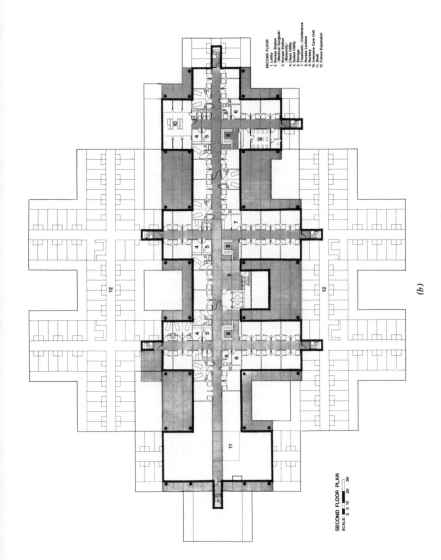

SECOND FLOOR
1. Lobby
2. Nurses Station
   (Medical-Surgical)
3. Nurses Station
   (Maternity)
4. Clean Utility
5. Soiled Utility
6. Storage
7. Treatment—Conference
8. Nurses Lockers
9. Nursery
10. Intensive Care Unit
11. Shell
12. Future Expansion

SECOND FLOOR PLAN
SCALE: 0 5 10 20 30

(b)

Figure 1lb. The add-on nursing unit is one approach to expansion that avoids the disruptions of vertical expansion (Madera Community Hospital, Madera, CA.; The Rex Allen Partnership, Architects).

225

to avoid blocking any such corridors with stairs or other fixed elements. Where such planning is impractical as, for instance, in small departments, soft space, that is space with minimal mechanical services such as office space or storage, should be planned adjacent to hard space. The soft space can be relocated relatively easily and will thus permit the required expansion.

A third principle is to develop circulation and utility arteries. Main circulation and utility distribution systems in a hospital are similar to those of a small city with the added complication that they should be conceived in three dimensions. Generally, maintaining a rectilinear pattern will provide the greatest amount of flexibility. Also, if they are consolidated, they will provide the greatest amount of free usable space.

A fourth principle is to separate, insofar as possible, the various kinds of traffic, pedestrian from vehicular and patient, staff, visitor, and service from each other. In a teaching institution, student and faculty should also be given special consideration. On the other hand, attempts to separate clean from soiled may be less justified. Maintaining an aseptic environment is of course essential, but traffic separation for clean and soiled can create both a false sense of security and some undesirable effects. For instance, operating rooms with two doors, one to a sterile area and one to a nonsterile corridor, tend to become passageways that introduce into the operating room traffic that has no business there, thus defeating the concept of sterility. Such architectural solutions tend to create a false sense of security that may result in a relaxation of administrative controls and also reduce flexibility of use.

A fifth principle is development of modular spaces, again to provide maximum flexibility. Room sizes are seldom so critical that a variation of 10 to 20% will make any difference in their usefulness. If a module can be developed that is acceptable for a large variety of occupancies, changes in use will require minimum alteration. With few exceptions, for instance, offices and examining rooms in an outpatient suite can be the same size. It may even be advantageous to rough-in plumbing in the offices so that they are easily converted to examining rooms should there be a change in program.

A final principle, particularly with the renewed interest in energy conservation, is to give careful consideration to orientation, sun control, and the materials used for the building envelope. The development of airconditioning and high levels of artificial illumination have had a significant effect on hospital planning. Dependence on natural light and air imposed limits on the width of buildings. When this was no longer necessary plans became more compact, both to reduce walking distances

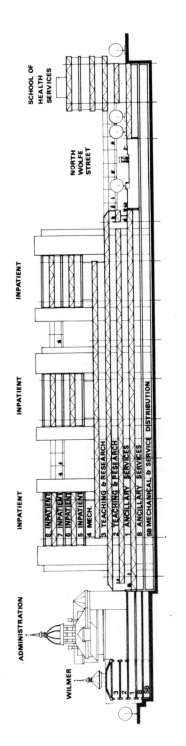
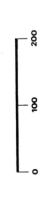

Figure 12. Separation of traffic—student/faculty, public/outpatient and service—is frequently accomplished by assignment of levels (Master Plan for Johns Hopkins Medical Institutions, Baltimore, Md.; Hugh Stubbins/Rex Allen Partnership, Architects).

227

and to expose less surface for heat loss or gain. However, the increasing reliance on an artificial environment also resulted in a growing disregard for the efficiency of the envelope. Although it is not suggested that there be a return to former planning concepts, it is recommended that there be a renewed concern for orientation, sun control, and the selection of exterior wall materials. In the temperate climates of the northern hemisphere, a north-south orientation generally provides the best opportunity for sun control. Using horizontal overhangs it is possible to shield glass areas from the high summer sun yet let in the low winter sun. By introducing saw-tooth windows or shielding fins similar results can be obtained with other orientations. In hot and humid climates a light-weight exterior material will give off latent heat quickly so that it does not continue to radiate heat at night. On the other hand,

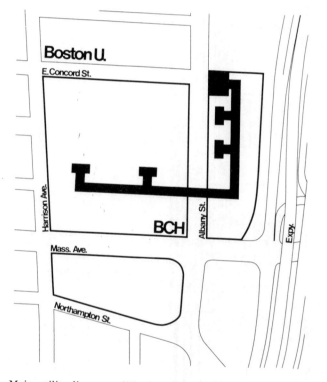

Figure 13. Main utility lines are difficult to move and, therefore, become fixed site elements that require careful consideration in the initial development of site plans (Boston City Hospital, Boston, Mass.; Hugh Stubbins/Rex Allen Partnership, Architects).

in hot dry climates, where days are generally hot and nights cool, thick walls will absorb the heat during the day and radiate the heat at night, and relatively small openings will reduce the glare.

10.2. SITE PLANNING

Many of the above principles will apply equally to site planning, particularly the development of circulation and utility arteries, and to the separation of different kinds of traffic. In addition, careful consideration must be given to site access for the public and staff and for service and emergency vehicles. A study of traffic density in the immediate vicinity may indicate problems and should influence the location of entrances. Screening of ambulance and service entrances (including morgue) from patient areas is desirable. Ambulances should not be required to pass

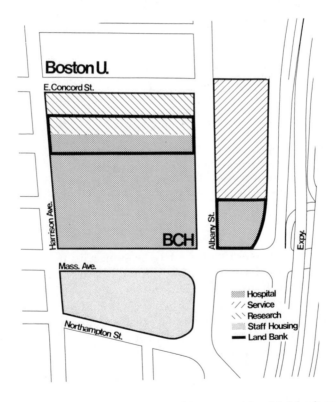

Figure 14. Site zoning to designate appropriate usage and a land bank provided it necessary by the demolition of obsolete structures will assure orderly development (Boston City Hospital, Boston, Mass.; Hugh Stubbins/Rex Allen Partnership, Architects).

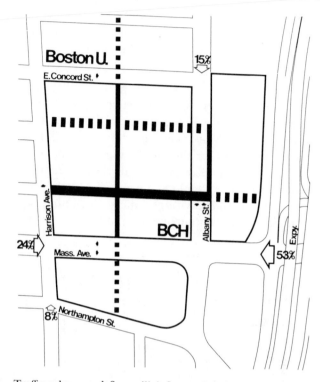

Figure 15. Traffic volume and flow will influence location of access for visitors, staff, emergency vehicles, and service; careful consideration should also be given to the establishment of principal internal circulation arteries that also tend to become fixed site elements (Boston City Hospital, Boston, Mass.; Hugh Stubbins/Rex Allen Partnership, Architects).

through parking areas where they may be subject to delay, and in wet climates they should have undercover approaches to the hospital.

For future growth any institution should have a land bank, an open area on which a future building or wing could be built without disruption of ongoing services. To maintain such a land bank it is essential that outmoded or obsolete buildings be demolished upon the completion of their replacements. If they are not and if they are simply converted to other occupancies, there will be no way of demolishing them in the future without disruption of service unless additional land is available or can be acquired.

A final principle to promote orderly site development is site zoning. Although particularly important for large teaching institutions where areas should be set aside for hospital, research functions, schools, housing, and so forth, even a small community institution should give careful consideration to site development to reserve land for such related functions as medical office buildings, extended care or skilled nursing, primary care, mental health, child care, or other health related facilities.

10.3. PLANNING FOR PARKING

Much of the data needed to determine parking requirements will be collected in the course of traffic studies necessary for general site planning. It will be necessary to determine broadly the number and characteristics of the several components of the hospital population including:

- How many persons, by categories, will be at the hospital during the peak daytime hours?
- How many within each category, can be expected to be using their own cars and will thus require parking space?
- Which of these groups will be at the hospital for less than a full day?

To do this, a survey may be taken of hospital employees, physicians, patients, and visitors as to the means of transportation they use. Hospital employee data may also be analyzed by the employee zip code or other geographical identifier and correlated with public tranportation maps to determine the likelihood of the employee's use of public versus private transportation. Surveys will still have to be made of physician and visitor traffic, however.

The issues surrounding the question of parking have become complex, and directions uncertain. Not very long ago it seemed clear that the directions being taken by municipalities was to require adequate parking to be built for the occupants of every new building. Environmental issues have recently turned this around, and the trend now is strictly to limit or even reduce the amount of parking that is allowed. Such strictures are often in critical conflict with reality: public transportation in most areas of the country is simply not adequate to replace the automobile at present, and in many areas populations are too scattered to allow car pooling to provide an adequate solution. Given this level of uncertainty about directions of public policy, it is hard to be sure that any parking plan drawn up today can be accomplished tomorrow. It is, however, possible to document the need as currently perceived and to use these data as a bases for discussion and negotiation with government authorities.

Institutional Parking Policy

The means by which parking places are assigned and controlled is an important part of initial planning. If the intention is to discourage parking, for example, will daily or monthly fees be charged to employees? Will these fees be set high in order to make the use of public transportation or car pooling more attractive? Are separate parking areas to be planned for different groups? This may serve to ensure that certain groups can be certain of finding a place but may also increase the vacancy rate and thus prove more expensive. Is the cost of parking to be absorbed or subsidized by the hospital, is the parking facility to be self-amortizing, or may it, perhaps, be contracted out to a private builder/operator? The last approach may be attractive in some ways, since the sensitive question of parking fees becomes somebody else's problem. However, the hospital does, in such a case, lose a degree of control, and this may create other kinds of problems.

Estimating the Need for Parking

Information needed

1. The number of hospital personnel by shift, with an estimate of how many in each shift (or day shift only, since this is the busiest time) arrive by car.

2. The numbers of attending and other physicians and an estimate of how many are present on a typical day, separately for mornings and afternoons.

3. The numbers of outpatients arriving by car separately for mornings and afternoons.

4. The numbers of visitors arriving by car, separately for mornings, afternoons and evenings. If visiting hours are restricted to after the day shift ends, parking requirements can be minimized.

5. An estimate of others visiting the hospital during the course of the day, including visitors to administrative and operational areas of the hospital.

Example

Assume that the several populations are distributed as follows and behave in the following ways:

- There are 900 hospital employees on the day shift, of whom 60% use their own cars and require parking space all day. (A detailed analysis might show that the absentee rate is sufficiently regular and large to reduce this number.)
- On the average, 150 physicians visit their patients per day—perhaps 120, or

about 80%, in the mornings and only about 20%, or 30, in the afternoons.
- On the average there is 1 visit for every 3 patients per day, occurring with only rare exceptions in the afternoon or evening hours. 90% of visitors arrive by car. Since the employee population drops sharply in the evening, only the afternoon visits are significant for the parking analysis. The afternoon visits amount to approximately 30% of the total. (Note that *visits* are counted in this instance, rather than visitors: Groups of two or three friends and relatives are most likely to arrive in a car as a group, rather than individually.)
- During a typical day, there are 80 clinic visits, divided fairly evenly between morning and afternoon hours. Presuming an 8-hour day and an average of 2 hours per visit, about a quarter of the patients will be at the hospital at any one time. A survey has indicated that only about 30% of these patients arrive by car.
- The emergency room has an average peak load (exclusive of patients arriving by ambulance) of 10 patients during the busy early evening hours, and as a matter of policy the hospital has decided that space must be reserved for this entire number, since a very high proportion arrive by cars driven by friends or relatives who will remain with the patient until he is released or admitted.
- Additional staff and other visitors account for an additional 30 places, according to the hospital's best estimates.

These data and estimates of parking place need can be summarized and tabulated as illustrated in the table on the next page.

The total tabulated represents the total requirements on hospital lots. There may be parking required in peripheral areas for specialized functions directly or indirectly related to hospital use. If there are residents, interns, and nurses quarters, for example, these may require their own parking facility. The number may usually be deducted from the total requirements, if distances are not great. Ancillary activities related to the hospital, such as research facilities, extended care units, and doctors office buildings will require a similar but separate analysis. Care should be taken to ensure that people engaged in activities in two separate facilities are not counted twice: A doctor engaged in research as well as being on the hospital staff needs only one parking place as long as the facilities are not at any great distance from each other.

Distribution of Facilities

The location of parking places can have a great impact on *internal* hospital circulation. People always seek out the shortest route, and no number of signs indicating where the outpatient entry is will force people to use that entry if there is an entry closer to where they have left their cars.

Average Daily Hospital Parking Requirements

Category	Total Numbers	Percent Requiring Parking	Maximum Day Shift (7a–3p)		Maximum Overlap (2:30p–3:30p)		Maximum Evening (3p–11p)	
			Percent	No.	Percent	No.	Percent	No.
Hospital Employees	1500	60	60	540	85	765	25	225
Visiting Physicians	150	100	80	120	50	75	20	30
Inpatient Visitors	135	90	30	37	30	37	70	85
Clinic Patients	80	30	25	6	25	6	25	6
Emergency	10	100	—	10[a]	—	10[a]	100	10
Other Hospital Visitors	30	100	20	6	20	6	20	6
Totals	1830	—	—	719	—	899	—	362

[a] Reserved parking

It seems self-evident but is sometimes forgotten that patients to clinics and to emergency rooms are often old and infirm, that they may require assistance in walking, and that parking spaces for these people should be as close as possible to the entrance they must use. Obstetric patients should also be provided drive-up and parking space close to the entrance. Healthy staff members and visitors can be asked to walk some distance from their cars. Physicians should be assured space by designating a specific area and perhaps restricting its use by a card-operated gate. With these exceptions, where a special need exists for immediate access, the use of parking space will be most effective when consolidated to the maximum.

Selected Bibliography

American Association of Hospital Consultants, *Functional Plannnig of General Hospitals*. New York: McGraw Hill, 1969.

American College of Surgeons, *Guidelines for the Design and Function of a Hospital Emergency Department*. Chicago: The College, 1970.

American Hospital Association, *AHA Guide to the Health Care Field*. Chicago: 1972 73.

American Hospital Association, *Food Services Manual for Health Care Institutions*. Chicago, 1972.

American Hospital Association, *Medical Records Departments in Hospitals*. Chicago, 1972.

American Hospital Association, *The Practice of Planning*. Chicago, 1973.

American Hospital Association, *Outpatient Hospital Care: A Complete Report*. Chicago, 1969.

American Hospital Association, *Rehabilitation Services in Hospitals*. Chicago, 1966.

Barnoon, Shlomo and Harvey Wolfe, *Scheduling A Multiple Operating Room System*. Health Services Research, Winter, 1968.

Bekey, George A. and Morton D. Schwartz, Eds., *Hospital Information Systems*. New York, 1972.

Bell, George H., *Hospitals and Medical School Design—International Symposium, Dundee*. Edinburgh: Livingstone, 1962.

Carner, Donald C., *Planning for Hospital Expansion and Remodeling*. Springfield, Ill.: Charles C. Thomas, 1968.

Clark, Virginia V., Ed., *Outpatient Services Journal Articles*. A collection. Flushing, N.Y.: Medical Examination Publishing, 1973.

Clibbon, Sheila and Marin L. Sachs, "Approaches to the Design of Health Care Facilities." *Health Services Research,* Fall 1970.

Collins, F. T., *Network Planning and Critical Path Scheduling*. Berkeley: Know How Publications, 1964.

DeBoer, John C., *Let's Plan*. Philadelphia: Pilgrim, 1970.

Douglas, Donald M., *Surgical Departments in Hospitals—The Surgeon's View*. London: Butterworth, 1972.

Drucker, Paul, *The Effective Executive*. New York: Grove, 1964.

Field, Herman, et al, *Evaluation of Hospital Design—A Holistic Approach*. Boston: Tufts New England Medical Center / USPH, 1971.

Francke, D. E. et al, *Mirror to Hospital Pharmacy*. Washington: American Society of Hospital Pharmacists, 1964.

Freeborn, Donald K., et al, Eds., "Determinants of Medical Care Utilization: The Physician's Use of Laboratory Services." *American Journal of Public Health,* 62:6, June, 1972.

Garrett, Raymond D., *Hospitals—A Systems Approach.* Philadelphia: Auerbach, 1973.

Gabrielson, I. W., et al, "Relating Health and Census Information for Health Planning." *American Journal of Public Health,* 59:7, July, 1969.

Ginzberg, Eli and Alice M. Yohalem, *The University Medical Center and the Metropolis.* Baltimore: Port City Press, 1974.

Glasscote, Raymond W., et al, *General Hospital Psychiatric Units—A National Survey.* Washington: Joint Information Service of the American Psychiatric Association and The National Mental Health Association, 1965.

Great Britain Department of Health and Social Security, *Hospital Building Notes.* London: A Continuing Series.

Hallan, Jerome B., et al, "Estimation of a Potential Hemodialysis Population." *Medical Care,* 8:3, May–June, 1970.

Hassan, William E., *Hospital Pharmacy.* Philadelphia: Lea and Febiger, 1965.

Henning, Dale A. and Preston P. LeBreton, *Henning-LeBreton Planning Theory.* New York: Prentice Hall, 1961.

Hudenberg, Roy, *Planning the Community Hospital.* New York: McGraw Hill, 1967.

Lindheim, Roslyn, *Changing Hospital Environments for Children.* Cambridge: Harvard University Press, 1972.

Lindheim, *Uncoupling the Radiology System.* Chicago: Hospital Research and Educational Trust, 1971.

Luce, R. D. and Raiffa, *Games and Decisions.* New York: John Wiley, 1957.

Mitchell, J. H., *A New Look at Hospital Case Records.* London: H. K. Lewis, 1969.

Nuffield Provicial Hospitals Trust, *A Balanced Teaching Hospital—A Symposium at Birmingham.* London: Oxford University Press, 1965.

Nuffield, *Studies in the Functions and Designs of Hospitals.* London: Oxford University Press, 1955.

Nuffield, *Towards a Clearer View—Organization of a Diagnostic X-ray Department.* London: Oxford University Press, 1962.

Nuffield Foundation: Division for Architectural Studies, *Research Laboratories.* London: Oxford University Press, 1961.

Nuffield, *Children in Hospitals.* London: Oxford University Press, 1963.

Owen, Joseph Karlton, Editor, *Modern Concepts of Hospital Administration.* Philadelphia, Pa.: W. B. Saunders Co., 1962.

Piore, Nora, et al, *A Statistical Profile of Hospital Outpatient Services in the United States.* New York: Association for the Aid of Crippled Children, 1971.

Pütsep, Ervin, *Planning of Surgical Centres.* London: Lloyd–Luke 1973.

Reinke, W. A. and Cathleen Williams. *Health Planning—Qualitative Aspects and Quantitative Techniques.* Baltimore: Johns Hopkins, 1972.

Rosenfield, Isadore, *Hospitals—Integrated Design.* New York: Reinhold, 1947.

Rosenfield, Isadore and Zachary Rosenfield, *Hospital Architecture and Beyond.* New York: Van Nos Reinhold, 1969.

Rosenfield, Isadore and Zachary, *Hospital Architecture: Integrated Components.* New York: Van Nos Reinhold, 1971.

Savage, L. J., *The Foundations of Statistics.* New York, 1954.

Scott, W. G., Ed., *Planning Guide for Radiological Installations.* Baltimore: Williams and Wilkens, 1966.

Shaffer, L. R., J. B. Ritter and W. L. Meyer, *The Critical Path Method.* New York: McGraw Hill Co., Inc., 1965.

Simmons, David A., *Medical and Hospital Control Systems.* Boston: Little Brown, 1972.

Smalley, H. E. and Freeman, J. R., *Hospital Industrial Engineering.* New York: Reinhold, 1966.

Smith, Warwick, *Planning the Surgical Suite.* New York: F. W. Dodge, 1960.

Spoerel, W. E. "Planning of Anesthetic Facilities." *Canadian Anesthesia Society Journal,* Vol. 16:1, January, 1969.

Souder, James J., Welden E. Clark, Jerome I. Elkind, and Madison B. Brown, *Planning for Hospitals.* Chicago: American Hospital Association, 1964.

Walter, Carl W., "Ventilation and Air Conditioning as Bacteriological Engineering." *Anesthesiology.* August 1969 (Vol. 31:2).

Wheeler, E. Todd, *Hospital Modernization and Expansion.* New York: McGraw Hill, 1971.

Wheeler, E. Todd, *Hospital Design and Function.* New York: McGraw Hill, 1964.

World Health Organization and International Atomic Energy Agency Joint Expert Committee, *Medical Uses of Ionizing Radiation and Radioisotopes.* WHO Reports 492, 1972.

Additional sources of information in planning for health services:

U.S. Department of Commerce: Bureau of the Census. *Directory of Non-Federal Statistics for State and Local Areas: A Guide to Sources:* 1969.

U.S. Department of Commerce: *Directory of Federal Statistics for Local Areas: A Guide to Sources:* 1966.

U.S. Department of Health, Education and Welfare: U.S. Public Health Service, *Comprehensive Health Planning: A Selected Annotated Bibliography.* PHS Pub 1753, 1968.

U.S. Department of Health, Education and Welfare: U.S. Public Health Service, *Annotated Bibliography on Vital and Health Statistics.* PHS Pub. No. 2094, Bibliography Series 82, 1970.

U.S. Department of Health, Education and Welfare: U.S. Public Health Service, *Health Statistics for Comprehensive Health Planning and Evaluation.* Vital and Health Statistics Series # 1000, 1970.

U.S. Department of Health, Education and Welfare: U.S. Public Health Service, Division of Hospital and Medical Facilities, *Procedures for Areawide Health Facility Planning—A Guide for Planning Agencies.* (Pub. No. 930-B-3). Washington, D.C., 1963.

Index

Reengineering Health Care

Building on CQI

John R. Griffith
Vinod K. Sahney
Ruth A. Mohr

Health Administration Press
Ann Arbor, Michigan   1995

99   98   97   96   95   5   4   3   2   1

Library of Congress Cataloging-in-Publication Data

Griffith, John R.
   Reengineering health care : building on CQI / John R. Griffith, Vinod K. Sahney, Ruth A. Mohr.
        p.   cm.
   Includes index.
   ISBN 1-56793-022-0 (hardbound : alk. paper)
   1. Health care facilities—United States—Administration. 2. Health services administration—United States. 3. Total quality management—United States. 4. Organizational change—United States—Case studies. 5. Health facilities—United States—Administration—Case studies. 6. Health services administration—United States—Case studies. 7. Total quality management—United States—Case studies.   I. Sahney, Vinod K.   II. Mohr, Ruth A.   III. Title.
   [DNLM: 1. Delivery of Health Care—organization & administration—United States. 2. Total Quality Management.   W 84 G816r AA1 1995]
   RA971.G755   1995   362.1'068'5—dc20   94-42697 CIP

The paper used in this publication meets the minimum requirements of American National Standard for Information Sciences—Permanence of Paper for Printed Library Materials, ANSI Z39.48-1984.   ∞TM

Health Administration Press
A division of the Foundation of the
   American College of Healthcare Executives
1021 East Huron Street
Ann Arbor, Michigan 48104
(313) 764-1380

Contents

List of Figures

Preface

This book tracks the implementation of Continuous Quality Improvement (CQI) in three leading health care organizations. Two of them, Henry Ford Health System of Michigan and Intermountain Health Care of Utah, are large integrated health care systems. The third, a smaller organization operating as a traditional hospital in a large southern metropolis, has chosen to be presented anonymously to protect against demands on its time.

All three organizations made an early commitment to CQI. As we observed them, their implementation of CQI concepts was successful, fulfilling many Baldrige Award criteria. They focused on management and physician education, customer mindedness, and process improvement. CQI gave them new energy, new ideas, a sense of employee involvement, and the motivation to identify and correct their weaknesses. Both Intermountain and Henry Ford made the investment of senior management time and resources needed to change the culture of these large and geographically dispersed institutions.

But interviews with more than 50 leaders within these dynamic organizations over a period of more than two years persuaded us that CQI, by itself, is not a sufficient response to the growing pressures in the marketplace for health care delivery reform. Additional measures are necessary to accomplish reengineering a health care delivery organization into the kind of customer-focused, low-cost provider demanded by a highly competitive environment. Powerful as it is as a concept and an implementation tool, CQI is not a replacement for sound strategy, effective financial planning, robust decision-making processes, information systems, and leadership. CQI may be the best way to begin reengineering; it is not enough to complete the process.

In comparison with the past, today's health care executives have less time to respond to market pressures for reforming health care organizations. We have written this book to share with readers the core skills they will need to begin the transformation of health care providers to lean, customer-focused, competitive organizations.

John R. Griffith
Vinod K. Sahney
Ruth A. Mohr

Acknowledgments

My coauthors join me in recognizing the real heroes of this book, the staff of the three systems we studied. Our roles were reportorial. They invented new methods, implemented them, and went beyond CQI to meet the challenges of the day. On top of that, they gave generously of their time that we might record the results.

Most of the figures are the work of case study institutions, invented by them to convey ideas important in continuous improvement and generated on commonly available spreadsheet and word processing software. We left them as they were to show what can be done.

I would like to extend a special thanks to Brent James, M.D., of Intermountain. His dedication to finding better ways, his commitment to principle, and his generosity in sharing his wisdom with others is exceptional.

I would also like to thank Kathy Sodt, my secretary, for her assistance with the manuscript. Even in this automated age, a book is a great deal of hard work, and her contribution made an enormous difference.

John R. Griffith

I am indebted to many colleagues for helping shape the ideas in this book. I have been fortunate to work with three giants in the health care industry, Edward Connors, Stanley Nelson, and Gail Warden. Each of these three individuals has held the CEO position in leading health care institutions and has served as Chairman of the American Hospital Association. Each has taught me much about management and leadership. My special thanks to Gail Warden, President and CEO of Henry Ford Health System, who in 1988 gave me the opportunity to lead the implementation of CQI at Henry Ford Health System.

Much of my thinking on CQI and learning organizations has been shaped by interactions with colleagues at the Institute for Healthcare Improvement (IHI), Quality Management Network (QMN), and the Group Practice Improvement Network (GPIN). I am especially indebted to Donald Berwick, M.D., and Paul Batalden, M.D., for their insights into CQI and intrinsic motivation.

I also wish to acknowledge my colleagues at Henry Ford Health System who read and commented on early drafts of the chapters. They include: Beth Anctil, James Blazar, Darlene Burgess, Peter Butler, William Conway, Jr., M.D., Annette DeLorenzo, Deborah Ebers, David Ellis, Kristen Gause, Tom McNulty, David Nerenz, Thomas Royer, M.D., William Schramm, Mark Stensager, James Walworth, and Anita Watson. My special thanks to Patricia Stoltz and Richard Wittrup, with whom I have had multiple discussions on CQI and who have helped shape my thinking. My thanks to Lynn Bonner and Brenda Carroll for typing and retyping the manuscript.

Finally, I wish to thank my wife, Gail, and my children, Mira and Vikram, for their constant encouragement and support on this project.

Vinod K. Sahney

1

Surviving the Revolution in Health Care Delivery

What Is This Book About?

Three Leaders and Their Progress

This book is a report and commentary on what three organizations with reputations for leadership are doing to meet the challenges of the health care field. Two of them are large, somewhat sprawling health care systems— Henry Ford Health System, of Detroit, and Intermountain Health Care, of Utah. The third is a smaller unit of a for-profit chain—Walke-Parker Medical Center, of Southern City. The objective record on these institutions supports their reputations: Their profit margins are solid, their market share is stable or growing, and they are developing new lines of business that look promising for the markets ahead. Intermountain Health Care was awarded the Healthcare Forum Witt Quality Award, and Henry Ford Health System received the 3M-Healthcare Forum Visionary Leadership Award.

In addition to leadership, we also tried deliberately for diversity. We wanted different sizes, geography, economics, and medical staff organization. Walke-Parker and Henry Ford Health System serve urban markets; Intermountain Health Care also serves a vast rural area. Henry Ford Health System and Intermountain Health Care are more advanced toward the managed care economic environment; Walke-Parker is just beginning the change. Walke-Parker and Intermountain Health Care have started from the prevailing U.S. pattern of independent medical staffs; Henry Ford Health System historically relied on a large employed group.

The case studies should not be considered "finished," and certainly not "final." None of the institutions themselves would accept such a designation, either in public or within their own walls. Rather, they are leading the way. Their achievements are worthy of study, though not of unthinking emulation. We have no way of knowing how many other institutions are leaders, or what we and these organizations might have missed. And, if you visit these organizations tomorrow, you will see things we did not see in 1993.

Organizations Advance by Integrating Technology

Organizations exist only because they facilitate transactions between people with different skills and needs, and they get bigger and better because they incorporate managerial technology of various kinds that allows them to facilitate more and better transactions.[1] The thesis of this book is:

Health care organizations will survive by reengineering—that is, by designing and implementing new ways of delivering care to meet changing customer demands. Critical management tasks supporting reengineering include the following:

- Providing professional leadership skills at all executive and management levels
- Helping physicians and other clinical personnel redesign care processes to improve cost and quality
- Developing effective and participative processes for all kinds of decisions
- Expanding information services to make them tools for clinical, managerial, and strategic problems
- "Walking the talk"—making continuous quality improvement (CQI) routine at all levels

Not accidentally, this list parallels the outline of the Malcolm Baldrige National Quality Award application, a detailed analysis of a company's commitment to quality. Health care organizations will be eligible for the award in 1996.

We expand these concepts in the next four chapters and in three detailed case studies. First, the four areas for reengineering that are management's unique responsibility are discussed. Chapter 2 identifies the steps managers and executives should take to fill the leader role; it breaks the global job of leadership down to seven functions and suggests specific steps for each. Chapter 3 emphasizes the critical contributions that doctors and other providers must make for an organization to become truly customer-focused; it describes how the case study institutions are helping their clinicians increase the quality of clinical processes and lower their cost. Chapter 4 shows how strategic decision processes like visioning and financial planning can be truly participative, and how operating decisions can be made responsive to strategic needs; it urges the deliberate dissemination of information and suggests a system of "accountable delegation" of specific decisions. Chapter 5 describes how the case study sites are using information services as a strategic weapon; it outlines the kind of data they are seeking, how they support decision-making teams, and how they are continuously improving their information capability.

Second, each of the three organizations are described, emphasizing CQI. Their environments, the origins of their CQI programs, the rollout of CQI principles to the workforce, and some of their unique achievements are discussed. There is a focus to the description of each case. For Henry Ford Health System (HFHS), the largest of the case sites, it is the decision processes, particularly the way HFHS uses them to build cohesion across many sites. HFHS's financial environment is in transition from traditional fee-for-service to cost-controlled and capitated. The history of CQI at HFHS illustrates how it integrates various performance measures, and how it balances local and central organizational issues. For Walke-Parker, it is an unusually thorough, well-coordinated measurement system, practical even in small institutions, that increasingly guides decisions, from the most detailed operations to major strategic questions. For Intermountain Health Care, the case focus is the extensive effort to understand and change the actual delivery of care, even in a market that remains mostly independent physician practitioners.

Is Health Care in a State of Evolution or Revolution?

Why the Answer is "Revolution"

Health care is in a revolution that involves the most basic beliefs of the people—patients, providers, and payers; it's a rapidly moving revolution that will create radical and permanent changes in the health care system.

It is not unparalleled. History shows at least two similar periods: around 1890, driven by anesthesia and aseptic surgery, and around 1950, driven by antibiotics and laboratory-based diagnosis. In those cases, changes in care technology drove social expectations and management technology.[2] The providers led; the customers followed. The revolution around 2000 is unique: social expectations will drive the care technology and the management technology. The customers will lead; the providers will follow.

Patients now want a say in their treatment, in areas ranging from acceptable waiting times to the selection of treatment itself. Payers now demand limits to health care expenditures, insisting that cost control is essential to our common economic survival. Both patients and payers are seeking "appropriate outcomes," rather than "appropriate care." The outcomes focus has already changed many assumptions about "good medicine." High-tech care is no longer viewed as an unmixed blessing. Prevention has been elevated to new importance. Integrated service to patients is becoming as important as excellence in a specialty or subspecialty.

The outcomes focus is slowly changing much of the workday. Teams and team participation are more important. The "lone cowboy" professional (and the solo practitioner) is a dying breed. The specialists—both physicians and clinical professionals like physical therapists—are no longer given unlimited authority. Care guidelines (also called "care plans," "critical paths," or "care protocols"—we will not make distinctions between these labels) will soon be routine for most referral care. Primary care doctors will not refer as quickly, and they will want a say in the care plans when they do. Their insistence, backed by the federal physician payment reform, will invert the pecking order of medicine. You can already see them taking the driver's seat and somewhat tentatively cracking the whip, particularly in the burgeoning health maintenance organizations (HMOs). Even the fee-for-service indemnity companies are using many of the same concepts, creating a concept of "managed indemnity."

These changes will affect every provider in health care. Radical shifts in demand are occurring, creating severe shortages in primary care and hidden surpluses of high-paid specialists. Care is moving to less expensive, less elaborate sites. Nursing is dividing into two very different professions—high-tech inpatient care and high-touch primary care. The authority, income, and work habits of several dozen other health care professions are changing. Young providers are approaching their work with radically different goals and attitudes from the post-war generations.

The traditional organization of community health care—the inpatient hospital plus independent physicians—is being replaced by a health care organization that integrates rather than separates the management of physicians, clinical professionals, and physical facilities. The new organization accepts episode payment (going at risk for a complete intervention) and capitation payment (going at risk for the patient's overall health). It will soon have more risk-sharing revenue than fee-for-service, and more outpatient revenue than inpatient. Because of its risk sharing, it will reward team performance more than individual excellence. It will delegate authority quickly and fully to teams who demonstrate success on outcomes and cost. Professional recruitment, credentialling, training, and motivation will be more important than beds, clinics, and high-tech facilities.

The Management Implications of Revolution

All institutions that deliver health care must adapt to these changes to survive. Most have already started; some seem to be in the lead. There are four major, interlocking tasks that successful institutions must accomplish. Accomplishing these tasks will require new approaches to traditional habits of operation, steady revision of care patterns, new responsibilities for many professionals, new systems of delegating and organizing care, and a new level of knowledge and information. They will also require substantial amounts of capital.

Task 1: Aggressively meet patient demands for service and quality

The survivors will have a very strong market orientation. They will accept a philosophy of care that is customer driven, rather than provider driven. They will pioneer in market analysis and outcomes quality measurement. They will recognize that excellence is essential to maintaining demand, and demand is essential both to control cost and to provide incomes for health care workers. They will attract patients by making sure the quality of each service is excellent by customer standards, beginning with primary care.

The primary care component of the organization will act in the customers' behalf, enforcing cost and quality performance standards on the referral providers. The effective customers for all types of tertiary referral care will be primary care providers. Thus, many existing organizations will be affiliated with "upstream" and "downstream" organizations. No matter what form their affiliation takes, they will retain the obligation to represent their customers to the downstream unit, while providing service and quality to meet upstream demands.

Task 2: Control costs in a capitation or insurance premium sense

Surviving organizations will accept the customer need for a new view of costs. They will strive to hold costs below published prices, and they will use cost advantages to attract new patients. Since there will be three levels of prices for the foreseeable future, the surviving institutions must manage three levels of price aggregation:

- Unit costs such as drug and diagnostic tests (less than fee-for-service prices)
- Episode costs such as DRG or ambulatory surgery (less than episode prices)
- Annual patient support costs such as HMO operations (less than capitation premiums)

The opportunity to reduce unit costs by expanding volumes of service will be curtailed. Insurers and purchasers will increasingly limit contracts to organizations that provide only necessary care. The combination of price and utilization controls will force centralization of low-volume services. Surviving organizations will provide no more services directly than they can support within cost limits. They will purchase low-volume services on behalf of their customers, making the transition between providers as painless as possible. Organizations will plan their production capacity based on epidemiological models. Both facilities and clinical human resources will be sized to meet demand.

Task 3: Attract the best doctors and individual health care providers

Surviving organizations will recognize that both excellent service and cost control begin with a core of well-qualified physicians and other providers, and that well-qualified providers will always have a choice of employment. They will make competitive incomes the foundation of their recruitment and retention efforts. They will recognize that the nonmonetary factors of job life are the most important incentives to recruitment and retention when pay is competitive, and they will build organizations that are maximally responsive to the workers' needs. They will create working conditions that make work itself the biggest reward.

Surviving organizations will remove the monetary and nonmonetary frustrations of the workplace. They will train and retrain their personnel—including doctors and clinical personnel—in the processes of CQI and the changing clinical needs. They will align pay incentives with corporate and group success. They will resolve conflicts among workers and professions quickly and evenhandedly. They will remove, when necessary, workers whose efforts fail to support the needs of their groups.

Task 4: Find capital to meet modernization and reform needs

Surviving organizations will recognize that new technology, the need for amenities, reorganization, and investments in cost saving will require a steady flow of capital. They will build capital needs into their cost-control programs, using profit and depreciation as the primary source of capital. They will make capital allocation decisions that provide for worker participation, but that achieve the organization's long-term success.

Surviving organizations will pursue affiliations and mergers that enhance their access to capital. They will recognize the importance of access to capital through reserves, borrowing, and equity. Organizations that evaluate their capital needs and act on them promptly will survive in leadership positions. Those who fail to master their capital situation will be subordinated to the more successful.

The search for capital will lead to a steady increase in scale of health care organizations. It is likely that an array of organizational devices including mergers, acquisitions, affiliations, alliances, and joint ventures will be used. Many organizations will grow closer together by sequential steps through several of these models; "permanent" organization structures may be a thing of the past. It is already clear that tertiary care can only be supported by a population of one million or more. In the larger urban areas, like Salt Lake City, Southern City, and Detroit, comprehensive integrated systems will emerge. The picture for smaller cities and rural America is less clear.

Is CQI the Essential Foundation for Survival?

The Contribution of CQI

The quality movement was led by W. Edwards Deming, Philip B. Crosby, and Joseph M. Juran, three independent thinkers whose perspectives have

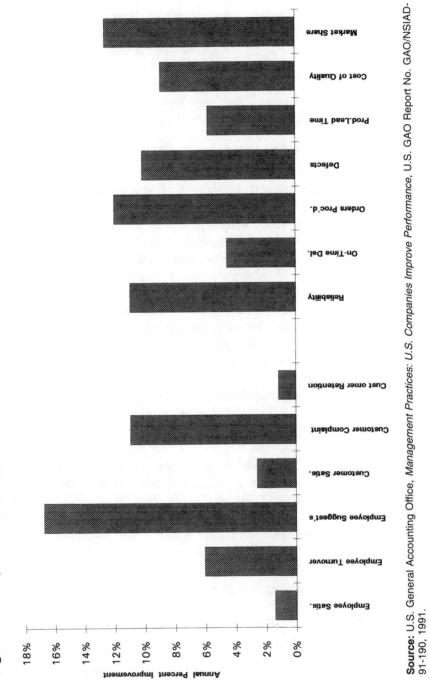

Figure 1.1   Improvement Reported by Baldrige Leaders

Source: U.S. General Accounting Office, *Management Practices: U.S. Companies Improve Performance*, U.S. GAO Report No. GAO/NSIAD-91-190, 1991.

generated a number of variations and styles. We will use the term "continuous quality improvement" (CQI) for all the versions of the quality movement because we think the principles, not the distinctions, are important.

CQI swept U.S. industrial leadership in the 1980s. A 1991 survey by Ernst and Young and the American Quality Foundation found that most large manufacturing organizations surveyed used some aspects of quality management and that U.S. performance was roughly comparable to German and Canadian, although somewhat behind Japanese.[3] According to the Ernst and Young survey, most U.S. respondents planned to increase employee participation, expand the use of technology to meet customer expectations, and increase reliance on quality and customer satisfaction data. The overall evidence supported the enthusiasm. A survey by the General Accounting Office showed that 20 companies that had competed well in the Baldrige Award, a national prize for quality movement success, had collectively done well on many important performance indicators, even just two-and-a-half years after starting (see Figure 1.1).[4]

Four fundamental concepts form the foundations of CQI in a successful application. Each of them was well established in management philosophy and management history before the quality movement; it is their integration that distinguishes the CQI contribution.

Customer focus

All commerce is transactions between customers (who pay money for service) and workers (who give service for money). Organizations exist only because they facilitate these transactions to the satisfaction of both. Research shows that institutions that recognize this truth thrive, and those that ignore it fail.[5] Both customers and workers voluntarily offer their resources (money or time) to a specific organization, and the enthusiasm with which they make that commitment determines the level of success. The better the organization fulfills customers' and workers' needs, the more customers will come, and the better the supply of workers. CQI explicitly gives the customer the dominant role in the transaction. Marketing, the study of all elements of the relationship between the organization and its customers—product, place, price, and promotion, including the narrower concept of advertising or sales—is built into the concept of an organization that is *customer-focused*.[6]

Employee (and physician) empowerment

Empowerment is the ability of the worker to change conditions of work to meet customer needs better. It implies that the worker, not management, will design the job procedures and the work environment. As such, it is a radical departure from the historical bureaucratic organization, ostensibly relinquishing control of the corporation to the lowest-ranking members. Empowerment and the related sense of personal achievement have long been recognized as the strongest motivation for worker performance.[7] Empowerment imposes three critical duties on management:

1. The duty to communicate customer demands and problems, rather than solutions, to the worker
2. The duty to answer all work-related questions that the worker raises
3. The duty to act as facilitator or coach, not decision maker

The concepts of modern human resources management—participation, worker training, supervisory training, shared incentives—are built into the concept of an organization that is *employee-empowered.*

Data-driven

Objective information is the linchpin of CQI because it permits workers to identify both customer needs and ways to improve performance. It is shared information that allows workers to form groups, to reach consensus on objectives, and to devise ways to respond. Quantitative data are inevitably preferred; they can be made more objective and they are more efficient to collect, report, and analyze. As a result, CQI stimulates a voracious and expanding appetite for information. It empowers workers to use facts, trains them to use them effectively, and enforces a search for greater precision and reliability. Information becomes the core resource of the CQI organization. Information services must themselves be subject to continuous improvement and rapid expansion. Although CQI starts with seven simple tools, the technology of twentieth-century management—marketing, financial, accounting, and statistical analysis—is built into the concept of an organization that is *data-driven.* This technology goes well beyond the simple tools.

Process focus

A central theme of CQI is to achieve quality improvement by focusing on process improvements. By identifying and improving key processes, an organization can change from an information and audit effort to a prevention strategy to improve quality.

Historically, in manufacturing as well as in health care organizations, quality assurance has focused on meeting minimum criteria. If the organization meets the minimum criteria, it is presumed to be a good-quality instrumentation. Examples include the criteria set by the Joint Commission on Accreditation of Healthcare Organizations. Once the organization is "anointed" or inspected, it is classified as "good" or "deficient." This approach has many deficiencies, including a focus on fixing problems instead of anticipating them. Focusing on continuous process improvement, on the other hand, reduces rework while constantly striving to improve quality at every level. Quality improvement does not stop if the institution meets the minimum level.

CQI in Health Care

Hospitals and health care systems began to adopt the quality movement about five years behind the industrial leaders. By the late 1980s, there were a number of institutions deeply committed to the concept, including the HCA hospital chain, Henry Ford Health System in Detroit, Intermountain Health Care in Utah, Bethesda Medical Center in Cincinnati, Rush–Presbyterian– St. Luke's in Chicago, Alliant Health Systems in Louisville, Harvard Community Health Plan in Boston, and the University of Michigan Medical Center. The concept was seen to have important implications for medical staff relations and clinical management and was strongly advocated by Paul Batalden of HCA[8] and Donald M. Berwick,[9] then of Harvard Community Health Plan. The Joint Commission on Accreditation of Healthcare Organizations (JCAHO) began incorporating CQI concepts into its standards in 1989.[10]

The three institutions in our case studies are all widely reported as health care leaders in CQI.[11] By 1992, the movement had swept the health care field. *Hospitals* magazine reported that almost 60 percent of hospitals, broadly distributed by size and geography, had a TQM/CQI program in place. Even among hospitals of 50 to 100 beds, almost half claimed programs. Of all those that had no program, 85 percent planned to start one, and only 3 percent said it was a fad.[12] (The rest said they had resource constraints of one kind or another.) The AHA survey showed that consultants were used modestly, but that CEOs took CQI seriously. Two-thirds spent more than 10 percent of their time at it, and 60 percent said it was the most important thing they'd ever done.[13]

Is CQI Enough? What Lies Beyond?

At the same time, it was becoming clear that CQI does not guarantee success. A survey by McKinsey and Company found that 20 of 30 programs had fallen short of goals.[14] Andrea Gabor, a prominent industrial writer investigating the effect of CQI on leading companies, noted that at least three prestigious companies—GM, IBM, and Xerox—had won Baldrige Awards, but had run into major business problems.[15] *Hospitals* interviewed Donald Berwick on the "TQM backlash." He conceded that "there is a voice in the country that's saying that quality management isn't fulfilling its initial promise." He also noted that there was a need for "a more solid base of consolidated information about who's doing what, what's working and what isn't working," and he noted the importance of basic management skills in successful TQM implementation.[16]

Pitfalls for the Unwary: Misconceptions about CQI

Analysis of the disappointments suggests that they stem from five mistaken beliefs and incorrect or incomplete actions based on those beliefs.[17]

Mistaken belief 1: TQM is a sufficient condition for success

It is a mistake to believe that any single aspect of management is a sufficient condition for success. Rather, the success of any organization depends on a wide range of factors, including the following:

- A proper fit between the need of the society, the environment, and the purposes of the organization
- Congruence of the organization's structure and the functions it is trying to perform
- The wisdom and skill of management
- Perceptivity, agility, and surefootedness in sensing and responding to changes in the needs of the marketplace

Excellence in one or two of these areas cannot guarantee success. It is the proper balance among all that makes the difference.

Mistaken belief 2: Crash implementation of CQI will accelerate results

CQI is as much a culture as it is a technique. It involves a new set of beliefs about management and organization—a "paradigm shift." It asserts, among other things, that top management does not really understand what goes on within the organization, and it is therefore incapable of doing very much to improve performance and is dependent on the initiative of the workers. That goes very much against the basic prejudices of most managers—and, for that matter, most workers. It is not likely to be accepted easily or quickly.

We do not understand much about how cultures change, but it seems clear that change cannot be commanded, it does not take place rapidly, and it cannot be brought about through technical instruction. Attempts at crash implementation are doomed to failure.

Mistaken belief 3: Staff or consultants can drive the quality process within an organization

The "outside-in" approach ignores the cultural dimension of CQI. The main determinants of staff behavior within an organization are not written down anywhere. They arise from the culture, from a set of expectations individuals share about each other and about the sorts of behavior that are and are not acceptable. CQI calls for major changes in those unwritten rules. Bringing in a group of outsiders with new tool kits misses that point and usually just adds cost.

Mistaken belief 4: Education is enough to achieve action and results

Regardless of how well the concepts are known, the secret lies in being able to do it. That means practice, with management providing the coaching and maintaining the morale of the team. Like the basketball coach, management has to accept that it cannot shoot the baskets or block the shots, but that it is responsible for advising those who do, for providing overall direction, and for having plans that allow the shooters and blockers to do their best.

Mistaken belief 5: Implementing CQI requires that performance evaluation be "trashed"

It may be true that in many companies performance evaluation is used only for determining salary increases and, on balance, does more harm than good. Some quality gurus have urged that performance evaluation be abandoned altogether. We believe that goes too far. Although most staff members sincerely want to do a good job, there are those who will take advantage of situations in which they are not held accountable for their performance, and most workers will do better with a measurement and a goal. So we continue to advocate performance evaluation, but more as a positive staff development tool than as an exercise in negative criticism. The emphasis in performance evaluation needs to be on continual feedback, team performance, and improving the system of work, and not just on individual evaluation.

The Concepts of Agility and Reengineering

What the customer wants in health care is not a mystery. The customer wants prompt access including the latest technology; convenient, effective, and comfortable service; and reasonable cost. There are inevitable trade-offs between these goals, but the trade-offs are at the margin. The customer wants them all and will support the organization that comes closest to delivering them all. The relative difficulty is also clear. The overwhelming issue for health care providers is cost control. President Clinton has articulated the goal in his health care reform plan—costs trends decreasing immediately to consumer price index (CPI) plus 1.5 percent, and declining in four years to the CPI. This decrease implies limiting current dollar growth of health care to something less than 5 percent per year. It has been averaging near 12 percent since 1970.[18]

The reduction must come mainly from ongoing productivity improvement. Customers will demand access and service, and they will include outcomes quality measures. The implications are more severe than most people realize. The health care CQI experiences reported to date have described a much more tolerant atmosphere, where any achievement is rewarded even if it has only a minor effect on cost. Not only does reform require greater effort, it requires providers to judge technology and personal service improvements more rigorously in the light of cost implications. It will force them to examine questions that threaten traditional autonomy and interprofessional relationships. The roles and authorities of physicians, nurses, and others will quickly come under scrutiny. Finally, it threatens job security, raising the specter of workforce reduction.

Ongoing improvements of this magnitude will not come easily. They will require ground-up redesign of most care processes, new and expanded job assignments for most workers, and new roles and authorities for most managers. First of all, they require a strategic thrust that CQI lacks, except in its most sophisticated applications. Whether you treat it as "Beyond CQI" or "Phase II" of CQI, it is the incorporation of more strategic direction that makes the three cases in this book likely winners in the twenty-first century. It's the skill of these organizations at answering questions that lie behind the four tasks:

- Who are the partners and collaborators with this organization, and who are its potential conquests?
- What are the future limits customers will accept, in terms of cost and quality performance?
- What are the services the customers value highest and least?
- What is the economically viable size of this operation and its major components? How many beds, doctors, nurses, outpatient care sites, and so on, do we need in the long run?
- How do we help our professional workforce (including doctors) adapt to changed demands?
- How much capital is needed to achieve the vision? What must we set aside to fund replacements, expansions, acquisitions, professional recruitment, and new product development?

The reality—not the buzzwords—of CQI is one step toward survival. In the chapters that follow, we identify four critical areas beyond CQI. We believe these areas are important capabilities of the surviving organization. They do not tell the shape of the twenty-first century health care organization; they tell how the organization will reengineer itself. The capabilities interweave the four tasks rather than paralleling them. They emphasize skills and actions that often relate to several tasks at once. It seemed to us that the case study organizations could most usefully be described by their excellence in these areas:

1. Leadership
   - The CEO's contribution: What are the unique tasks that the CEO and senior managers must do, and what are the measures that they should track?
   - Using a shared vision: How do you gain consensus around a vision, and how do you keep the vision a vital and persuasive force in your organization?
   - Fostering empowerment: How do you use job achievement to build job satisfaction, and how do you allay anxieties that erode self-confidence and initiative?
2. Customer-focused clinical care
   - The lessons from Intermountain Health Care: How do you build effective clinical quality improvement teams?

- Redesigning work: How can process improvement be used to take major costs out of health care delivery organizations?
- The role of clinical guidelines and clinical expectations: How does clinical CQI differ from traditional QA?
- Motivation and education: What steps help physicians and other clinicians use clinical paths to achieve high-quality care?

3. Decision-making structures
   - Planning for decisions: What are the recurring topics where consensus must be built, and how do you address them effectively?
   - Integrating multiple efforts: How do you coordinate many different activities into one program, and how do you make that program good enough to meet customer needs?
   - Dealing with the "smokestacks": What is the emerging organizational structure for health care organizations, and how do you build it?

4. Managing the information explosion
   - Making information the linchpin of CQI: What are the core measures and how do you build an information system around them?
   - Using expectations to achieve accountability: How can you use information to encourage rather than control, and what does that entail for information systems?
   - Building clinical information: What are the special needs of clinical quality improvement task forces, and how do you supply these?

How Can You Use This Book?

This book is mainly useful as a source of conceptual benchmarks—snapshots of things that worked for our case studies in CQI, in leadership, in clinical care, in other decision processes, and in information strategies. We hope those who read the book straight through will come away with a comprehensive vision of twenty-first century management technology that they can use to plan their own organization's path and priorities. At the same time, since some readers may have more specific goals, we have tried to write each chapter so it will stand on its own. Readers with the following interests may skip to the appropriate chapters:

- *CQI:* Chapters 3, 6–8
- *Leadership:* Chapter 2 and the opening sections of Chapters 6–8

- *Customer focus and clinical care:* Chapters 2, 3, and 6
- *Decision processes:* Chapters 4 and 8
- *Information systems:* Chapters 5 and 7

Finally, if you are interested in one case study organization, note that we have tried to identify the major quotes in the first four chapters by indenting them. It should be a quick scan to pick out the remarks of people from the organization you are interested in.

Notes

1. These concepts are developed in depth by several sources listed in the Suggested Readings section. Specifically, see Chandler 1977 and Pfeffer and Salancik 1978 regarding organizations in general; see Griffith 1992 and Fottler et al. 1989 regarding applications to health care.
2. See Suggested Readings: About Previous Health Care Revolutions.
3. Ernst and Young, American Quality Foundation. 1991. "International Quality Study." Cleveland, OH: Ernst and Young. (Available by writing Ernst and Young, 1600 Huntington Building, Cleveland, OH 44115.)
4. U.S. General Accounting Office. 1991. *Management Practices: U.S. Companies Improve Performance through Quality Efforts.* Report No. GAO/NSIAD-91-190. Washington, DC: Government Printing Office.
5. Kimberley, J. R., and E. J. Zajac. 1985. "Strategic Adaptation in Health Care Organizations: Implications for Theory and Research." *Medical Care Review* 42 (Fall): 267–302.
6. Kotler, P. 1987. *Marketing for Health Care Organizations.* Englewood Cliffs, NJ: Prentice-Hall.
7. Revans, R. W. 1972. *Hospitals: Communication, Choice, and Change: The Hospital Internal Communication Project Seen from Within.* London: Tavistock.
8. Batalden, P., D. Smith, J. Bovender, and D. Hardison. 1989. "Quality Improvement: The Role and Application of Research Methods." *Journal of Health Administration Education* 7 (3): 577–83.
9. Berwick, D. M. 1989. "Continuous Improvement as an Ideal in Health Care." *New England Journal of Medicine* 320 (5 January): 53–56.
10. Joint Commission on the Accreditation of Healthcare Organizations. 1989, 1990. "Standards Development Addresses Quality Improvement, and Quality Improvement Standards Address the Role of Leaders." *Joint Commission Perspectives* 9 (November–December), 10 (March–April).
11. See the Notes and Suggested Readings sections at the end of each case study, Chapters 7, 8, and 9.
12. Eubanks, P. 1992. "TQM/CQI: The CEO Experience." *Hospitals* 66 (5 June): 24–36.
13. Ibid.

14. Fuchsberg, G. 1992. "Quality Programs Show Shoddy Results." *Wall Street Journal* (14 May).
15. Gabor, A. 1991. *The Man Who Discovered Quality*. New York: Penguin Books.
16. Eubanks, P. 1992. "TQM Backlash Prompts Questions." *Hospitals* 66 (5 June): 30.
17. Sahney, V. K., R. D. Wittrup, and G. L. Warden. 1992. "TQM: Observations from the Trenches." *The Quality Letter for Healthcare Leaders* 4 (July–August): 13–16.
18. Fuchs, V. R. 1990. "The Health Sector's Share of the Gross National Product." *Science* 247 (2 February): 534–38.

Suggested Readings

About previous health care revolutions

Starr, P. 1982. *The Social Transformation of American Medicine*. New York: Basic Books.
Stevens, R. 1989. *In Sickness and in Wealth*. New York: Basic Books.

About the role of organizations

Chandler, A. D. 1977. *The Visible Hand: The Managerial Revolution in American Business*. Cambridge, MA: Belknap Press.
Fottler, M. D., J. D. Blair, C. J. Whitehead, M. D. Laus, G. T. Savage. 1989. "Assessing Key Stakeholders: Who Matters to Hospitals and Why?" *Hospital & Health Services Administration* 34(4): 525–46.
Griffith, J. R. 1992. *The Well-Managed Community Hospital*. 2d ed. Ann Arbor, MI: Health Administration Press. See Chapter 3.
Pfeffer, J., and G. R. Salancik. 1978. *The External Control of Organizations: A Resource Dependence Perspective*. New York: Harper and Row.

About continuous quality improvement

Deming, W. E. 1986. *Out of the Crisis*. Cambridge: Massachusetts Institute of Technology Center for Advanced Engineering Study.
Imai, M. 1986. *Kaizen: The Key to Japanese Competitive Success*. New York: Random House.
Gabor, A. 1991. *The Man Who Discovered Quality*. New York: Penguin Books.
Juran, J. M. 1989. *On Leadership for Quality: An Executive Handbook*. New York: Free Press.

CQI in health care organizations

Conrad, D. A., ed. 1993. "Seeking Health Care Quality: The Implications of Medical Practice Guidelines." *Frontiers of Health Services Management* 10(1).

Issue includes B. C. James, "Implementing Practice Guidelines through Clinical Quality Improvement," pp. 3–38; M. R. Chassin, "Improving Quality of Care with Practice Guidelines," pp. 40–45; H. I. Goldberg, "Should We Be Implementing Untested Guidelines?" pp. 45–47; J. G. King, "The Relevance of Practical Experience to American Hospitals," pp. 48–50; J. S. Todd, "Quest for Quality or Cost Containment," pp. 51–53; and B. C. James, "Reply," pp. 54–55.

Gaucher, E. J., and R. J. Coffey. 1993. *Total Quality in Health Care.* San Francisco, CA: Jossey-Bass.

Joint Commission on Accreditation of Healthcare Organizations. 1991. *An Introduction to Quality Improvement in Health Care: The Transition from QA to CQI.* Chicago: JCAHO.

Leebov, W., and C. J. Ersoz. 1991. *The Health Care Manager's Guide to Continuous Quality Improvement.* Chicago: American Hospital Publishing.

Marszalek-Gaucher, E., and R. Coffey. 1990. *Transforming Healthcare Organizations: How to Achieve and Sustain Organizational Excellence.* San Francisco: Jossey-Bass.

Melum, M. M. 1992. *Total Quality Management: The Health Care Pioneers.* Chicago: American Hospital Publishing.

Mozena, J. P., and D. L. Anderson. 1993. "Quality Improvement Handbook for Health Care Professionals." Milwaukee, WI: ASQC Quality Press.

Sahney, V. K., and G. L. Warden. 1991. "The Quest for Quality and Productivity in Health Services." *Frontiers of Health Services Management* 7(4): 2–40.

2

The Role of Leadership

Personal leadership by CEOs and clinical leaders will start and sustain the process of developing tomorrow's lean and agile health care system. The larger and more successful the organization, the more critical the leader's task. The health care industry can learn valuable lessons from its counterparts in the automobile and manufacturing industries. Organizations that were considered successful a decade ago, like IBM, GM, and Sears, are now fighting for survival. In the auto industry, General Motors once commanded more than a 50 percent market share. But it was the least able among U.S. auto companies to respond to Japanese competition, and today its market share has fallen below 35 percent. Ford and Chrysler, on the other hand, made the painful but successful transition under the leadership of Don Peterson and Lee Iaccoca during the 1980s. Both aggressively reduced excess capacity and personnel while improving their products and manufacturing processes. Ten years ago, it took Chrysler more than six years to bring a new car from initial concept to the show room; now it has reduced this period to under three years. It took GM seven years to develop the Buick Regal which it introduced in the spring of 1988[1] after spending $7 billion. Honda, on the other hand, launched its 1989 Accord within three years of initiating the project. Two other companies present contrasting examples of leadership: IBM was slow to adapt to the changing marketplace and to shift from mainframes to PCs; AT&T, on the other hand, made the transition from a fully regulated industry

to an unbundled, highly competitive telecommunication industry with fly-
ing colors.

If we had to identify a single key essential skill of a leader, it would
have to be the ability to be a change agent. Successful leaders are quick
to assess the current and future environment and are able to set a process
in motion that transforms the organization to the desired future. Abraham
Zaleznik[2] argued that managers and leaders are different. Leaders adopt
an active attitude toward goals. They worry about ideas and how ideas
affect people. They relate to people in intuitive and empathetic ways to
seek change. They create a sense of urgency. Managers, on the other hand,
tend to adopt impersonal goals and view them as a means of getting the job
done. They react to people in a hierarchical way, with an emphasis on the
sequence of activities that needs to be undertaken. They consider their key
tasks to be making compromises among different groups to solve problems
and getting the job done. Managers worry about compliance; leaders worry
about commitment.

John Kotter[3] states that leadership and management are two distinctive
and complementary systems of action. Both are necessary for success:
"Leadership complements management; it does not replace it." Leadership
is involved in bringing change into the organization. It is the process of
motivating and inspiring people and, through this process, aligning them
to the corporate strategy. Management, on the other hand, is focused on
bringing order and getting things done in a cost-effective manner. In an
organization with a high proportion of professionals, every manager has
to develop the skills of a leader to get things done effectively. It is very
important that professionals making critical resource allocation decisions
buy into the changes conceptualized by leadership.

In this chapter, we explore some of the critical skills and abilities
demonstrated by leaders who have successfully led their organization
through major changes. It is not our intent to imply that every leader has
all of these skills in equal measure, but studies have found that successful
leaders demonstrate their effective use of these skills to accomplish change.

Seven Key Abilities of Successful Leaders:

1. To think strategically and create a vision
2. To communicate and develop a shared vision
3. To create an organizational culture focused on customer service
4. To create an organization capable of continual improvement

5. To create organizational agility

6. To create employee commitment to the organization

7. To focus and produce results.

Successful leaders make things happen. They have the skills to create, not just to convince. They think strategically and create a personal vision of the organization. They create an environment for change; it does not just happen automatically. In addition, skilled leaders have a great ability to focus and produce results. In our case studies, Gail Warden (CEO, Henry Ford Health System), Scott Parker (CEO, Intermountain Health Care), and Charles Christiansen (CEO, Walke-Parker Medical Center) accomplished all of these things. These three organizations have benefited significantly from their leadership and face the uncertainties of the future well equipped to survive and thrive.

Ability to Think Strategically and to Create a Vision

"Strategic thinking" is thinking that goes on within the mind of the CEO, to shape and clarify the organization's future strategic profile.[4] It is the process by which the CEO develops a picture of what the organization should look like and its profile at some point in the future. Ask yourself: "What is the aim of the organization?" What is the need for the organization? Who are the key customers? What is the need in the community and the society as a whole for this organization? Many organizations confuse strategic planning with strategic thinking. "Strategic planning" is the process by which the organization plans to accomplish the strategic vision of the organization. It is the process by which an organization wins over key individuals. Strategic thinking involves four analytical steps: understanding customer needs, understanding competitors, understanding the organization's core strengths, and understanding environmental changes.

Understanding Customer Needs

The key to understanding customer needs in health care is to free yourself from the provider perspective and the products and services currently being offered. Role-playing is a helpful exercise to define what kinds of products and services you would like as a customer. Customer surveys and focus groups of customers are valuable tools for understanding customer needs. A common mistake made here is to lump all customers into a single category.

Additional insights can be gained by segmenting the customers into as many distinct groups as possible and to think about the unique needs of each of the groups. In health care, middle-income groups may want low out-of-pocket costs and may be satisfied with an HMO with tighter controls on the provider network. Higher-income groups may be willing to pay a premium for physician choice and access to specialists. Children under the age of five years have very different needs than elderly patients over the age of 80. The task in the customer segmentation process is to constantly force yourself to define new ways to segment customers. Customer analysis must also consider the role of benefit managers in major corporations. What are the needs of those who buy health care on behalf of major corporations or governmental units?

Finally, visualize unmet customer needs. What can we learn from other service industries, for example, hotel chains or airlines? One hospital welcomes the patients and their families in a reception lounge with tea and cookies served by a hostess while the admitting paperwork is done. Patients and their families find the wait much more tolerable and tend to form a good first impression. Many hospitals are now offering valet parking services, a simple service unheard of a few years ago. At one hospital, patients are given preoperating instructions both in a written pamphlet and on a cassette tape. A customer-oriented organization not only meets the current needs of the customer, but it actively identifies future needs.

Understanding Competitors

As part of the strategic planning process, most health care organizations perform a competitor analysis. This analysis usually lists the services offered by competitors and their market shares in the primary and secondary service areas. Rarely does this analysis include an analysis of competitors' strategies. What are the key strengths of the competition? What are their core competencies? Why do patients prefer to go to competitors for services? Are competitors especially strong in a particular market segment? Does a competitor have any alliances that give it a marketplace advantage? What future strategies are likely to be pursued? What strategies will it not be able to pursue? Competitor analysis requires you to role-play and treat a competitor as an active and smart organization. What will be the new competitive products? What areas are vulnerable to carve-outs by entrepreneurs with low-cost solutions?

Understanding the Organization's Core Strengths

As an important step in the strategic thinking process, you must clearly see and analyze the core strengths of the organization. Core strengths may reflect the location of the organization. Many health care organizations are burdened by poor location and indigent care; a health care organization located in an affluent suburb has the differential advantage of a good payer mix. The Mayo Clinic, Cleveland Clinic, and the Henry Ford Health System enjoy another kind of core strength: These organizations have large multi-specialty group practices with salaried medical staff as an integral part of their organization; most community hospitals are struggling to integrate their medical staffs with a health care organization. A third type of core strength may be a low-cost structure, which allows an organization to compete based on price. As managed care spreads, organizations with a low-cost structure will have a differential advantage over their competitors. In the era of managed care, those health care organizations that have sophisticated information systems that allow them to track cost of service by diagnosis and by providers will also have a marketplace advantage.

Understanding Environmental Changes

Understanding environmental changes that may affect the organizational strategy requires a study of demographic, economic, technological, and political changes. Understanding demographic changes requires studying the shift of the population from one region of the country to another and from cities to suburbs, and studying age groups and their shifting needs for health care. Understanding economic changes requires studying the growth or decline of businesses and the job creation capacity of the community. It requires understanding the business climate. Will businesses move into the service area or will the existing businesses move out? Understanding economic changes requires studying the likely changes in health care benefit packages offered by employers. What is likely to be the effect of a cafeteria or flex benefits offered by employers on the strategy of the health care organization? And what about the technological changes in the industry? What will be the effect of new medical technology—for example, of radial keratotomy on the optometry business, of a shift to ambulatory surgery on inpatient beds, or of gene therapy on surgical services? Finally, under-standing environmental changes requires an understanding of the political climate. How will national health care reform affect the organization? What about universal health insurance? What will happen if the state mandates Medicaid beneficiaries to enroll in HMOs?

Strategic thinking requires leaders to analyze four areas—namely, the customers, competitors, the core strengths of the organization, and environmental changes—in order to define the future vision of the organization. What should the organization optimally look like? What would be the nature of its products, services, and customers? In which market segments does it plan to compete, and in which segments does it not plan to compete? In which geographical areas does the organization plan to expand?

In 1974, Henry Ford Hospital's former CEO, Stan Nelson, changed the character of the organization when he convinced the trustees to invest in the development of suburban ambulatory care centers. Nelson was able to identify correctly his organization's core strengths as a multispecialty group practice. He used this model to enter the suburban market and establish large ambulatory care centers. Community hospitals at that time were focused on building inpatient capabilities. Many were not able to open ambulatory care facilities because they were afraid to antagonize their community physicians. Today, Henry Ford Health System has 35 ambulatory care centers located in the greater Detroit metropolitan area. This distribution system gives it a unique advantage in its market.

Gail Warden, president and CEO of Henry Ford Health System, arrived in Detroit in April 1988. He found that his predecessor, Stanley Nelson, had systematically built or acquired key components of a health system— community hospitals, ambulatory care centers, a psychiatric hospital, substance abuse treatment centers, an HMO, physician group practices, nursing homes, and home health care agencies—adding them to the existing tertiary care teaching and research institution. All were combined under one parent organization called Henry Ford Health Care Corporation. Warden conceived and conceptualized an integrated system and began describing his vision of Henry Ford as a regional health system in which all of the components of the system worked together. Responding to an environment beginning to demand cost discipline, Warden saw a leading system model for the future that could align the clinical, teaching, research, and charitable missions of the organization with the market-based imperatives, and he began to create a vision of survival through service integration. He envisioned a seamless health care delivery organization in which patients—as customers of the system, rather than customers of an individual component—could go from one entity to another with the least number of barriers. Adopting the patient's perspective, he envisioned a system with all of its components meshing with one another like a fine-tuned machine. This vision of an integrated health system able to provide comprehensive services in a seamless fashion is very attractive to health care professionals who are constantly dealing with barriers to patient care created by fragmented systems.

The crafting of mission and vision statements must follow the process of strategic thinking: "A mission statement (or vision statement) has meaning only to someone with a 'sense' of the mission being described. We, therefore, see mission statements as being most useful after a sense of mission has been created, not before. . . . As we see it, mission statements frequently do more harm than good because they imply a sense of direction, clarity of thinking and unity that rarely exists" (9).[5]

Ten Key Steps to Thinking Strategically and Creating a Vision

1. **Define current profile**
   Identify the organization's current profile including its current products, services, customers, and market share. Examine trends over the past five years.

2. **Identify customer needs**
   Define customer segments and the needs of each of the segments. What needs are currently unmet? What may be some of the future needs of the customer?

3. **Understand competitors**
   Define strategies of key competitors. What are their differential advantages? Why do customers select your competitors over you?

4. **Define the organization's core strengths**
   Identify core strengths of the organization. Core strengths may reflect location, technology, organizational structure, cost advantage, information systems, or some other key advantage.

5. **Understand environmental changes**
   What changes in the environment are expected in the near future? These may include legislative or regulatory developments or changes in payment policies. What new technologies are likely to appear and influence the delivery system?

6. **Involve senior leadership**
   It is important to use a strategic thinking process that involves key stakeholders. Their involvement will facilitate implementation. The

strategic thinking process requires an open dialogue, and an outside facilitator may be needed to force an open discussion.[6]

7. **Examine strategic alliances**

   Are there organizations that offer an opportunity to form a strategic alliance? Explore potential alliances with a partner who offers a unique strength.[7]

8. **Develop future strategic scenarios**

   Develop alternative strategic scenarios based upon environmental changes and the organization's key strengths. What will be the key strategies of the organization for each of these alternative scenarios?

9. **Develop competitor reaction**

   For each of the future strategic scenarios, define the reaction of each of the competitors. How is the competitor likely to react? Evaluate your strategies in view of the competitor's reaction.

10. **Define strategic vision**

    Select and define the strategic vision of the organization. Be specific and define what the organization will look like and what its key products, customers, and core strengths will be.

Ability to Communicate and Develop a Shared Vision

> A shared vision brings people together. It unites and provides the link between diverse people and activities. Shared visions are expressions of what people have in common, of what they in the community are committed to. People with shared visions are more likely to take responsibility.
>
> *Marjorie Parker* (63)[8]

The most critical leadership skill needed for implementing an effective change process is to create and nurture a shared vision among all of the members of the organization. Peter Senge, in his classic book *The Fifth Discipline*, states:

> A shared vision is not an idea. It is not even an important idea. It is not even an important idea such as freedom. It is rather a force in people's hearts, a force of impressive power. It may be inspired by an idea, but once it goes further—if it is compelling enough to acquire the support of more than one person—then it is no longer an abstraction, it is palpable. People begin to see it as if it exists. Few, if any, forces in human affairs are as powerful as shared vision (206).[9]

Effective leaders have an ability to communicate their personal vision within the organization in such a way that over time it becomes a shared vision. This is a task of immense proportions. It requires constant communication at all levels of the organization. It involves an active dialogue among the members of the organization to clarify and evolve their thinking. If members of an organization do not spend sufficient time discussing and evolving their own mental models in interactions with their leaders, conflicting and competing visions begin developing within the organization. These alternate visions slow down the speed with which the organization can move forward and interfere with the vision developed by the leadership.

The single most critical factor in translating personal vision into organizational vision is leadership time spent in dialogue with members of the organization. In many organizations, senior leaders go away for a weekend retreat with a consultant and develop a statement of vision for the organization. This statement is approved by the board of trustees and is published in the employee newsletter. Leaders then get busy with their daily work and assume that the rest of the organization shares in this vision. Although this type of exercise is a necessary part of the process, by itself it is rarely successful. Although the people attending the retreat may accept the vision statement and may even change their behavior to align themselves with the vision, within the rest of the organization there is, at best, a formal compliance and, at worst apathy. Under formal compliance, people do the minimum to keep their job and no more. Under apathy, people show no interest and no energy and may even actively sabotage the vision. Usually resistance or apathy shows up in questions raised by employees: Where is this organization going? Why are we investing in this new product or acquisition? Why are we not told what is going on? Senge[10] (219) has categorized the buy-in of employees into three possibilities: (1) enrollment/commitment, (2) compliance (various types), and (3) apathy.

Gandhi was able to take a personal vision of freedom for India from British rule and make it the shared vision of the masses of Indian people. He spent over 20 years speaking to illiterate villagers in thousands of villages and, at the same time, writing about his vision in articles and books for the educated. He translated his personal vision of a free India through nonviolence to a shared vision among the people. He went on a hunger strike every time violence broke out in order to convince his followers that his strategy was nonviolence. Ultimately, masses were willing to lie down in front of armed police, withstanding beatings without fighting back. The vision of freedom was so compelling that people were willing to accept grave personal risks. Martin Luther King, Jr., used similar tactics in the United States. Through marches, speeches, and rallies, he was able to enlist the African-American community in developing a shared vision of freedom. His "I Have a Dream" speech at the Lincoln Memorial in Washington described his vision; through numerous other speeches he made it the dream of millions of both black and white people in this country.

In a private conversation, Alan Gilmour, vice chairman of Ford Motor Company, said:

> In the early 1980s, Ford developed its vision statement, which said we want to be the lowest-cost, highest-quality manufacturer of cars and trucks. This simple vision, which certainly is not very profound, has been constantly reinforced within the company. In the latest J. D. Powers consumer survey, Ford placed six cars in the top ten cars rated for quality. Ford has also achieved the distinction of being the lowest-cost producer of cars in North America.

Health care organizations present special challenges when it comes to developing a shared vision. First, the highly educated professionals who staff these organizations, including physicians, nurses, physical therapists, and many others, are often trained to give their primary loyalties to their professions and to their patients rather than the organization. They have great job mobility and, for them, career development often requires frequent relocation from one employer to another. Consequently, their personal visions and the vision of the organization can easily diverge, making it difficult to achieve focus in the organization's purpose or to change its general direction. Second, a great deal of the difficulty in developing a shared vision in health care organizations results from the focus of clinical professionals on the treatment of individual patients. These professionals value highly the care of each patient and find it difficult to relate this to a vision of the business enterprise.

Four Key Steps in Communicating and Developing a Shared Vision

1. Description

The first step in developing a shared vision is to translate the vision statement and to write a simple description of the desired future state.

What will the organization look like? What will be its key products and strategic initiatives? What values will the organization accept?

2. Strength and weakness analysis

Once the vision is written, it needs to be reviewed with a careful eye to evaluate its strengths and weaknesses. What are some of the potential outcomes of the new vision? Under the best scenario, how will the organization perform using this vision? What are some of the worst possibilities?

3. Defining critical success factors

As the vision and its strengths and weaknesses are analyzed, key factors and external variables that will shape the vision should be identified. Factors that are critical to the successful implementation of the vision may include critical resources such as key people and their skill levels, available capital, and buy-in of key stakeholders.

4. Planned implementation

Accomplishing the vision requires that key tasks to effect the changes and their sequence of implementation be defined. As each task is scheduled, the effect of the task and likely reactions within the organization must be evaluated.

An illustration of communicating and developing a shared vision

Gail Warden used the four key steps to communicate and engage the whole organization in developing a shared vision:

Step 1: Description. As a first step, the board of trustees accepted Warden's recommendations to appoint a "Futures Committee" of the board, which was charged with developing a vision for what he defined as the "Henry Ford Health System" (HFHS) in the year 2000.[11] Warden discussed his vision with the Futures Committee, which, after considerable discussion and further refinement, accepted it.

Step 2: Strength and weakness analysis. Gail Warden convened a retreat involving 80 senior managers and physicians and shared his vision of HFHS endorsed by the Futures Committee of the board. Break-out groups analyzed the specific gaps between the vision and current reality. These groups were also asked to analyze the strengths and weaknesses of HFHS. Meanwhile, the Futures Committee also discussed existing strengths and weaknesses, key products, and significant competitors of each operating entity within the organization.

Step 3: Defining critical success factors. The Futures Committee defined over twenty key requirements for the system to reach its vision, which were narrowed down to six (see Figure 2.1).[12]

Step 4: Planned implementation. Recognizing the importance of labels and clarification of responsibilities, Warden also identified the need for changes in the name and governance structure of Henry Ford Health Care Corporation. Henry Ford Health Care Corporation thus became "Henry Ford Health System" to emphasize its new focus. A governance consultant with expertise in the nonprofit sector was engaged to assist in defining a new governance structure with improved working relationships and alignment among the different components of the health system. The key

Figure 2.1

Key System Requirements for HFHS

1. Develop a cohesive, vertically integrated health care system that demonstrates a commitment to excellence and the process of continuous quality improvement.

2. Pursue an organizational focus that combines advanced clinical care delivery through managed care.

3. Continue to grow to serve a broad range of people in the region, achieving the benefits of scale for all constituencies of Henry Ford Health System.

4. Strengthen the position of Henry Ford Health System in health care insurance by providing a range of desired products that meet the needs of employers and consumers.

5. Provide the necessary funds to support (a) the Henry Ford Health Sciences Center, (b) continuous quality improvement throughout the system, and (c) continued growth.

6. Effectively communicate the Henry Ford Health System vision to all constituencies—health care users, medical staff, other employees, business and labor leadership, the national health care community, government, regulators, the financial community, and philanthropists.

recommendations of the governance consultant were implemented. Those that deal with alignment specifically are the following:[13]

- Increase the number of elected trustees from 20 to 25.
- Increase the number of ex officio positions on the board to 12: the president/CEO, Henry Ford Health System; the chair, Board of Governors, Henry Ford Medical Group and two other specified physicians; the chairs of each of the six legal subsidiary boards, representing those operating entities; one member selected by the board from among the chairs of the other advisory governing boards within the system.
- Appoint a systemwide Nominating Committee with responsibility for overseeing the recruitment, selection, and retention of all volunteers within the system's governance structure.
- Formally establish a Chairman's Council and make it responsible for the exchange of critical information among business units, the consideration of key policy issues facing the system, the orientation of new volunteer leadership, and the annual trustee caucus.

The objective of all of these efforts was to improve the buy-in of all of the trustees in the vision of the Henry Ford Health System and to engage the trustees in the active dialogue in the development of the system.

Warden moved quickly to shape the vision internally. Each of the 11 operating entities was asked to build on the system vision by developing its own vision statement with the help of its medical staff, board, and management. Each was also asked to prepare a three-year strategic plan and to present it to the system leadership for discussion and approval.[14] The objective of this effort was to have operating managers identify the key steps necessary to achieve the system vision, the resources needed, and the barriers at the operating level. In order to gain external knowledge and to provide external benchmarks, Henry Ford Health System joined the "Integrated Health System Study" being conducted by Steven Shortell at Northwestern University in cooperation with KPMG Peat Marwick and eight other health systems.[15] The key focus of this study was to engage in shared learning to accelerate the development of integrated health systems. Other external comparisons were made available through the CRISP study, which focuses on essential characteristics and identifiable performance measures for integrated systems.[16]

The following additional steps were also taken to achieve a shared vision during Warden's first five years:

- Changes in governance to increase further consolidation
- Systematic development of the board, management, and medical staff commitment to the vision
- Systemwide strategic planning process that tied the individual planning processes of each of the system entities to the vision of the system
- Systemwide operational budgeting and capital budgeting process that integrated and rationalized the capital allocation based on system priorities
- A new focus on a systemwide clinical information system to enable patient data to be accessible throughout the system
- A new flexible employee benefits program that brings all operating unit employees into a common structure, making it easier for employees to move to new jobs in different entities within the system
- A systemwide total quality education process to create a common culture and a common systematic improvement methodology throughout the system
- A systemwide biweekly CEO newsletter that is sent to all trustees and senior leadership of the system, highlighting key events that occurred within the system during the past two weeks
- Participation in the Health System Integration Study to develop shared learning and benchmarking with eight other leading integrated health systems
- A bottom-up discussion of the system's mission, vision, and guiding principles at every level of the organization (see Figure 2.2).
- Appointment of a Senior Operating Team consisting of chief operating officers of the operating divisions to discuss key systems initiatives and to give their advice to the senior leadership of the system.

These initiatives and many others resulted in the selection of Henry Ford Health System for the Twenty-First Century Innovators Award[17] by 3M and the Health Care Forum at the 1992 Visionary Leadership conference. This award recognizes health care organizations for the creation and implementation of a strategic vision.

The development of a shared vision in a health care organization depends on the ability to harness the energies of the people within the

Figure 2.2

HFHS Mission, Vision, and Value Statements Review Process, 1993

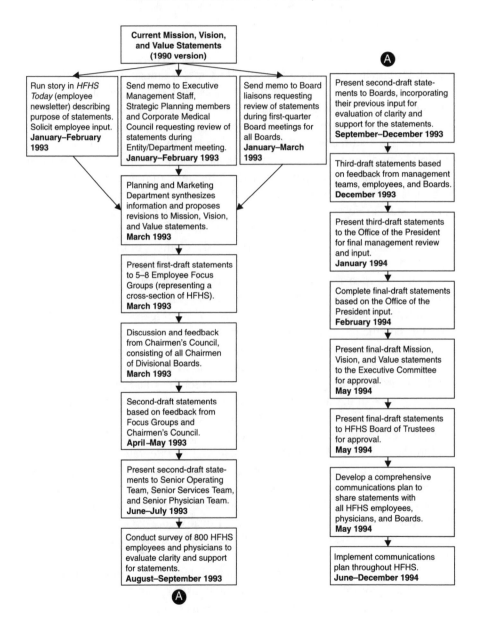

organization. It requires an alignment of the goals of the board of trustees, the senior management leadership, the medical staff, and all employees of the system. This type of alignment is not possible without a very powerful organizational vision that becomes a personal vision for each of the members of the system.

Visionary leaders not only position their organization to constantly move toward the new vision, but they also identify and work to influence key environmental factors that may affect the organization adversely. Lee Iaccoca recognized this when he took over as the CEO of Chrysler. He knew that he had to develop new products, cut manufacturing costs, and improve quality so that customers would perceive value in the cars produced by Chrysler. He also recognized that he had to buy time. Thus, he launched an external campaign to slow down the Japanese push to capture the American automobile market. He persuaded the president of the United States to negotiate voluntary quotas with the Japanese for cars imported into the United States. He knew that such a move would not only buy time, but would also galvanize support from UAW members toward a common cause. He would then use this UAW support to make changes in his manufacturing operations that would lower costs and ensure the company's survival.

Gail Warden realized that his vision of developing an integrated regional health system could be accelerated by effecting changes in health care licensing regulations within the state of Michigan. As early as 1988, Warden saw the growing demands of business and government for cost discipline as an opportunity to promote integrated health systems in the public policy arena. He created a Government Affairs Department and focused its work toward educating state government executives and legislators on the advantages of integrated regional health systems as a reform strategy. He took time to chair a governor's statewide task force on cost containment and steered their recommendations toward developing integrated health systems within the state. He championed the potential of integrated regional health systems as an acceptable and responsible reform strategy with leadership of the American Hospital Association, the American Medical Association, the American Group Practice Association, the Institute of Medicine and numerous other professional groups.[18] Locally, he began to discuss the vision of regional health systems with business and labor leaders and other provider and insurance executives.

Building a shared vision requires a high level of communication skills within the organization itself. It is more than just explaining. It is advocating and convincing. A cultural change is required. Two key barriers to the full buy-in of a system vision are a lack of understanding of the vision and a reward system that is solely based upon individual or divisional performance and not linked to system performance. A broader understanding can be created only when the system vision is crafted and articulated regularly and with great clarity. Clarity involves making the company objective relevant and understandable to each of the operating division leaders as well as to all employees. Just because the vision makes sense to leaders, doesn't mean it will to workers. A fear of losing their job or position may play a key part in the buy-in process by employees. The visions of complex organizations like Intermountain Health Care and Henry Ford Health System require a stretch. It forces people to develop a broad view of self and the group, to look beyond the immediate, the near, and the expedient.

A key ingredient for developing a shared vision within any organization is for the leaders to be recognized as scrupulously honest and trustworthy. Leaders need to recognize the power of nonverbal communications—or "walk the talk." The vision has to be interpreted by all levels of employees as one that will benefit the organization as well as the customers, rather than just make things easier for the leaders.

Ten Key Steps in Communicating and Developing a Shared Vision

1. Describe the vision
Describe and articulate a vision of the future for the organization. Describe how customers will interact with the organization and what role the employees will play.

2. Identify critical success factors
Identify the key requirements and success factors that are critical to accomplishment of the vision.

3. Advocate the vision
Strongly advocate the reasons why the vision is the right thing to do from a customer perspective and why it is in the best interest of the organization.

4. Interpret the vision
Interpret the vision with easy-to-understand examples and scenarios that illustrate key elements of the vision.

5. Engage in dialogue
Interact with all levels of the organization to present and discuss the vision with employees and to learn about their concerns.

6. Remove barriers
Constantly work on removing the barriers expressed by the employees in accomplishing the vision.

7. Focus on interrelationships
Constantly relate the key initiatives and the work of the organization to the vision.

8. Communicate
Remain the chief spokesperson for the vision and constantly describe it at every opportunity both internally and externally.

9. Recognize milestones
Give periodic updates to the organization with specific accomplishments and presentation of key tasks ahead. Recognize individuals who assist in moving the vision forward.

10. Measure progress
Evaluate the success of the organization by measuring the progress made by the organization toward the vision.

Ability to Create an Organizational
Culture Focused on Customer Service

Improving service is about as difficult a job as a company can undertake, because it means reforming attitudes and practices in nearly every department.

"Companies That Serve You Best,"
Fortune, *December 7, 1987*[19]

Service quality improvement does not happen by accident. It requires and demands professional management and measurement systems. It requires that business decisions be continuously assessed in terms of their impact on quality. It requires a special and deeply ingrained commitment, sustainable over the years.

"The Strategic Management of Service Quality,"
Produced by the Strategic Planning Institute[20]

As discussed earlier in this chapter, an organization's vision is shaped by the leaders' understanding of customers' and the community's needs. The leaders then need to get the organization focused on who these customers are and how to meet their needs. The customers of a health care organization are the patients, families of patients, payers, employees, and the community as a whole. This section focuses on the leadership implications for creating an organizational culture that has its roots in customer service. In subsequent chapters, we will discuss specific tools and techniques to enable the organization to improve customer service.

Leadership and commitment by senior management are crucial to developing a customer service culture in any organization. To develop such a culture, management needs to drive a cultural transformation to place the customer first. Anywhere from five to ten years may be required, even with the full attention and resources of senior management. In the beginning, many employees will be skeptical of the changes and will devise new ways to test the sincerity of management. This is where the leadership of the CEO and senior management is crucial. Senior management must convince employees of the need for change and to accept individual responsibility for implementing change, in order to develop the new culture that measures success by customer satisfaction.

An organization that provides poor customer service suffers in many ways. The first and most apparent result is the loss of revenue when customers switch to competitive products or services. In the past, physicians and hospitals have been insulated from this penalty because patients have been reluctant to switch providers. They have endured poor service and long waiting times or inconvenience. With the emergence of market competition and increased choice due to the excess supply of beds and the growing number of physicians, consumers are increasingly willing to switch providers as well as their insurance carriers. In addition, purchasers are defining the choices for their employees based upon measures like customer satisfaction, access, and cost. In many HMOs the voluntary disenrollment rate exceeds 20 percent a year. A major reason given is poor customer service, including the inability to see a physician in a reasonable time when sick.

The second key loss is the deterioration of the organization's image due to adverse publicity connected with poor service. A study conducted by the White House Office of Consumer Affairs found the following:

- An average business never hears from 86 percent of its unhappy customers. For every complaint received, the average company has 26 customers with problems, 6 of which are serious.
- Of the customers who register a complaint, between 54 and 79 percent will do business with the company again if their complaint is resolved. This figure goes up to a staggering 95 percent if customers feel that the complaint was resolved quickly.
- The average customer who has a problem tells 9 or 10 other people about it.[21]

The third loss is the added cost of recruiting new customers, which may include additional spending for advertising and sales as well as price discounts. The organization also incurs the cost of fixing the problems created by a poor service delivery process. Crosby refers to these costs as the "cost of nonconformance."[22] Examples include the cost of internal failures (e.g., the cost of reinspection, retesting, scrap, rework, repairs, and lost production) and external failures (e.g., legal services, liability, damage claims, replacement, and lost customers). Crosby estimates that nonconformance can account for as much as 25–30 percent of an organization's operating cost.

Lou Gerstner, the new CEO of IBM, summarized his assessment of the lack of customer focus at IBM and its culture after six months on the job as follows:

> I have never seen a company that is so introspective; caught up in its own underwear, so preoccupied with internal processes. . . . People in this company tell me it is easier doing business with people outside the company than inside. I would call that an indictment.[23]

Ten Key Steps in Becoming a Leader Focused on Customer Service

1. Create vision

Leaders develop a clear vision of customer service including underlying values and beliefs. What does excellent customer service mean in your organization?

2. Develop the framework

Leaders develop a customer service framework including customer service guidelines. Guidelines should include acceptable as well as unacceptable behavior toward customers. For example, at the Ritz Carlton, when a customer asks for directions to a meeting room, the acceptable behavior for employees is to escort the guest to the room and not simply point to the room or give directions.

3. Actively listen

Leaders must be actively involved in listening to customers and understanding their requirements. Gail Warden created the function of Business and Labor Relations to strengthen dialogue with these customers. He meets with the CEOs of major customer employers face to face. The purpose of these meetings is to engage in a dialogue and to learn the needs of the customer. In addition, Warden takes time out to talk with patients, including those receiving care in their homes.

4. Promote the concept of internal customers

Leaders must also create an environment of fostering the needs of internal customers. The best way to view the organization is to look at the organization chart upside down. The frontline employees are there to serve the customers. The job of the supervisors is to help the frontline employees do their job by providing coaching and necessary resources. The job of managers is to serve the needs of the supervisors (83).[24]

5. Encourage participation

Leaders create an environment of participation. They encourage employee suggestions for customer service improvement. They make themselves available to listen to employees and remove barriers to customer service. Leaders build interdisciplinary teams to break down barriers between work units. They work on developing a senior management team that is able to work together in a cooperative fashion.

6. Measure results

Leaders encourage development of quantitative measures of changes in customer satisfaction that can be monitored over time. They encourage departments to define key customer service measures and set goals for improvement. They share customer feedback with employees for the purpose of identifying processes to improve. They create urgency in fixing customer-related problems.

7. Train all employees

Leaders focus on improving the skills and abilities of their employees to improve processes and to interact with customers. They invest in training and development of all levels of employees. Leaders actively participate in training as well as improving their own skills.

8. Manage complaints

Leaders create an environment in which prompt attention is paid to resolving customer complaints. Leaders take time out to listen to customer and employee complaints. They use their resources and position to resolve these complaints by focusing the resources of the organization on improving processes whose failures lead to customer complaints.

9. **Communicate**

Leaders spend a great deal of energy communicating with all levels of the organization directly. Besides formal meetings, leaders spend time walking around the organization and interacting with frontline employees. They create situations in which workers feel comfortable discussing their individual concerns as well as those issues facing the organization. Leaders take these opportunities to communicate organizational goals.

10. **Provide recognition and rewards**   .

Leaders freely give credit and recognition to employees for a job well done. They rarely miss an opportunity to recognize an employee for customer service improvements.

Ability to Create an Organization
Capable of Continual Improvement

In the medical profession, experimentation and testing of new concepts and theories have resulted in steady and dramatic improvements since the 1800s. Most of the advances made in clinical care are the result of advances in technology and clinical science—or what may be called "expanded professional knowledge." When the production and service delivery process rely on a single individual, a physician conducting a routine physical, this type of learning is sufficient to produce output of good quality.

But as the process of care comes to involve a team of providers from multiple disciplines, the design and operation of the service delivery process becomes a complex task. The coordination of the work among individuals with differing professional backgrounds becomes the key to success. Additional improvements can be made, when professional knowledge is linked to improvement knowledge. Deming[25] has called this "a system of profound knowledge." Paul Batalden and Patricia Stoltz[26] have expanded on Deming's knowledge for improvement to include the following four elements: knowledge of a system, knowledge of variation, knowledge of psychology, and theory of knowledge.

Knowledge of a System

A health care delivery system consists of a group of people representing different professional backgrounds, multiple processes, materials, and methods who work together to achieve a common purpose. In a complex health care delivery system, the relationship of each of the elements to the common purpose is not direct and, in fact, may seem very remote. For example, the relationship of cleaning a patient room to infection control is not usually clear to a housekeeper unless a leader explains it to him or her. The role of a leader is to effectively communicate the relationship of an individual's work to the common purpose. Batalden and Stoltz[27] suggest that leaders must be able to answer, and help others to answer, three basic questions:

1. Why do we make what we make?
2. How do we make what we make?
3. How do we improve what we make?

"Why do we make what we make?" refers to the aim of the system. To answer this question, you must be able to link the services produced to the defined needs of the customers. In the case of health care services, this means understanding the needs of the patients, families, and payers. It is the role of the leaders to clarify the linkage of an individual's work to the aim of the system.

"How do we make what we make?" refers to the means of production. What are the steps to deliver a given service? Drawing a flow process chart[28] clarifies these steps. Leaders do not produce physical objects, but they do make decisions. Clarifying how strategic plans are made and the role of each level of the organization in the plan, as well as how capital budgets are decided, are some of the tasks that leaders must work on.

"How do we improve what we make?" refers to the process of developing knowledge to improve the current system of delivery. Juran refers to this step as "quality improvement" in his quality trilogy.[29] It is Juran's contention that most organizations pay attention to planning for quality as a new service is designed. Most organizations also put a quality control (assurance) process in place to monitor the performance of specific clinical processes. But very few organizations plan for a systematic way of improving processes.

At Walke-Parker Medical Center, Joe Corrigan, the chief financial officer, observed:

> TQM tools are a way to redesign the operation, to change the processes we use. Walke-Parker always has been efficiently run if you look at the current processes we are using. But we gain improved efficiency by redesigning the process and eliminating rework. Our plan is to try to eliminate specialization. We will go to a much smaller list

of job classifications. For example, we will redesign the process of respiratory therapy to reassign jobs to nurses on the floor.

Peggy Hanford, who holds the dual jobs of chief operating officer and chief nursing officer at Walke-Parker said:

> Managers are beginning to come to grips with the fact that with staff reductions we cannot continue the way we have always done things. They have come to the realization that they have to look at changing how they look at their jobs, how they staff their jobs, what the current processes are, how they can reduce handoffs, and eliminate waste and complexity. In 1988, when we began TQM, we had a chief nursing officer, assistant directors and four coordinators. We have elimintated the jobs of the assistant directors and the coordinators. We now have nurse managers on the unit reporting directly to me.

Knowledge of Variation

Variation is present in almost all health care delivery systems. Understanding variation over time is central to improving the performance of the system. Shewhart[30] suggested that variations can be divided into two categories—chance and assignable. Deming defines "chance variation" as common cause variation, and "assignable variation" as special cause variations. Special cause variations occur due to a specific reason or set of circumstances not usually present in the process; for example, the waiting time in the emergency room is long today because one of the two x-ray machines broke down. Special causes are relatively easy to fix. Removal of special causes makes the process stable. Common cause variation, on the other hand, occurs due to multiple reasons regularly present within the process.

Understanding the two types of variation is critical in improving a process. Each type of variation requires a different type of action. If action is taken under the assumption that a common cause variation is the result of a special cause, one usually makes the process more variable. Batalden and Stoltz[31] give the following illustration: "If the appointment of a VIP patient is mistakenly erased when a computer terminal goes down, setting up a parallel scheduling process is a costly and inappropriate improvement that could very well cause as many errors as it protects against" (430). Most quality experts recommend that action be first taken to remove special cause variation. The next step in improvement is fundamental process change.

The best way leaders can develop knowledge of process variation is to plot quality characteristics of processes over time on a run chart or a control chart. When particular patterns are seen or values fall outside the control limits, there is a high probability that the variation is due to assignable causes. On the other hand, variation within the control limits are due to common causes. Performance of processes with common cause variation can only be improved through fundamental changes in the process. Almost all quality experts recommend that action to make fundamental process change be led by management with input from process knowledgeable workers. Often this means, particularly with processes that cross departmental lines, formation of a team to study the process and to actively make changes to improve the process using a step-by-step methodology known as PDCA—"Plan, Do, Check, Act" (see Chapter 3). The contribution of the leaders may be the insistence on empiricism, celebration of achievements, and focus on the potential of improvements made.

Knowledge of Psychology

The third dimension of improvement knowledge includes the study of human motivation and understanding the process of change. Psychologists and organizational behavior experts have studied this in detail; thousands of papers have been written on the subject. Success in an organization greatly depends upon the abilities of the leaders to motivate the employees to do their best and give the organization their best efforts. There are no foolproof formulas for motivating employees, but a few general guiding principles can be given:

- Most employees want to provide good service but don't know how and may lack the training, the proper equipment, or other resources.
- Every employee is an individual. What may motivate one employee may not motivate another.
- Many factors cause loss of motivation (e.g., poor working conditions, discrimination, inequities in pay). Herzberg[32] calls these factors "dissatisfiers." These factors may diminish motivation, but providing more of them does not provide increased motivation; for example, inequities in pay leads to workers' dissatisfaction but equity in pay does not lead to increased motivation among workers.

Theory of Knowledge

The process of building knowledge and learning is fundamental to continual improvement. A simple method for developing increased knowledge within the organization is to teach workers to design tests of change using a systematic approach or to use process improvement teams, especially cross-functional teams, to work on well-defined projects. Teams can be encouraged to use a process improvement method[33] that includes knowledge building[34] experiments. PDCA is a powerful tool to conduct experiments at the operational level.[35] Using the PDCA cycle allows employees to apply a scientific method to the improvement process.

Batalden and Stoltz[36] have developed a framework for the continued improvement of health care. They have described their framework as follows:

> Transforming a health care organization so that it is capable of continued improvement requires
>
> - development of new knowledge;
> - creation of a leadership policy that fosters a shared sense of purpose and promotes organizational learning;
> - mastery of tools and methods that accelerate improvement of work;
> - application of systematic strategies for building and using knowledge to the process of daily work (424).

Figure 2.3 summarizes their framework. For an organization to make progress and to improve continually, leaders must focus on each of the elements on this table.

Ten Key Steps to Create an Environment of Continual Improvement

1. Educate and train employees

Teach all employees the basic tools of continual improvement. All employees should view their jobs as not only to perform the tasks assigned to them, but also to improve their work processes.

2. Practice

Encourage all employees to use these tools in their own daily work. Leaders should serve as role models of continual improvement by learning, practicing, teaching, and reviewing improvements within the organization.

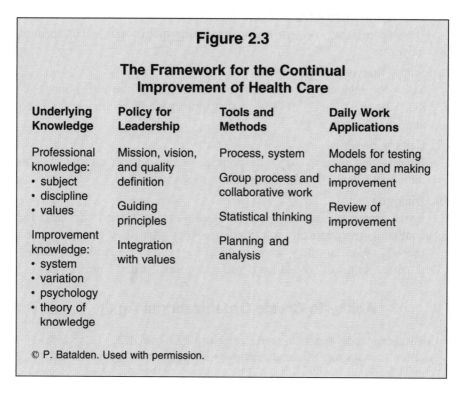

Figure 2.3

The Framework for the Continual Improvement of Health Care

Underlying Knowledge	Policy for Leadership	Tools and Methods	Daily Work Applications
Professional knowledge: • subject • discipline • values	Mission, vision, and quality definition	Process, system Group process and collaborative work	Models for testing change and making improvement
	Guiding principles	Statistical thinking	Review of improvement
Improvement knowledge: • system • variation • psychology • theory of knowledge	Integration with values	Planning and analysis	

© P. Batalden. Used with permission.

3. **Charter teams**

    Charter quality improvement teams to improve specific work processes. Focus the work of these teams on key processes.

4. **Provide recognition**

    Develop an environment in which quality improvement efforts are recognized.

5. **Benchmark**

    Use benchmarking as a strategy to evaluate key processes, adopting the best practices learned from other organizations.

6. **Provide role models**

    Charge senior leadership with responsibility for acting as role models for the organization by participating in quality improvement projects and serving as educators. Leaders should review the progress of teams and help them to move forward by servicing barriers and providing guidance and resources.

7. Develop a quality framework

Develop a framework for quality including quality guidelines for employees.

8. Stress the cost of quality

Stress the relationship of quality to the success of the institution; candidly discuss the cost of poor quality and its effect on the organization and loss of customers.

9. Review policy

Identify and review corporate policies to make them consistent with the corporate framework for quality.

10. Dialogue

Speak frequently to all levels of employees and stress the need for continual improvement. Ask the employees what they have improved recently. What are they working on to improve now? How is it related to customer needs? What have you as leaders learned from customers?

Ability to Create Organizational Agility

Management today has to think like a fighter pilot. When things move so fast, you can't always make the right decision—so you have to learn to adjust, to correct more quickly.

Fred Wiersema (76)[37]

An agile organization is one that can respond quickly to threats as well as to marketplace opportunities. An agile organization knows its current and future customers, the needs of the community, and its own internal process capabilities so well that it can reshape itself very quickly. It knows which process needs to change, how, and to what degree. An agile organization uses each threat as an opportunity to adapt the organization to prepare for the future. At Henry Ford Hospital (the organization that preceded HFHS), Stanley Nelson served as CEO from 1970 to 1988. During this period, he systematically developed a management team and prepared the organization for change. As a result, the culture at Henry Ford Health System has evolved to value versatility and adaptability. Henry Ford was a leader and an early adapter of such ideas as ambulatory care centers, substance abuse treatment facilities, HMOs, Medicare risk contracts, and health care integration. When Gail Warden joined HFHS as its CEO in 1988, he continued the emphasis on change. He initiated the Center for Clinical Effectiveness to focus on outcomes and clinical efficiencies and the Center for Health System

Studies to focus on performance improvement of integrated health systems. He developed a close linkage with Case Western Reserve University to connect medical education and research with the clinical and market-based imperatives and aggressively pursued community hospitals to join HFHS through acquisition, collaboration, or both. He positioned the organization for increased philanthropy and expanded the named chair program as a strategy to recruit good clinical chairs to Henry Ford. Through constant monitoring of the environment and anticipating future changes, both CEOs were able to position their organization for success in a changing market and for the future.

Organizational agility will be the key to success for every corporation in the future. Without agility, responses will be too slow, too late, or just wrong. The pace of change resulting from market and reform pressures will be too fast for any organization that resists change or that takes too long to carry it out.

Developing organizational agility requires an attitude of experimentation. No organization can play it safe, be mistake free, and become agile. Innovation and versatility require organizational leadership to be willing to accept new ideas and failures. It is the job of the leadership to create an environment in which failures are viewed as a means of learning for the future. It is the leadership's responsibility both to permit mistakes as well as to see that the organization does not make the same mistake twice. An agile organization constantly monitors the environment and its competitors to anticipate change and to develop new products and services that will position the organization for the future. Agile organizations create an environment of learning while changing. People within agile organizations learn more than people in organizations that stick to tradition. 3M Corporation has set as a corporate goal that 25 percent of its revenues must come from products that have been introduced in the past five years.[38] By stating its goals in a measurable fashion, the leaders at 3M have sent a clear message within the organization that they value innovation and new product development. At General Electric (GE),[39] Jack Welch took over as CEO in 1981 at a time when GE was already a successful organization. Welch then set a goal of making GE a leaner organization and took 100,000 jobs out of the company in ten years. He set a goal that all company divisions would be number one or two in their industries in profitability and market share or they would be sold. This action forced each division to become customer responsive, lean, and agile.

Examples abound of institutions that have been unable to adapt. In the computer industry, IBM and Digital failed to adapt to the fast moving micro-computer industry and today are still recovering. Not long ago, Compaq Computers was considered a lean, dynamic company, successfully battling IBM. But then the arrival of Dell and Northgate made Compaq look sluggish. In the auto industry, Ford and Chrysler moved in the early 1980s to become lean and agile organizations; GM did not. In the department store business, Sears failed to adapt to upscale merchandising and lost significant market share during the last 20 years. And in health care? In market after market, we can see the penetration of managed care, a trend that many hospitals ignored and are now paying a price for, in terms of lost patient volume. Many failed to adopt strategies to change organizational focus when the paying population moved to the suburbs. Many health care organizations located in cities closed, unable to handle the burden of indigent care with too small a base of paying patients. In Detroit, Henry Ford Hospital invented a survival strategy in 1974 by developing suburban ambulatory care centers in order to balance its patient mix between paying and nonpaying patients.

Agility is more than responsiveness. It is being proactive to introduce change and innovation. It is aggressively selecting the next change, solving the customer's problems before the customer articulates them. It is understanding the organization's customers at such a deep level that the organization can come up with innovative solutions that are customer delights but that the customers have not even thought of yet. What does agility mean in health care? It means reorganizing physicians, developing ambulatory care, downsizing inpatient facilities, developing and using care protocols, preparing the organization for risk contracts, learning the rudiments of insurance, improving customer service—and doing all this while maintaining a community focus. These are not easy tasks. It is the leader's role to actively lead this change process through the development of vision, financial and staff support, encouragement, and education.

Organizational agility can only be developed when the whole organization adopts a continuous learning culture. Garvin[40] has defined a "learning culture" as "an organization skilled at five main activities: systematic problem solving, experimentation with new approaches, learning from their own experiences and past history, learning from the experiences and best practices of others, and transferring knowledge quickly and efficiently throughout the organization" (81).

Ten Key Steps for an Organization to Become Agile

1. Adopt a customer focus

An agile organization anticipates the customer's needs before the customer does. It builds market research capabilities. It monitors the needs of key customers. It understands what customers want. It helps shape their demands and provides solutions.

2. Stretch goals

Leaders must set aggressive targets for performance.

3. Prune costs

Focus on examining low value-added items. Target areas for review and learn to eliminate some of the current activities.

4. Keep staff lean

Keep staff lean and targeted on serving key internal customers.

5. Decentralize

Functionally decentralize and focus the work in operating divisions. Economies of scale is an overrated concept in service industries.

6. Focus on core competencies

Define the core competencies of the organization and build on them.

7. Benchmark

Study core processes and benchmark their performance to industry leaders and key competitors.

8. Reengineer

Focus on reengineering core processes as well as nonperforming processes.

9. Flatten the organization

Take out layers of the organization. Increase the number of personnel reporting to managers from current levels to between 12 and 15.[41]

10. Give rewards

Pay above-average wages in comparison to industry norms; recognize and reward high performers. A lean organization must be tolerant, not punitive, when new ideas do not work. Leaders must work to create a safe environment for risk taking and solving customer problems.

Ability to Improve Employee
Commitment to the Organization

Most employees are sophisticated individuals, who raise families, buy and sell real estate, and design complex activities. But many times these employees are treated like children on the job.

Gordon Dveirin and Kenneth Adams[42]

People don't work just to have a job. Everybody strives for meaning in what they do beyond just a paycheck.

Norman Blake[43]

Consider two health care institutions, A and B. When frontline employees are interviewed in organization A and asked about patients' complaints, they say that they cannot serve the customers because the telephone systems do not work and the supervisors will not give them more resources. Supervisors blame the lack of resources on managers, who in turn blame it on top management. When frontline employees of organization B are interviewed and asked about patients' complaints, they say that they are familiar with the problem and have discussed it with their supervisors. They say that they have formed a process improvement team to study the problem with the help of their supervisors and department heads and hope to solve the problem soon. Which organization has the potential for succeeding? An organization in which employees are engaged in their work and can contribute their knowledge, intelligence, and thinking in a constructive way will have the edge in a competitive environment.

Most employees will not give full commitment to their work unless they feel that they will benefit from doing so. A recent survey[44] revealed that only 13 percent of U.S. workers believe that they will personally benefit from improved company performance, in contrast with 95 percent of Japanese workers who believe they will. A key role of leadership is to help create an environment in which employee goals are aligned with those of the organization.

Fortune magazine publishes an annual list of "America's Most Admired Corporations"[45] and how they earn their winning reputation. One of the eight key factors used in this evaluation is the "ability to attract, develop and keep talented people." Among some of the top companies are Merck, Wal-Mart, 3M, and Levi Strauss. The most admired companies treat their employees exceptionally well, which is both a factor in and a result of their success. They are very mindful of the workers' whole quality of life (e.g., on-site child care), creative needs (e.g., flexible schedules), and so forth. Robert Haas, CEO of Levi Strauss, thinks employee engagement and satisfaction are fundamental to running a strong business: "You have to create an environment where everyone feels like a representative of the company. Unless you have people who know what you stand for and want to make every transaction the best, you are going to stub your toe."

Jan Carlzon, president of Scandinavian Airlines System popularized the concept of "moments of truth." He defined this as any time a customer comes in contact with an employee of the organization in person, by phone, or by fax. In the course of an average day, a service organization encounters thousands of these "moments of truth." In the case of a 500-bed hospital, you can easily imagine thousands of moments of truth every day: A patient calls to make an appointment. A patient waits to see a physician. A patient is x-rayed. A nurse gives a shot. A physical therapist teaches a patient new exercises. A patient may come in contact with 500 moments of truth, and if just one of these encounters is with a rude employee, the patient leaves the institution with a bad impression. The key to success in the health care industry, therefore, is to constantly work with all employees to help make each encounter a positive patient experience.

At Henry Ford Health System, focus groups are conducted on a regular basis with frontline employees to understand how customer services can be improved. The responses of the frontline workers match the concern expressed by the patients in the patient satisfaction surveys. The key question then is, How do you improve employee commitment to the organization? An important way is to remove the barriers encountered by employees in their daily work. The concepts are easy to understand, but not easy to implement; commitment and trust are built only over a long period of time.

Another important way to increase employee commitment is to have a continual dialogue with them about what they perceive as customer expectations, and how they believe that these expectations can be met. A one-time training or exposure is not enough. Continual coaching by supervisors and managers is the key to success. Behavior changes and skill development take constant practice. Positive reinforcement is also an important catalyst in improving employee commitment. Recognition is a reward in itself. If a frontline worker asks a question, will he or she get a constructive answer? It is the denials, brush-offs, and evasions that destroy morale and commitments. Leaders have a role in reducing fear and increasing feedback.

Motorola made a major turnaround that it attributed to training and retraining its workers.[46] The company spent $120 million (3.6 percent of payroll) on education and training in 1992 and calculates that every $1 spent on training delivers $30 in productivity gains. Motorola University delivered 102,000 days of training to employees and suppliers in 1992 and concedes that there is heavy up-front cost in training but that the payback is impressive.

Organizational commitment and loyalty are key factors in creating a mutually beneficial working environment. In a recent survey,[47] 87 percent of the readers of an industrial trade journal said that there is generally less company loyalty than five years ago, and only 12 percent said there is more. For the same period, 77 percent said that their company is less loyal to them, and only 21 percent said that the company is more loyal to them. Most employees in such an environment take an attitude that they are temporary. They admit that they are not working as hard as they could, and they no longer think that there is an explicit or implicit social contract between them and their employers. It has been estimated that with a full-court press, an organization needs one year for every layer of management to develop an employee commitment. Most organizations develop slogans like "People are our greatest asset," but they do not back it up with any action. Leaders can ensure progress only if they are willing to spend the time. Some techniques to consider to build the commitment of employees include education and training, improving skills of employees, listening to workers' concerns, removing barriers from employees' work activities, and participating in process improvement teams. At HFHS, quality management education is used as a mechanism for building employee skills. At the same time, employees are pleased that the organization is investing in them, and they get a greater sense of self-esteem and loyalty because they think that the organization values them. In addition, they enjoy learning and networking with their peers. Key questions to ask include, Suppose frontline employees encounter a customer problem—will they be able to solve it? Will they know where and when to get help? Are processes designed to enable the employees to serve the customer? So, what fosters the loyalty and commitment of employees? Honest and open communications, the chance to be part of a decision-making process, and the ability to better themselves and be recognized in front of their peers.

**Ten Key Steps to Improve Employee
Commitment to the Organization**

1. **Create a shared vision**

   Employees participate in a dialogue to create a shared vision. Leaders regularly involve employees in deciding how to achieve the organizational vision. The questions each employee must ask are, Does the vision statement makes sense? How does it relate to my work? How will it help my patients?

2. **Foster empowerment**

   Employees have a clearly established level of resource control that allows them to exercise judgment in improving processes and service to customers. Their questions get answered and their ideas are heard.

3. **Conduct education and training**

   A continual process of employee training and education is conducted to improve skills and to develop self confidence. People need and value the skills to do the job well and opportunities to continue to grow and learn new skills.

4. **Provide feedback**

   Employees are given continual feedback on their individual performance, as well as their team and company performance, especially on customer service measures.

5. **Generate trust**

   Leadership creates an environment of trust among the employees and the leadership. It constantly clarifies for employees how they are going to deal with issues that confront the welfare of the employees as well as of the organization.

6. **Offer preferences for promotion**

   Employees are given preference for promotions before recruiting from the outside. Employees are given opportunities to improve their skills in order to move up within the organization.

7. **Charter teams**

   Management relies on teams to improve key processes and to encourage cross-functional problem solving.

8. **Improve recruitment**

   The right people are hired, matching the skills and values of the employee to the organization.

9. Give recognition

Employees are given recognition for a job well done in front of their peers and their families.

10. Promote rewards

Employees have a clear signal that they will benefit from the success of the organization. Gain sharing or employee stock ownership plans are encouraged.

Ability to Focus and Produce Results

It is wonderful how much is done in a short space, provided we set about it properly, and give our minds wholly to it.

William Hazlitt[48]

Leaders are results oriented. The six essential abilities discussed above are necessary building blocks for success. Leaders create a process for developing these abilities within the organization, together with well-defined goals and objectives to create the urgency for change and focus essential to move the organization. In 1987, Motorola set a stretch goal for 1992 of 6 σ quality, or less than 3 defective parts per million. (Motorola called its Quality Initiative 6 σ goal where 6 standard deviations at or less than 3 defectives per 1 million parts.) For the next five years, Motorola initiated education programs and project teams all focused on achieving this goal and reached its target.

Leaders take long-term goals and translate them into short-term specific objectives that employees can focus on and use as measures to gauge their performance. Leaders communicate these objectives clearly throughout the organization, and they empower and inspire management and employees to accomplish the objectives. Leaders define specific objectives and then make sure that they provide the resources, coaching, and inspiration necessary to accomplish them.

It is the role of leadership to focus the organizational improvement effort on major processes of the organization. It is easy for employees to drift into improvement projects that are nonstrategic, although requiring improvement (e.g., parking, the cafeteria). It is critical that leaders communicate—using organizational management processes like planning, budgeting, and operational reviews—major objectives in specific terms. Operational initiatives must be linked to these strategic terms. As an example, at Henry Ford Health System, Gail Warden set access improvement as a key initiative for the organization for 1993. Each of the operating divisions was asked to clearly outline what initiatives they planned to take to improve patient access. The Henry Ford Medical Group included in its 1993–1995 three-year strategic plan a number of initiatives: recruitment of additional physicians; major changes in the phone system for appointment making; installation of a nurse call system in every region; reengineering of the primary care physician delivery system; and an access innovation fund by which physicians, managers, and employees submitted innovative ideas for pilot testing. Ten projects were funded in 1993. Other divisions, including the Metro Medical Group and the Health Alliance Plan (HMO division), had similar initiatives to address this key area for improvement.

Charles Christiansen, CEO of Walke-Parker Medical Center, when asked about his role as chief executive, said:

> My role is a strategist. My job is to make sure that the proper framework is in place in the organization and to help everybody understand their role in the strategic vision of the organization. It is my job to put pressure points and celebration support points in place, and to remove as much variability in pursuit of the strategic vision as possible. I must make sure that the strategic vision is understood and shared. You, as a leader, have to know what you want to happen in terms of the specific measures that are displayed on a chart we call the "radar chart." This is our strategic vision expressed in a measurable way. We identify what measures are needed to achieve the vision. We then try to identify what the "drivers" are that will make it happen, and what the "inhibitors" are that will prevent us as an organization from reaching our vision. Drivers include not only the specific measures we need to improve, but also the system changes like our new merit pay system that will affect outcomes. In 1993 we abandoned all individual merit increases in favor of a system of group pay incentives based upon overall quality scores and cost per statistic. Then we look at the employee education we need. Last, we monitor what we do. We celebrate when we make our goals and develop an action plan when we are falling behind.

Leaders have an uncanny knack for producing results. In a recent article, Schaffer and Thompson[49] argue that successful change programs begin with the clear articulation of results: "Most corporate change programs mistake means for ends, and process for outcome. The solution: focus on results, not activities." Schaffer and Thompson's warning is very timely.

Boards of directors hire CEOs to accomplish results. If the organization is showing operating losses, the board will be interested in hearing the initiatives being taken to turn the organization around, but ultimately the leadership of the CEO will be questioned if these initiatives do not produce results. Remember the changes in CEOs made by the boards at such companies as GM, Kodak, and IBM after several years of unacceptable results.

Achieving results requires not only an ability to think strategically, but also an ability to focus on and execute the strategy. It requires all of the abilities that have been discussed above: creating the vision, communicating and developing a shared vision, being clear about the needs of customers and the community for the vision to be achieved, building the capabilities for continued improvement, keeping the organization lean and agile, having employees committed to the organization. All are necessary for results. What's more, the leader needs to keep the focus on what the organization must achieve by continually articulating the improvement priorities in terms that people understand, and to work on removing barriers. Focus requires undivided attention to details and a comprehension of barriers and facilitators to implement the strategies. Achieving results requires a clear focus on organizational energy and a concentration of resources on the critical details that will allow it to implement the change. It is easy to get sidetracked by unrelated activities. No organization has unlimited resources to do everything. It is the role of leaders to focus the organization, its resources, and its people on a few key results that are necessary for success.

Ten Key Steps to Create Focus and Produce Results

1. Define organizational vision
Develop and articulate a vision for the organization.

2. Define specific objectives
Define specific objectives that will allow the organization to achieve the vision. Further define the objectives and describe them in short-term accomplishments.

3. Define critical processes
Identify core processes that need improvement.

4. Identify process owners
Identify core process owners who will be responsible for leading the necessary improvements. Do you have the right talent?

5. Identify process improvements

Identify improvements for implementation. Provide key resources to facilitate implementation.

6. Educate and train

Educate and train employees in new methods and processes.

7. Identify barriers and facilitators

Identify barriers and facilitators to accomplishing the objectives. What resources would be necessary? Are organizational changes necessary? Are certain groups within the organization not cooperating?

8. Communicate the objectives

Speak out and look for opportunities within the organization to share the vision and specific objectives.

9. Measure progress

Measure progress toward key objectives and identify the gap between the objectives and the current performance. Keep all employees apprised of progress made toward the objectives.

10. Provide recognition and rewards

Identify individuals and teams for recognition as specific accomplishments are achieved.

Conclusions

During the next decade, health care organizations across the country will face significant pressures to improve the quality of their services while reducing the rate of cost increases. Under various health care reform scenarios, the political leadership of this country is focused on reducing annual expenditure increases in health care experienced in the past decade, from the current 12–15 percent, to a number close to the consumer price index (3.5 percent in 1993). Many businesses are not satisfied with this reduction. They want total expenditures to decrease, and not just the rate of increases to decline. In Detroit, the three major auto manufacturers asked their major health care suppliers to roll back the health care expenditures for their companies in 1994 by 10 percent from 1993 levels.

Total quality management has been implemented successfully by many organizations—3M, Xerox, Motorola, and Federal Express, just to name a few—as an effective tool to manage productivity and to cut operational costs. However, it is likely that TQM by itself will not be sufficient for the health care industry to face the magnitude of change required to survive in the coming decade. Just as the auto industry had to adapt the practice of lean manufacturing, the health care industry will need bolder steps to survive. Incremental process improvement as a tool for managing productivity and reducing operational costs cannot alone produce changes of sufficient magnitude in the time required. Bold leadership, focused on creating an agile and lean organization driven by customer knowledge, will be essential.

The change required for survival can only be accomplished with a determined and focused leadership effort, one that is determined to take the fat out of the organization and to create a culture of a lean organization focused on the needs of the customer. This chapter has discussed seven key skills that the health care leadership must develop to be successful in the next decade.

Health care delivery is at a crossroads in this country. Old ways are exhausted and can't help meet customer demands or competition. Like every other industry, health care has to prepare itself for a transformation. In 1933, Franklin Roosevelt said in his inaugural address, "This generation of Americans have a rendezvous with destiny." We believe that the current health care leaders have a rendezvous with destiny. Health care expenditures cannot keep rising at the current rate. Health care leaders have the opportunity and the moral responsibility to lead in the restructuring of the industry.

In the following chapters, we will describe some of the management technology that is necessary to support the kind of radical change that is required. All these processes and methods depend upon leadership to get started and to keep them on track.

Notes

1. Womack, J. P., D. T. Jones, and D. Roos. 1990. *The Machine That Changed the World*. New York: Macmillan.
2. Zaleznik, A. 1977. "Managers and Leaders: Are They Different?" *Harvard Business Review* 55 (May–June): 67–78.
3. Kotter, J. P. 1990. "What Leaders Really Do." *Harvard Business Review* 68 (May–June): 3–11.
4. Robert, M. 1993. "The CEO's Vision: The Starting Point of Strategic Thinking." *The Strategist* 4 (4): 5–9.
5. Campbell, A., and L. L. Nash. 1992. *A Sense of Mission*. Reading, MA: Addison Wesley.
6. Robert, M. 1993. *Strategy Pure and Simple: How Winning CEO's Outhink Their Competition*. New York: McGraw Hill.
7. Ibid.

8. Parker, M. 1990. *Creating Shared Visions*. Clarendon Hills, IL: Dialog International.

9. Senge, P. 1990. *The Fifth Discipline: The Art and Practice of the Learning Organization*. New York: Doubleday/Currency.

10. Ibid.

11. Sahney, V. K., and G. L. Warden. 1991. "The Quest for Quality and Productivity in Health Services." *Frontiers of Health Services Management* 7 (4): 2–40.

12. Sahney, V. K., and G. L. Warden. 1993. "The Role of CQI in Strategic Planning." *Quality Management in Health Care* 1 (4): 1–11.

13. Henry Ford Health Care Corporation Board of Trustees. 1989. *Governance Recommendations*.

14. Sahney and Warden, "The Role of CQI."

15. Shortell, S. M., D. A. Anderson, R. R. Gillies, J. B. Mitchell, and K. L. Morgan. 1993. "The Holographic Organization." *Health Care Forum Journal* 30 (2): 20–26.

16. Nerenz, D. R., B. M. Zajac, and H. S. Rosman. 1993. "Consortium Research on Indicators of System Performance (CRISP)." *Joint Commission Journal on Quality Improvement* 19 (12): 566–75.

17. Rauber, C. 1993. "Getting a Jump on the 21st Century." *Healthcare Forum Journal* 36 (1): 74–78.

18. *Hospitals and Health Networks*. 1993. "The AHA's New Chairman-Elect Designate: Gail Warden." 67 (5 August): 30–37.

19. *Fortune*. 1987. "Companies that Serve You Best." (7 December): 44–47, 53.

20. Clemmer, J. 1990. *Firing on All Cylinders*. Toronto: MacMillan of Canada.

21. Albrect, C., and R. Zemke. 1985. *Service America*. Homewood, IL: Down-Jones-Irwin.

22. Crosby, P. B. 1979. *Quality Is Free: The Art of Making Quality Certain*. New York: NAL Penguin.

23. *Business Week*. 1993. "Rethinking IBM." (4 October): 87–96.

24. Clemmer, *Firing on All Cylinders*.

25. Deming, W. E. 1993. *The New Economics for Industry, Government, Education*. Cambridge: Massachusetts Institute of Technology Center for Advanced Engineering Study.

26. Batalden, P. B., and P. K. Stoltz. 1993. "A Framework for the Continual Improvement of Health Care: Building and Applying Professional and Improvement Knowledge to Test Changes in Daily Work." *Joint Commission Journal on Quality Improvement* 19 (October): 424–52.

27. Ibid.

28. Freedman, D. H. 1992. "Is Management Still a Science?" *Harvard Business Review* (November–December): 26–38.

29. Juran, J. 1988. *Quality Control Handbook*. New York: McGraw Hill.

30. Shewhart, W. A. 1939. *Statistical Method from the Viewpoint of Quality Control*. Washington, DC: Graduate School of the U.S. Department of Agriculture. Reprinted by Dover, 1986.
31. Batalden and Stolz, "A Framework for Continual Improvement."
32. Herzberg, F. M. 1968. "One More Time: How Do You Motivate Employees?" *Harvard Business Review* (January–February). Reprinted 1987, *Harvard Business Review* 65 (5): 109–20.
33. Garvin, D. A. 1993. "Building a Learning Organization." *Harvard Business Review* 71 (4): 78–91.
34. James, B. C. 1989. *Quality Management for Health Care Delivery*. Chicago: Hospital Research and Educational Trust.
35. Ibid.
36. Batalden and Stolz, "A Framework for Continual Improvement."
37. Stewart, T. A. 1993. "Welcome to the Revolution." *Fortune* (13 December): 66–68.
38. Mitsch, R. A. 1990. "Three Roads to Innovation." *Journal of Business Strategy* (September–October): 18–21.
39. Beckham, J. D. 1993. "The Merits of Intentional Scarcity." *Healthcare Forum Journal* 36 (4): 56–61.
40. Garvin, "Building a Learning Organization."
41. Beckham, "The Merits of Intentional Scarcity."
42. Dveirin, G. F., and K. Adams. 1993. "Empowering Health Care Improvement: An Operational Model." *Joint Commission Journal on Quality Improvement* 19 (7): 222–32.
43. *Chief Executive*. 1992. "Getting to Team." (April): 44–58.
44. Ibid.
45. Reese, J. 1993. "America's Most Admired Corporations." *Fortune* (March): 62–75.
46. Henkoff, R. 1993. "Companies that Train Best." *Fortune* (March): 62–75.
47. Moskal, B. 1993. "Company Loyalty Dies, A Victim of Neglect." *Industry Week* (March): 11–12.
48. Hickman, C. R., and M. A. Silva. 1984. *Creative Excellence: Managing Corporate Culture, Strategy, and Change in the New Age*. New York: New American Library.
49. Schaffer, R. H., and H. A. Thomson. 1992. "Successful Change Programs Begin with Results." *Harvard Business Review* (January–February): 80–89.

3

Customer-Focused Clinical Care

A test result lost, a specialist who cannot be reached, a missing requisition, a misinterpreted order, duplicate paperwork, a vanished record, a long wait for the CT scan, an unreliable on-call system—these are all-too-familiar examples of waste, rework, complexity, and error in the doctor's daily life. . . . For the average doctor, quality fails when systems fail.

Donald Berwick[1]

Hospitals and other health care organizations are no different from their manufacturing counterparts when it comes to organizational structure. Almost all health care organizations are organized functionally. This vertical organization with authority and responsibility flowing up and down (Figure 3.1) creates chimneys that act as barriers for information flow and cooperation across the boundaries. The leaders of these chimneys are usually more concerned with protecting their territory than the quality of the aggregate experience—patient care—as a patient travels from one department to another.

Consider the traditional approach to a basic routine process in every hospital, the admission of an elective patient. In many hospitals, in the case of an elective surgery, the process might go like this: Physician and patient agree that the patient is going to be admitted. The patient is given an admitting order and stops at the desk of the physician's secretary, who calls the operating room and gets a surgical time that fits the schedule of both the patient and the physician. The secretary then calls the hospital admitting department for a room. If no room is available, the secretary must call

Figure 3.1

Traditional Chain of Command for Clinical Services

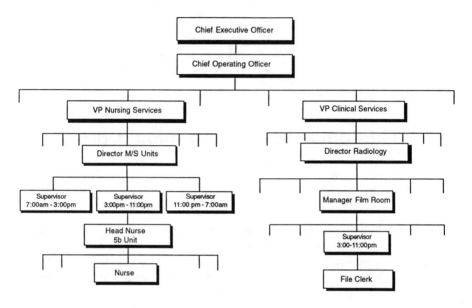

the operating room again to reschedule the surgery on an alternate date. Once the room and surgical time are fixed, the patient is asked to call the business office at the hospital to provide preadmission information, including insurance information, and receive instructions for preadmission testing. On the day of admission, the patient is asked to come in at 11 a.m. for preadmission testing. The patient finishes the routine tests and arrives at the admitting office by 12:30 p.m. In most cases the patient waits for one to four hours to be taken to a room. The usual reason for the delay is that rooms are unavailable because physicians did not promptly write discharge orders for patients who were supposed to leave, sometimes because diagnostic testing results were delayed in transit. Other reasons for the delay could include rooms left uncleaned because housekeeping was busy elsewhere or the failure of the unit clerk on the floor to inform admitting that the room was ready, thus postponing the admission workup to the afternoon shift. This simple routine process, still carried out many times each day in every hospital, shows how responsibility is diffused in the typical organizational structure. Each department—admitting office, business office, housekeeping, nursing, operating room, discharge planning, physicians, and others—is a chimney, responsible for its own small portion of a series of tasks. No one department is in charge of the process from beginning to end. There is no one to measure or to know that the results of all the small failures in the interdependent system are not a summative function. Rather, the failure of the system's performance is a product of the performance of each part multiplied by the performance of each other part. Workers are often more concerned about protecting themselves from additional work than about working together to improve the process. Leaders often rely on financial measures alone to understand the organization's work. Patient wait and inconvenience usually is the department's last concern. It is rare to find a hospital that routinely monitors defined quality measures for this process. Empty beds made available by 50–70 percent occupancy rates have reduced waiting times and solved this process management problem for many hospitals. Other institutions, however, have formed quality management teams to reduce waiting times through process improvement. A University of Michigan Hospital team reduced the average wait time for patients by more than 80 percent, from more than 125 minutes to less than 24 minutes[2] (433).

Examining the Process through the Eyes of the Customer

Many industrial organizations have changed their organizational structure from vertical chimneys to a horizontal structure that recognizes the interdependencies of the "parts" and to renew the focus on the needs of the customer and to study and improve processes. These changes involve identifying key processes within the organization and assigning responsibility to improve and monitor the performance of the processes to individuals and clearly defined teams.

Ryder System[3] recently converted its "purchasing a vehicle for leasing" process from the traditional departmental organization to a new horizontal model. In the old process, purchasing a vehicle for leasing required 14 to 17 handoffs of a document that wended its way from one functional department to another, first at a local and then a national level. By viewing this paperwork flow from purchasing the vehicle to providing it to a customer as a single process, Ryder has reduced the handoffs to two and cut its purchasing cycle time by one-third, to less than four months.

AT&T Network Systems Division has reorganized into 13 core processes, each with an owner and a champion.[4] The owner's job is to focus on the day-to-day operations of a process. The champion ensures that the process is linked with overall business strategies and goals.

At Kodak, direct responsibility for 15,000 employees producing 7,000 different black and white products rests with a single team, which has named itself the "Zebra Team."[5] The team has defined its mission as "to produce high-quality products that can delight their customers." The Zebra Team has further specified performance objectives in the areas of cycle time, work-in-process inventory, total production costs, on-time deliveries, and customer satisfaction. The Zebra Team regards its job as building capabilities and teamwork among members and removing obstacles or resolving handoff issues.

The literature includes a number of examples of health care organizations that have used horizontal process–focused teams to improve outcomes and patient satisfaction while simultaneously lowering cost by reducing waste, duplication and error. Dartmouth Hitchcock Medical Center is a member of the Northern New England Cardiovascular Group, a consortium of five organizations that have reduced the regional mortality rate for bypass surgery from 6 to 3 percent by examining the complete process for treatment of cardiovascular surgical patients.[6] "At first, we brought the mortality rate down primarily by studying it," says William Nugent, M.D., chairman of the Medical Center's cardiothoracic surgery. "Once we knew the mortality rate, we could start learning more about the system that produced it. In doing that, we put together a critical path. Then we tried to look at cost and utilization and how we could be more efficient in terms of the care we provided" (10).[7] The overall length of stay has dropped from 9.9 days to 7.1 days. Fully 97 percent of elective surgery patients are admitted to the hospital on the morning of the surgery. Patients often are operated on within 45 minutes of the admission. Using focus groups, Nugent identified as patients' key concerns the following concepts: caring, comfort, certainty, convenience, communications, and cost. These six concepts now provide the framework for the organization's improvement efforts in other patient care areas.

In another hospital, a quality improvement team focused on eliminating waste in major joint replacement procedures. A main reason for an average ten-day length of stay was found to be scheduling conflicts because major tests, rehabilitation therapy, and posthospitalization care had not been scheduled in advance of the hospital admission. Through process improvements and preadmission coordination of major tests, rehabilitation therapy, and posthospital care, length of stay was reduced from ten to five days.[8] Examining the process from a patient's view, and not just as a surgical process, allowed the team to see all aspects of the process, including preadmission activities, inpatient activities, and postadmission activities, as part of a single process.

At Henry Ford Hospital, a cross-functional team consisting of medical oncologists, nurses, management services analysts, and home health care personnel examined the inpatient chemotherapy process.[9] It studied approximately 200 of the hospital's patients treated with a high dose of cisplatin, a drug that attacks tumors of the lungs and neck. The two major side-effects of this drug are severe damage to the kidneys and vomiting. To reduce these effects, patients are asked to drink large amounts of fluids before the drug is administered. A typical patient undergoing this treatment spends three to four days in the hospital for the complete treatment, including hydration and follow-up laboratory tests. The team documented every step of the process using flow charts. In its study, the team found that the hospital stay could be reduced by two days if the patient drank the required fluids at home before entering the hospital and if laboratory test times were changed to meet the needs of the patient. The project team developed patient eligibility criteria for patients who could hydrate at home, wrote instructions for patients and family members, educated the nursing staff to teach patients pretreatment care routines, set up outpatient follow-up care, and analyzed the potential financial effect. Through proper study and understanding of the customer needs, the team was able to introduce the changes and reduce patient stays to less than two days (18).[10]

Process Improvement

A "process" can be defined as the activities carried out to transform inputs (workforce skills, financial entitlements, knowledge, supplies, methods, equipment) into outputs (products, services). This transformation adds value in one of three aspects—time, place, or form.[11] Time value is added when something is available when needed (e.g., a presurgical test result is available to the surgeon just prior to the surgery). Place value is created when something is available where it is needed (e.g., a sterilized instrument is available to the surgeon on an OR cart in the operating room). Form value is created when something is available in the form it is needed (e.g., patient medication is available in measured doses). A "process" can then be defined as a grouping of all tasks in sequence, directed at accomplishing one particular outcome.[12] A central theme of continuous quality improvement (CQI) is to define the processes used to produce a service and to focus on improving the quality of services by improving the performance of the processes. Joiner[13] has identified six sources of problems in a process:

1. Inadequate knowledge of how a process does work
2. Inadequate knowledge of how a process should work
3. Errors and mistakes in executing the procedures
4. Current practices that fail to recognize the need for preventive measures
5. Unnecessary steps, inventory buffers, and wasteful measures
6. Variation in inputs and outputs.

"Process improvement," then, is defined as "the continuous endeavor to learn about the cause-and-effect mechanisms in a process to change the process to reduce variation and complexity and improve customer satisfaction."[14] Many different process improvement methodologies have been reported in the literature; two are summarized in Figure 3.2. Each attempts to introduce an orderly way by which a team of employees can work together step by step to improve any process.

These process improvement methodologies have also introduced the scientific process of an orderly exploration for improvement. Almost all of the methodologies for process improvement end with a variant of the Plan-Do-Check-Act (PDCA) cycle. The PDCA cycle allows a process improvement team to plan a change, make the change, and test whether it leads to improvement. If it leads to improvement, the final step is to plan how to hold the gains made. It is important for every organization to pick a methodology for process improvement and to train all employees in the use of the methodology so that all employees speak the same language. Training in the use of the same process improvement methodology will accelerate the work of teams as they struggle to improve processes. It will reduce the arguments as to how to proceed and what steps to take first that are commonly observed when a group is put together to improve a process.

Shewhart[15] and later Deming[16] introduced a very important concept for process improvement, the two types of variation observed in the outcome of a process. Deming labeled the first type of variation as *common cause* variation—the variation inherent in the process at all times, day after day. Common cause variation is typically due to the interaction of a large number

Figure 3.2

Process Improvement Methodologies

Hospital Corporation of America

FOCUS-PDCA

1. **F**ind a process to improve

2. **O**rganize a team that knows the process

3. **C**larify current knowledge of the process

4. **U**nderstand causes of process variation

5. **S**elect the process improvement

6. **P**lan improvement and data collection

7. **D**o improvement, data collection, and data analysis

8. **C**heck data for process improvement, customer outcome, and lessons learned

9. **A**ct to hold gain, to reconsider owner, and to continue improvement

Joiner Associates Consulting Group

Five Stage Plan for Process Improvement

1. Understand the process
   - describe the process
   - identify customer needs and concerns
   - develop standard process

2. Error-proof the process

3. Streamline the process

4. Reduce variation
   - reduce variation in measurement systems
   - bring the measurement process under statistical control
   - reduce variation in the process
   - bring the process under statistical control

5. Plan for continuous improvement
   - plan for monitoring of changes
   - do the monitoring
   - check the results
   - act to make improvement continuous

Sources: Batalden, P. B., and P. K. Stoltz, "A Framework for Continual Improvement of Health Care," *Joint Commission Journal on Quality Improvement* 19 (October 1993): 424–52; Scholtes, P. R., *The Team Handbook*, Madison, WI: Joiner Associates, 1992.

of small sources of variation. These small variations can add up to cause large variations observed in the process. The second type of variation is called *special cause* variation—the variation not part of the process all the time. Special cause variation arises due to a specific event—for example, one of three emergency room physicians calls in sick, thus leading to

Figure 3.3 Ten Secrets of Managing Care for Improved Value

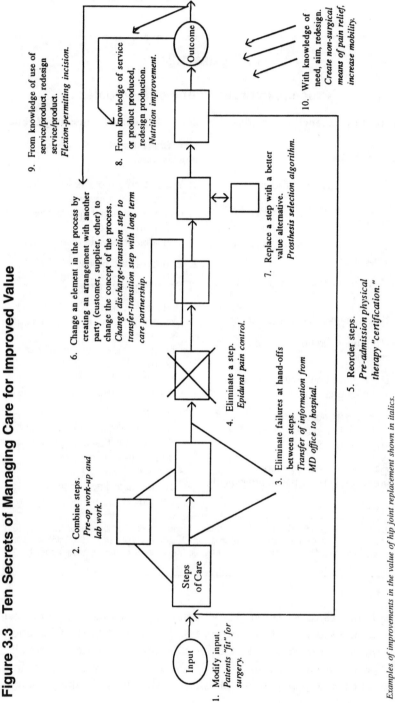

Examples of improvements in the value of hip joint replacement shown in italics.

© P. Batalden. Used with permission.

long waiting times for patients in the emergency room. Addressing each cause of variation requires different approaches. For process improvement it is important to remove the special causes first. Once the special causes are removed, the process is called a "stable process." The performance of stable processes can be predicted. The capabilities of a stable process can be measured and compared to customer requirements. If the customer requirements are not met, this will prompt a process improvement strategy.

The first step is to identify areas for improvement. Some of the areas that may need improvement and provide opportunities include the following:

- Knowledge of customer needs
- Root causes of the problem
- Areas of delay
- Areas of unnecessary movement and transportation
- Handoffs between areas
- Appropriate skills needed versus those available.

Some of the methods for improving a process are the following (see Figure 3.3):

- Combining steps
- Developing a standard process
- Developing methods to prevent commonly occurring mistakes in the process including training and building foolproof methods into the process
- Streamlining a process by eliminating unnecessary steps, reducing inventory
- Eliminating causes of variation in the process
- Redesigning the process and reassigning responsibilities to eliminate handoffs
- Reordering
- Eliminating steps.

Batalden[17] and his colleagues have illustrated the use of many of these strategies using hip-joint replacement as a model (see Figure 3.3). Examining the clinical processes in any medical center, it is clear that much opportunity lies ahead in improving processes and reducing the costs incurred when things are not done correctly. These are Secrets 2, 3, 5, and

Figure 3.4

Framework for Customer-Focused Process Improvement

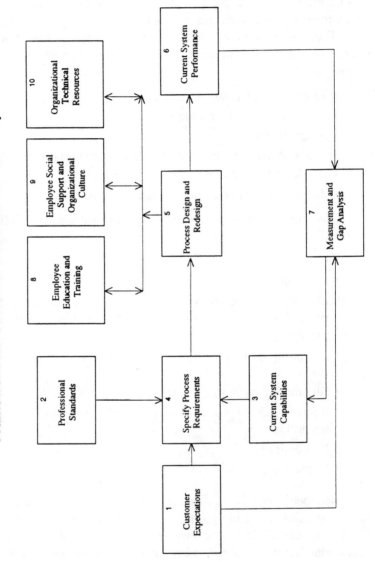

sometimes 4, shown in Figure 3.3, where nonmedical systems fail, leading to redundancy and waste. There are many examples of waste in the process of health care delivery: physicians keeping duplicate copies of medical records because they cannot be certain that medical records will be available on time when they are ready to see their patients; x-rays retaken because the patient was not positioned correctly; surgery delayed because presurgical clearance is not available; and physicians ordering a test "stat" because they want to get test results back on time. In one hospital, the postsurgical wound infection rate was found to be 8 percent while the national average was 3 percent. Patients with infection ended up being readmitted and remained in the hospital for an average of six days. For each patient admitted, the cost of poor quality added $10,000. Only by systematic study and examination of the process can we improve the performance of the system.

The second area for process improvement is in unnecessary variation in clinical practice, Secrets 6 to 10 of Figure 3.3. Physicians are trained in many different medical schools and residency programs, and receive training under many different mentors. The empirical, scientific knowledge underpinning daily clinical care is very limited. As a result, it is not unusual to find a high degree of variation in clinical care even among physicians practicing in the same hospital. Process improvement methodologies give us a scientific method by which we can pool together the wisdom and knowledge of a group of care providers and by which we can build new knowledge to develop improved and new processes. Clinical process improvement holds great opportunities for improving both quality and cost-effectiveness of care.

Conceptual Framework for Customer-Focused Process Improvement

Figure 3.4 presents a conceptual framework for customer-focused process improvement in a health care organization. This process is illustrated with an example of the experience of a patient in an ambulatory clinic. The simplified flow diagram is shown in Figure 3.5.

Customer Expectations

The first step in any process improvement is to understand customer expectations. It is important to define the customers of the process under study. For most processes there are multiple customers, and the expectations of

Figure 3.5

Key Components for an Ambulatory Care Encounter

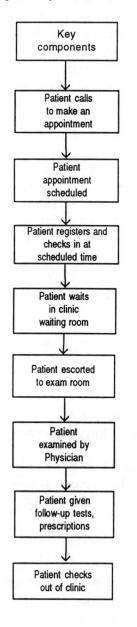

| Key components | • Possible process improvements |

Patient calls to make an appointment
- Sufficient phone lines
- Sufficient staffing
- Appropriate patient triaging

Patient appointment scheduled
- Appointment availability
- Physician schedules
- Telephone etiquette

Patient registers and checks in at scheduled time
- Patient registration system
- Medical records availability
- Patient greeting

Patient waits in clinic waiting room
- Keeping patient informed of delays
- Patient education

Patient escorted to exam room
- Clear patient instructions
- Patient greeting

Patient examined by Physician
- Examination and History taking
- Answering patient questions
- Clarity of patient follow-up instructions

Patient given follow-up tests, prescriptions
- Scheduling follow-up tests
- information for tests

Patient checks out of clinic
- Scheduling follow-up
- Payment collection

each group of customers must be documented. For example, patients who call for appointments want to see their physician relatively soon. But a customer calling to make a routine physical appointment has expectations that are very different from a patient calling because he or she is ill. In the first case, the patient may be willing to wait two weeks. In the second case, the patient expects to be seen the same day. Segmenting the patients and defining the requirements of each group will help to identify process improvements and means to better design the process and meet patient expectations.

Professional Standards

The second step is to clearly understand the professional clinical standards. Physicians may have set a standard that requires a patient complaining of a head injury to be seen by a physician immediately. Similarly, patients coming for a complete physical may be required to fast for 12 hours before certain tests.

Current System Capabilities

The next step is to understand and define the capabilities of the current system. For example, does the appointment system allow the staff of one clinic to book appointments in another? Can the appointment system be queried to find the first open appointment on a Wednesday? How early are the appointment calendars made available (e.g., 60 days, 90 days).

Specification of Process Requirements

Based on a knowledge of customer requirements, professional standards, and current system capabilities, the key process requirements must be specified. For example, patients calling in ill will be given an appointment with a physician within 24 hours, or the appointment calendars of all physicians will be available for appointments at least 90 days in advance, or 95 percent of the patients will wait less than 15 minutes in the clinic to see their physicians. Specifying process requirements depends on the process of balancing customer needs with current system capabilities while being cognizant of professional standards.

Process Design and Redesign

The process is designed and redesigned to meet customer specifications. This design and redesign process is the focus of the CQI process. Figure 3.5

shows a list of associated process improvements to improve each of the steps in the ambulatory care encounter. For example, to reduce the time patients attempting to reach the clinic by telephone are kept on hold, a clinic needs sufficient telephone lines, sufficient staffing, appropriate patient triaging guidelines, and statistical data to respond to (e.g., the actual time on hold). Similarly, there are potential improvements at each of the other key steps in the ambulatory care encounter. Both technical improvements, in the form of process improvement and changes in equipment and facilities, and also employee training and skill development are important.

Current System Performance

The next step is to develop a detailed system that accurately measures quality characteristics over a period of time. In this example, measures begin with patient satisfaction. They may be expanded to include patient wait time on the telephone when making appointments, availability of appointments, patient wait time in the clinic, availability of medical records, and cancellation rates.

Measurement and Gap Analysis

For each of these quality characteristics, operational definitions and a measurement system to gather data are needed. For example, patient wait time may be defined as the interval between the actual time of the appointment and the time a patient is seen or between the time of patient arrival in the clinic and the time the patient is seen. Careful definition and special studies may be necessary when collecting the data. Later, the most valuable measures may be built into information systems. In some cases, patients may be asked to subjectively evaluate performance. For example, patients may be surveyed about staff courtesy and helpfulness and about their perceptions regarding how long they waited for an appointment and how long they feel they should have waited.

Employee Education and Training

Employees need training to learn how to perform a job correctly. Too many times employees are hired and put on the job with little orientation to the organization or to their specific assignment and processes they work within. Employees also need to learn specific customer service skills. What is the proper way to greet customers? What should an employee do when a customer is upset about a service? What are appropriate subjects to discuss with a patient? Employees also need training on how to work with their colleagues to improve processes.

Employee Social Support and Organizational Culture

Work performance levels are highly dependent on whether employees feel they are part of the organization. Are employees valued members of the team? Are employees encouraged to study and test improvements in their own work processes? Does management listen to their ideas? What barriers do employees face in doing their jobs? Periodic employee surveys should be conducted to expose areas for improvement and to systematically gain insight into employees' views about the environment for work and learning.

Organizational Technical Resources

The ability of an organization to serve customers will depend on its technical capabilities. Is there an easy-to-use information system that allows employees to look up patient information? Is there a patient appointment system that meets the needs of the clinic? Is the telephone appointment system user-friendly? Are management reports easy to use? Do leaders and employees get information about patient complaints and specific areas that need improvement?

Illustration of the Conceptual Framework

This conceptual framework may be illustrated with the help of the ambulatory care encounter shown in Figure 3.5. Data from a Henry Ford Medical Group (HFMG) survey showed that patients were very satisfied with care provided by physicians (Figure 3.6). Over 60 percent of the patients were very satisfied with physician competence, physician concern, and overall; less than 10 percent were dissatisfied or very dissatisfied. On the other hand, patient access criteria measures did not score as well. As shown in Figure 3.6, 20 percent of patients surveyed were dissatisfied or very dissatisfied with their time in the waiting room. Management at HFMG decided that access improvement would be its major target area for the next three years. Let us examine the actions of leadership at Henry Ford Medical Group using the framework described earlier.

Figure 3.6

Satisfaction Levels: The Henry Ford Medical Group Patient Satisfaction Survey

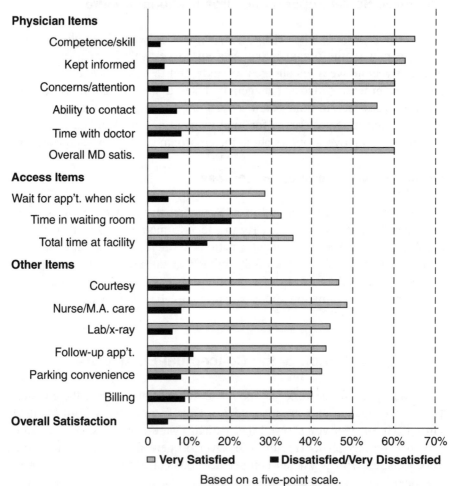

☐ Very Satisfied   ■ Dissatisfied/Very Dissatisfied

Based on a five-point scale.

Customer Expectations

Using external customer (patient) survey data and focus groups as well as internal customer (physician and support staff) focus groups, management was able to identify three key areas of improvement: (1) the patients prefer to see their personal physician when seeking care; (2) patients expect around-the-clock availability of information and advice over the telephone (from a knowledgeable person); and (3) when needed, primary care and specialty appointments should be available in a timely manner.

Professional Standards

Each of the specialty clinics was asked to define professional standards for care that could affect making appointments or reporting test results. In primary care, physicians have been approving telephone guidelines to be used by registered nurses to give advice and to triage patients based on their needs to be seen at specific levels of care. In specialty areas, physicians have been working on clinical guidelines for appropriate referrals to subspecialties.

Current System Capabilities

In those areas that surfaced as priorities—in particular phone services, appointment availability, and the specialty referral process—the HFMG spent considerable time understanding the current reality, including detailed knowledge of the processes and sources of variation in them. This exercise was fundamental in providing the knowledge necessary to launch a redesign of primary care services.

Specification of Process Requirements

After examining the customer expectations data, professional standards, and the current system capabilities, the leadership identified the key strategies (leverage points) that would close the gap between the current situation and the vision for primary care that will meet both internal and external customer expectations:

- Improving telephone systems, nursing triage, and advice services
- Developing patient panels (patients aligned with a personal physician) with a focus on improving appointment availability for patient populations
- Improving specialty referral processes
- Employee training.

Process Design and Redesign

Physician-led subgroups were developed to oversee the process changes to be made on each of the four key strategies to be implemented. Each

Figure 3.7

Market Measurement Access Study, Overall Patient Satisfaction and Dissatisfaction Rates, Henry Ford Medical Group

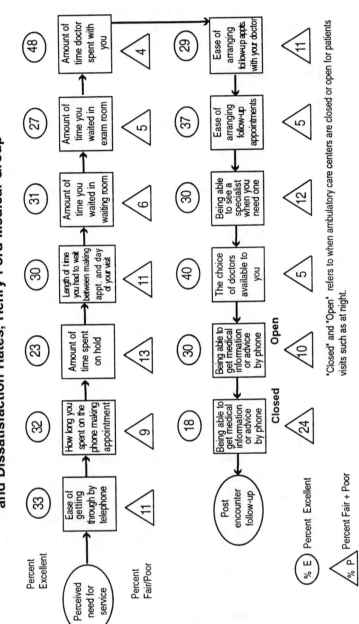

strategic area identified pilot areas where quality improvement teams met to design the improvements. These pilot areas worked to implement the strategies and move toward a "best method" using evaluation criteria. A number of process changes have already been introduced.

Current System Performance

Developing system performance indicators for both customer satisfaction and process variables related to the key strategies helps to track improvement efforts. HFMG has focused its attention on customer satisfaction with access variables, appointment availability waits, and phone service standards.

Figure 3.7 demonstrates the satisfaction with key access variables for the HFMG. This data is collected on a routine basis on all primary care points of services within both HFMG and Metro Medical Group and is useful in targeting concerns of patients as well as specific clinic locations to focus improvements on. Likewise, tracking next-available appointments helps isolate areas in need of better appointment availability.

Measurement and Gap Analysis

Understanding current system performance and having a customer-focused vision for primary care helps identify corrections or short- and long-term needs that if met will accelerate the key strategic improvements. Figure 3.7 shows the detailed analysis of customer satisfaction with the encounter process. Each of the 13 boxes represents a specific patient question and the response. At this early stage of process improvement, there was only one impressive activity—time spent with the physician.

In the short term, it is important to have the type of phone equipment that will provide process information data regarding quality service indicators (such as the length of time to answer, length of call, or abandonment rates) and to have an appointment scheduling system that facilitates the reporting of appointment wait times and that is able to capture no-show rates for all physicians, which is very valuable in pinpointing the need for improvement. The use of such information and measurements will, in the long run, drive the behavior changes necessary to sustain improvements.

Employee Education and Training

One of the other key strategies identified as critical to move the HFMG closer to its vision is training and education. Although many areas are in need of training, the decision was made to focus on the training needed to implement the other three strategies: training on telephone systems, computer skills, and telephone nursing advice skills. Training on the physician selection process and training on the use of panel report information are also important educational needs for physicians, support staff, and medical group leadership and has been launched recently.

Employee Social Support and Organizational Culture

The next step includes continued efforts toward reaching a shared vision around the stated priorities. The various pilot projects are working toward a best practice that will shorten the time frame for widespread changes in the group. "Best practices" demonstrate that a much better method can be developed and hence encourage people to undertake changes in their own work. The various quality improvement teams must feel supported and that they are part of a learning organization. Teams must be encouraged to try new approaches and continually learn what will impact the customers' expectations and satisfaction.

Organizational Technical Resources

Finally, resources must be allocated toward the implementation of identified strategies that will improve customer service and satisfaction. The technical infrastructure must be created to support the clinical practice. Data regarding the quality of telephone services is critical for influencing the needed staffing to meet customer demand. Similarly, physicians require information and feedback about their patients' utilization and clinical status in order to enhance clinical quality of care. At HFMG both internal resources and corporate resources (management services and corporate planning and marketing) were provided to implement the identified strategies.

Customer satisfaction improvement requires understanding every step of the processes in detail, designing appropriate measures of customer satisfaction, linking those results to key processes, and making improvements where needed. Figure 3.8 shows a hierarchy of measures. The overall customer satisfaction measure may include a question like, "Would you recommend Henry Ford Medical Group to a friend?" The key to improvement lies in understanding the systems and processes related to key outcomes of satisfaction. Further, for each of these systems specific measures, such as patient satisfaction with time on hold when making an appointment, must be tracked. As work teams pinpoint and improve their understanding of specific processes as well as their own capabilities, they are better able to respond to and improve service to patients.

Improving Physician Involvement in CQI

It is critical that physicians be actively involved in improving processes in health care. In every significant process, the physicians are involved as customers, as suppliers, or as processors. Very often the physicians are all three. In the admission and discharge process, a physician is a "supplier" in his or her role in providing information to the admissions and discharge

Figure 3.8

Relationship of Process Measures to Customer Satisfaction

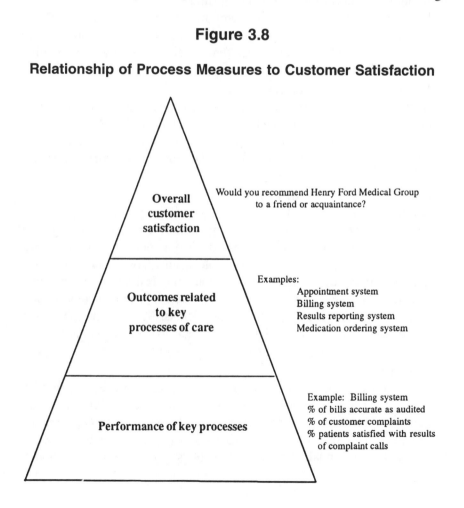

Overall customer satisfaction — Would you recommend Henry Ford Medical Group to a friend or acquaintance?

Outcomes related to key processes of care — Examples: Appointment system, Billing system, Results reporting system, Medication ordering system

Performance of key processes — Example: Billing system, % of bills accurate as audited, % of customer complaints, % patients satisfied with results of complaint calls office about discharging a patient. The inability to discharge a patient on time—say, before the 11 a.m. target—is often because the physician has not written the discharge order. On the other hand, when a new patient is being admitted, the physician is a customer. He cannot do the admitting workup unless the patient has been admitted and is in the unit. As a processor, the physician is involved in planning patient care, treating, and monitoring changes in the patient's condition while the patient is in the hospital. Thus, physicians must also be engaged in the improvement of clinical work. Berwick[18] has recommended the following eight methods to promote physician involvement:

1. **Reallocate committee and meeting time**
   Physicians serve voluntarily on many medical staff committees. By reallocating this committee time to learning CQI methods, to project team work, or to developing new cross-functional efforts, physician involvement can be increased.

2. **Invite physician volunteers to help**
   In the early stages, hospitals can look for physicians who are champions of CQI. At Intermountain Health Care, Walke-Parker Medical Center, and Henry Ford Health System, almost all early participants were physicians who were attracted to the CQI concepts through exposure at seminars.

3. **Formalize the involvement role**
   Hospitals can take small steps to recognize the physicians when they come forward. This recognition may include financial and logistical support in attending short courses or visiting other health care organizations. At Henry Ford, over 300 physicians have taken the six-day quality improvement course. At Intermountain Health Care, Brent James has offered a course over two years focused on CQI and outcome studies, which have been popular with the physicians. Many of the physicians participating in this course have gone back to their areas and applied CQI processes to improve clinical processes in their specialty.

4. **Use data**
   Physicians are comfortable with data, and it can be used to stimulate physician curiosity. Showing data on variation among clinicians, in patient outcomes, or in cost/efficacy drug studies is a strong stimulant to action. The key here is not to accuse a physician; phrases such as "economic credentialing" and "losing physicians" are an invitation to disaster.

5. Watch for interested specialties

In hospitals or group practices, some physicians may quickly embrace CQI. It is important to provide support in the form of learning opportunities, data analysts, facilitators, and recognition of the progress made by these physicians. At Henry Ford Health System, an orthopedic surgeon and a medical oncologist were the leaders of the early clinical teams. As these two teams made progress, the CEO invited the leaders of both of these teams to present their work to the board of trustees. Assistance was provided to help in writing a journal article,[19] which led to an interview and a lead story on the front page of the *Wall Street Journal* highlighting the work of the chemotherapy team.[20] Recognition by peers helped these groups to continue their work and to study additional processes.

6. Include physician leaders from square one

It is better to involve top physician leaders from the beginning in the efforts to implement CQI. At Henry Ford Health System, all clinical department chairs and division heads participated in the six-day CQI course within the first year the courses were offered. The head of Henry Ford Medical Group was a member of one of the first improvement teams launched. Many other physicians from the Henry Ford Medical Group leadership were appointed members of the Quality Technology Council that guided the implementation of CQI within Henry Ford Health System.

7. Define involvement specifically

Asking physicians to get involved without providing specific invitations to participate in key activities will not produce results. Some ways to specifically involve physicians are inviting them to attend a course on CQI, appointing them to project improvement teams, providing opportunities to facilitate improvement teams, and arranging for service part-time as fellows in quality improvement. At Henry Ford Health System, several physicians have spent one day a week as fellows at the Center for Clinical Effectiveness with their salary for that day being supported by the institution. This action has resulted in some physicians becoming very knowledgeable and actively engaged in clinical improvement projects.

8. Connect quality management to guidelines and critical paths

Clinical guidelines usually produce fear among physicians; many are afraid of cookbook medicine. Combining CQI and clinical guidelines can help physicians focus on the process of patient care instead of the individual outlier provider, as a means of reducing unnecessary variation.

CQI verses Quality Assurance

Historical efforts to systematically improve quality of hospital care can be credited to many, including Florence Nightingale[21] and A. E. Codman.[22] The first efforts to set quality standards were led by the American College of Surgeons as early as 1917.[23] The methodology used as part of this early quality process was to specify minimum quality standards and to perform a retrospective care review and peer discussion. These early efforts by the American College of Surgeons led to an increasingly broad acceptance of quality assurance (QA) concepts. In 1951, the American College of Surgeons was joined by the American Hospital Association, the American Medical Association, and several other groups to form the Joint Commission on Accreditation of Hospitals (JCAH).

The QA effort from 1950 to 1985 was driven mostly by health care organizations. It focused on the quality monitoring and evaluation process prescribed by the JCAH. This process required specification of important aspects of care, identification of clinical indicators, and establishment of thresholds for evaluation. Data were collected and compared with these preestablished thresholds (e.g., medication errors of less than 1 percent). If the data showed fewer errors, then no action was taken; otherwise, a study was launched that focused on correcting the problems identified.

Merry[24] has pointed out the drawbacks of the QA approach (see Figure 3.9). He points out that the quality results of a specific process can be expected to be distributed in a bell-shaped curve shown in Figure 3.9. For example, the medication errors in hospitals are distributed in a bell-shaped curve. A small section of the curve marked A can be labeled as an area of negligence or risk management. For quality problems in this area, QA case review works quite well. Most physicians will agree that minimal standards were not adhered to. In the zone B, or the QA zone, however, there is considerably less agreement among the reviewers. Finally, in zone C, or what he calls the quality improvement zone, the monitoring and evaluation approach has not challenged health care organizations to improve and provide the best care. Instead, most organizations have been satisfied in meeting the minimal standard.

CQI, on the other hand, focuses the attention of the organization on continually improving all processes. As organizations mature in their ability to improve processes, they compare their processes against best practices through a process called "benchmarking." By learning from the best, an organization constantly improves its performance. As an example, if the

Figure 3.9

The Total Quality Spectrum

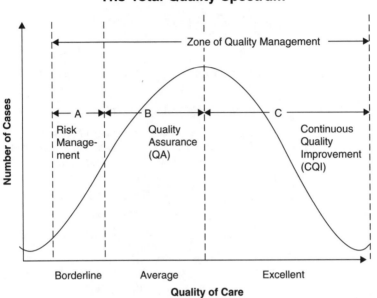

Reprinted with permission from Bader & Associates, as it appeared in *The Physician Leader's Guide.*

minimal standard for nosocomial infection rate is 4 percent, a hospital with a QA approach to quality that achieves a 3.8 percent infection rate will be satisfied that it passed the minimal standard. A hospital whose approach is one of continuous improvement will seek ways to reduce its infection rate further, to 3.5 percent or less. The hospital may identify other institutions that have consistently reached low rates and learn from them in an effort to become the best. CQI and QA are compared in Figure 3.10.

Outcomes Management and CQI

Outcomes measurement refers to the process of evaluating what happens to patients as a result of receiving medical care. Examples of outcome studies include comparison of end-results for patients receiving two drugs for the

Figure 3.10

Comparison of QA and CQI

	QA	CQI
Aim	To pass accreditation or required by regulation	Continuous improvement as a business strategy
Scope	Individual departments	Hospitalwide
Focus	Finding outliers; solving problems; identifying individuals whose performance is below threshold	Improving processes; benchmarking against the best to learn and improve processes
Employee involvement	Quality assurance coordinators	QI teams knowledgeable in the process
Methods	Inspection, audits	Prevention, scientific process improvement
Senior management involvement	Very little	Driven by senior management
Activity	Minimum required	Continuous at all levels

treatment of a medical condition or comparing treatment using drugs with a surgical treatment. Outcomes data may show the performance of two hospitals for cardiac bypass operations. Outcomes measurement is one of the hottest topics in medicine today.

Recently, much has been written about both outcomes management and CQI. There are people who believe that the only way to improve health care is to measure outcomes. In many cities and states, large financial investments have been made to compare health care institutions based on outcomes. Since 1989, Pennsylvania has required every hospital in the state to submit mortality and morbidity data for approximately 68 diagnosis-related groups (DRGs). In the three years of data collection, very few hospitals have been flagged as good or bad hospitals in terms of performance. In fact, only 2 percent of the cases were identified as poor care, and 0.6 percent as good care. This data also showed that significant variation in outcome occurs in only a few DRGs, and in one-half of the 68 DRGs tracked, no hospitals were flagged.[25] For 20 of the DRGs, 0–5 percent of the hospitals were flagged for poor outcomes; in 13 DRGs, 5–10 percent of the hospitals were flagged. In addition, of the hospitals flagged in one year, only 25 percent were flagged the following year. Kathleen Lohr[26] has summarized it best, "In practice, the knowledge base for both efficacy and effectiveness of many health care services is weak, our understanding of the links between the process and outcomes of care and of the relative importance of the science and art of care is incomplete." The Health Care Advisory Board[27] has made the following conclusions based on an in-depth study of the current status of outcome measurement:

- Measures are not statistically meaningful or accurate.
- Results are not comparable across institutions.
- Measures are not severity-adjusted (for patient acuity).
- Measures are not risk-adjusted (for patient demographics).
- Indicators have no direct link to provider action.
- Data cannot be calculated (due to technological constraints).
- Results are easily "gamed" or manipulated.

Yet it is clear that the demand for outcomes data will continue to gain momentum. Later, some of the report cards currently being developed will be discussed.

Clinical Practice Guidelines and CQI

Wide variations in clinical practice have been documented by many medical researchers all over the country. Wennberg and Gittelsohn[28] have identified wide variation in surgical rates; Brooks and Lohr[29] have detailed wide degrees of variations in physician practices; and James[30] has stated that "variations in clinical practice is the core problem. There is a tremendous variation in how individual physicians diagnose and treat similar patients."

One means to encourage the reduction of inappropriate or needless variation is to use clinical practice guidelines (CPGs). The Institute of Medicine (IOM) defined CPG as "systematically developed statements that assist practitioners and guide patient decisions about appropriate care for specified clinical circumstances."[31] The American College of Physicians states that guidelines "are simply a means of providing knowledge, derived from a scientific analysis of the practice of medicine, in a useful format to physicians, patients and others about the best use of health care resources."[32]

James[33] has described the use of clinical guidelines at LDS Hospital in Salt Lake City. Fourteen internists generated an extensive flowchart (over 40 pages in length) for the management of adult respiratory distress syndrome (ARDS). The process for improving the protocol required that if a clinician failed to follow the protocol at some point, the corresponding protocol element was automatically placed on the agenda for the next clinical team meeting. The clinician who had disagreed with the protocol step had an opportunity to present his or her reasoning. The team observed the following benefits as the clinical protocol was increasingly used:

- Physician time to manage these complex cases was reduced.
- For patients who survived, those under the protocol had a shorter length of stay.
- Patient survival increased from a historical 10 percent to more than 40 percent.
- The cost of treatment decreased by 25 percent.

CPGs are a good mechanism by which outcomes research, as well as group learning, can be translated into practical recommendations. Proponents of CPG believe that guidelines help in reducing variation and lead to improved quality.

CPG research emphasizes the need to reduce variation. Berwick[34] distinguishes "intended variation from unintended variation": An example of intended variation is when a physician treats two patients with the same condition differently because of knowledge of the patients. For example, a senile patient could not reliably take oral drugs without supervision, so an IV or an inpatient facility might be used for this patient. Intended variation may also be due to planned variation, introduced in order to study the impact of changes. For example in a PDCA cycle, a team may introduce changes in the process to study if the changes improve performance.

Burbas, McLaughlin, and Schultz[35] have presented several barriers to the development and use of CPGs:

- Clinicians fear that the guidelines represent prescriptive cookbook medicine and will become rigid standards for reimbursement and legal purposes.
- Clinicians fear that guidelines will quickly become outdated, yet be hard to change.

- Clinicians criticize the guidelines developed by academics because they do not relate to day-to-day practice.
- Clinicians fear that guidelines will be used as the basis for performance reviews.

These fears are realistic, but they can be addressed by well-designed approaches. Lessons learned from the CQI and change management literature suggest ways to increase the likelihood that CPGs will be accepted and used by physicians:

- First the American College of Physicians defines CPGs, to be viewed as simply a means of providing knowledge derived from scientific analysis of the practice of medicine.
- CPGs should be developed and used as a learning tool and a mechanism to reduce variation. In the management of ARDS patients at LDS Hospital, as previously described, every intensivist could override the guideline but was required to present his or her reasoning to peers in order to improve both learning and improving the guideline.
- Participation in developing and modifying the guidelines is an effective way to gain acceptance.
- Eddy[36] has recommended that the guidelines be characterized as "standards" or "options." To designate a guideline as standard, there must be substantial and valid data. "Options," which are less well-understood and documented, permit greater freedom.
- Using CPG and process performance information to identify processes with the greatest variation can help focus improvement work. Using CPG and provider variance information to identify outliers can lead to defensive behaviors that can impede improvement.

The Role of Benchmarking

Camp[37] defines benchmarking "as the continuous process of measuring products, services, and practices against the toughest competitors or those companies recognized as industry leaders." Benchmarking is most often misunderstood. It is not uncommon to hear statements like, "We benchmarked our billing system against five other hospitals and found that we were doing fine; our billing errors were no worse than the average." Benchmarking is not a process to compare against peers or the average, but a method to improve a process by learning from the best. Benchmarking helps an organization to become externally focused and to identify the gaps it has to close between itself and the organization with the best practices. Take the example of hip replacement surgery, which illustrates how benchmarking fits into a process and can be used to improve the operation:

1. Document your own process. Define the beginning and end of the process. The process may begin with the decision by a surgeon that a patient needs hip replacement and end six months after surgery.

2. Flowchart and completely document the internal process.

3. Form a team composed of orthopedic surgeons, nurses, home health care professionals, and physical therapy and rehabilitation technicians.

4. Ask this team to define the key quality characteristics of this process and their measurements using customer interviews, existing records, and if necessary, special studies.

5. Measure performance of the different surgeons. How much variation is there? What does the distribution look like? Are leaders on one measure also leaders on others? What can we learn from internal comparison? Many improvements are usually identified by learning from each other from within an organization. Perhaps the heart surgery solutions can be used for hip replacement.

6. Study the process as suggested by Batalden or Joiner Associates (see Figure 3.2 or Figure 3.3). Look for process changes to reduce errors and redundancy.

7. Develop CPG with standards and options. Review systematically as a continuing medical education program.

8. Identify external organizations to be benchmarked. This usually requires reviewing the literature and calling colleagues at other organizations. Identify organizations that have achieved superior results.

In effect, the first eight steps put the internal process in order, teach people how to improve, processes consensus on goals and methods, and recover the "easy money." That done, an institution is ready to achieve benchmark. Benchmarking is a valuable tool in the continuous improvement process only if it begins with the right attitude. Participants must visit a "benchmark" institution with an open mind and willingness to learn. A benchmarking team must be familiar with its own processes and areas that experience problems. Only then can they properly engage people in the visiting institutions to ask them the right questions. Finally, benchmarking is not a one-time process. It should be repeated at periodic intervals of time to see what new developments have taken place. Subsequent benchmarking becomes much easier because the participants become comfortable with the process of benchmarking and are also knowledgeable of the process to be benchmarked.

Customer-focused clinical process improvement offers a major opportunity for improvement in health care systems. To harvest this opportunity will require management and medical leadership to create an environment of trust and support within the health system. Leadership will have to develop an educational process to begin training medical, nursing, and other clinical leadership to examine clinical processes with a focus on improvement and customer service. Technical assistance must be provided to assist physicians in improving processes. Henry Ford Health System has established a Center for Clinical Effectiveness with physician leadership to work with physicians collaboratively to improve clinical processes. Intermountain Health System has also developed The Institute for Health Care Delivery Research under the leadership of Brent James. This center is engaged in teaching, training, and assisting clinicians in improving clinical processes. This institute has four goals:

1. To recommend strategic priorities regarding health care delivery and clinical research based on community needs
2. To provide data, statistical analysis, and coordination to internal and external health care delivery research efforts that advance IHC strategic objectives
3. To provide research and technical support for IHC TQM strategy
4. To seek external collaborations and funding to achieve the above objectives.

In Minneapolis, Health Partners has established an Institute for Clinical Systems Integration to develop clinical protocols and perform outcomes study. This institute is jointly funded by Health Partners and Minneapolis Business Health Care Action Group. At Dartmouth, Jack Wennberg has organized the Center for the Evaluative Clinical Sciences, which offers specific graduate study opportunities at the master's and doctoral level linking outcome measurement and clinical process improvement.

The role of leadership is to work with physicians to set priorities for clinical improvement. Finally, leadership needs to encourage physicians to use the benchmarking processes to learn and continuously strive to make improvements to the system.

Quality Report Card

All health care organizations produce a financial report produced on a standard basis and displaying the financial status of the organization. Most financial statements show the performance of the organization during the period and compare it against the budget as well as against the previous period. These statements are shared with the board of trustees and the senior management of the organization. If financial performance deviates from the plan, management begins investigations and action steps are planned to correct the situation.

But what about a statement summarizing the quality performance of the organization? Such a statement would show the progress an organization is making on key organizational quality characteristics. Unfortunately, this type of statement is not produced routinely in health care organizations. In the past few years, a number of health care organizations have been piloting a quality report card that is routinely produced in a standardized format. Henry Ford Health System and Sharp Health System are two organizations that have been producing a quality report and sharing it with their boards of trustees. Figure 3.11 shows the key dimensions of the report produced at Henry Ford Health System. Initially, a systemwide task force produced a draft report and presented it to the system board of trustees as well as the trustees of all subsidiary operating entities. Based on the feedback, the report was modified. The key design principles of the report were that the customer of the report was defined as Henry Ford Health System Board of Trustees and that the number of indicators was intentionally limited to serve the needs of the board.

Several managed care organizations have also developed a quality report highlighting their performance of the health plan on key indicators. Kaiser Permanente of Northern California produced its first report card in 1993; Figure 3.12 summarizes the indicators used by Kaiser.

The National Committee on Quality Assurance (NCQA) has designed a quality report called the Health Plan Employer Data and Information Set (HEDIS) to help employers understand the value of health plans and to provide a means of comparing health plans based on a common set of quality indicators. Figure 3.13 shows the HEDIS quality indicators.[38]

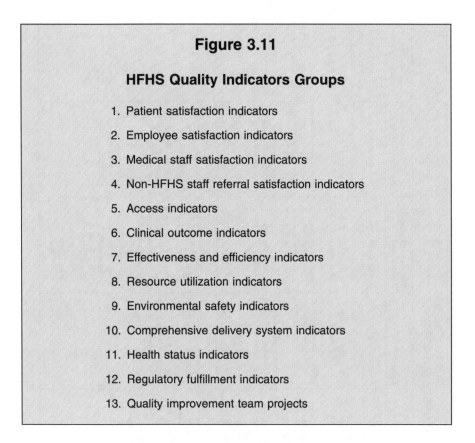

Figure 3.11

HFHS Quality Indicators Groups

1. Patient satisfaction indicators

2. Employee satisfaction indicators

3. Medical staff satisfaction indicators

4. Non-HFHS staff referral satisfaction indicators

5. Access indicators

6. Clinical outcome indicators

7. Effectiveness and efficiency indicators

8. Resource utilization indicators

9. Environmental safety indicators

10. Comprehensive delivery system indicators

11. Health status indicators

12. Regulatory fulfillment indicators

13. Quality improvement team projects

Although at this point, only scattered examples exist of specific measures, this project has attracted wide attention. Many of the measures will be adopted as standard, and many new ones will emerge.

Henry Ford Health System started a project in 1989 focused on developing a set of indicators that could be used to evaluate a vertically integrated regional health system. A consortium of 25 health care systems nationwide has been participating in this project, called "The Consortium Research on Indicators of System Performance (CRISP)."[39] Ninety-one indicators were developed, all based on a generic mission statement for vertically integrated health systems. In this innovative project, consortium members have developed a shared learning laboratory to define operationally each of the indicators and to use a standard, commonly acceptable measurement system.

Figure 3.12   Kaiser Permanente Quality Indicators

Childhood Health	Maternal Care	Cardiovascular Disease	Cancer	Common Surgical Procedures	Other Adult Health	Mental Health/ Substance Abuse
• Childhood immunizations (% of 1- and 2-year-olds immunized) • Disease outbreak rates (number of people with disease per 1,000,000) • Asthma hospitalizations (number of children discharged per 100,000) (number of ER visits per 1,000,000)	• Low birthweight (% of live births weighing < 2,500 grams and < 1,500 grams) • Prenatal care in first trimester (% of pregnant women for whom prenatal care began in first trimester) • Prenatal screenings (% of pregnant women screened for infectious diseases) • Cesarian delivery rate (% of women delivering by cesarian section)	• Cholesterol and hypertension screening (% of members screened for each disease) • Myocardial infarction (number of people discharged per 100,000) • Coronary artery bypass graft (number of people discharged per 100,000) • Heart disease and stroke mortality (number of people who died of each disease per 100,000) • Hypertension screening followup (% of hypertensives seen within one month of screening)	• Mammography screening (% of 50- to 65-year-old women screened in last 2 years) • Pap smear screening (% of women age 18 to 64 who had test) • Cancer stage at diagnosis (% of cancers diagnosed at 3 different stages, for breast, cervical, colorectal) • Mortality rates (number of deaths per 100,000 for each cancer: breast, cervical, and colorectal)	• Laminectomy rate (number of members who underwent treatment for lower back pain per 100,000) • Appendix rupture rate (% of appendectomy discharges when rupturing occurred) • Gall bladder rate (number of people per 100,000 who had surgery) (% of operations performed laparoscopically) • Hysterectomy rate (number of women per 100,000 who had surgery) (% of hysterectomies performed vaginally) • Average length of stay (number of hospital days for each procedure: laminectomy, appendectomy, gall bladder, hysterectomy)	• Diabetes discharge rate (number of members discharged per 1,000,000) • Diabetic eye disease (% of diabetics who had retinal eye exam) • Flu shot rates (% of adults > age 65 vaccinated) • Pneumonia/pleurisy discharge rate (number of members discharged per 1,000,000) • Adult asthma discharge rate (number of discharges per 100,000) • AIDS survival (average length of survival since diagnosis)	• Outpatient follow-up rates for major affective disorder (MAD) (% followed up) • Suicide rate (number of suicides per 100,000 people)

Source: Kaiser Permanente of Northern California.

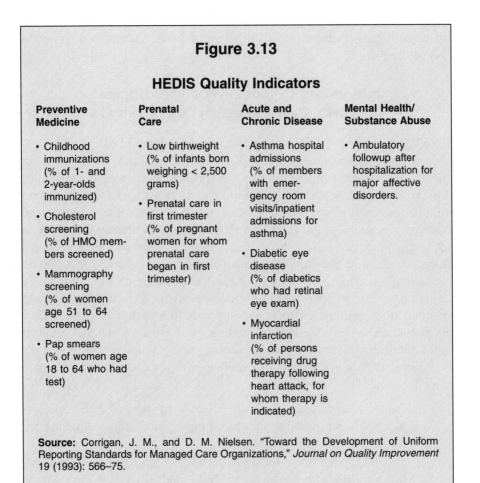

Figure 3.13

HEDIS Quality Indicators

Preventive Medicine	Prenatal Care	Acute and Chronic Disease	Mental Health/ Substance Abuse
• Childhood immunizations (% of 1- and 2-year-olds immunized) • Cholesterol screening (% of HMO members screened) • Mammography screening (% of women age 51 to 64 screened) • Pap smears (% of women age 18 to 64 who had test)	• Low birthweight (% of infants born weighing < 2,500 grams) • Prenatal care in first trimester (% of pregnant women for whom prenatal care began in first trimester)	• Asthma hospital admissions (% of members with emergency room visits/inpatient admissions for asthma) • Diabetic eye disease (% of diabetics who had retinal eye exam) • Myocardial infarction (% of persons receiving drug therapy following heart attack, for whom therapy is indicated)	• Ambulatory followup after hospitalization for major affective disorders.

Source: Corrigan, J. M., and D. M. Nielsen. "Toward the Development of Uniform Reporting Standards for Managed Care Organizations," *Journal on Quality Improvement* 19 (1993): 566–75.

Dennis O'Leary[40] observes: "Report cards are coming because there is now a social mandate for performance measurement. Report card is only a catchy term, but the mandate is real. Almost every reform proposal being introduced at federal and state levels includes a requirement for measuring performance outcomes and reporting performance information."

Although health systems will be required to produce externally mandated indicators of quality like HEDIS, in the meantime each organization needs to define for itself key quality characteristics covering 15–20 specific areas that it can now measure and that it considers essential for success.

These indicators should then be used just like financial reports to focus the attention of the organization and to serve as broad measures of progress against the plan.

Integrating Customer-Focused Clinical Care with New Physician Organizations

Simultaneously with the development of customer-focused care, many organizations will face reorganization of their medical staff and the development of physician-hospital organizations (PHOs), medical service organizations (MSOs), or other new forms. Henry Ford may have had an advantage arising from its historical structure as a salaried group practice. But the advantage is not as big as one might think. As Henry Ford grew during the 1980s, it acquired not one but three groups, plus a number of physicians on affiliated hospital staffs in its Health Alliance Plan network who were in solo or single specialty partnerships. As Mark Young notes in the Henry Ford case study (see Chapter 9), the Henry Ford physicians have had to struggle steadily to integrate all these practice organization forms. The other two case studies, Intermountain and Walke-Parker, continue to have conventional medical staff arrangements, yet they, too, have made progress on the clinical agenda.

Here are a few thoughts on handling both the quality and economic reorganization:

1. Pursue both at once. Both are essential to succeed in the marketplace. It's not possible to wait to finish one before beginning the other.

2. Try to keep the two discussions separate. Clinical care is something that has to be addressed anyway. If it is addressed well, there will be rewards to make the economic reorganization more palatable, and doctors can be reassured about some of the real concerns reflected, as in Burbas, McLaughlin, and Schultz.[41]

3. Shift as soon as possible from a QA to a CQI mentality. If a few doctors are consistently flirting with unacceptable minimums, now is the time to solve the problem. Negotiate the solution, buy the solution, or just remove the privileges of the offenders. The result is a staff that is oriented toward winning, not losing.

4. Focus CQI on the first four steps in Figure 3.2, addressing problems that do not directly change medical decisions yet make practice easier and more profitable. Develop a clinical support staff that

is customer-focused and process improvement–oriented. When lab, x-ray, ICU, and OR work right, it is an advantage for doctors, and they will quickly recognize it.

5. Expand the arenas where doctors participate in the decisions, starting at the top of the decision hierarchy described in Chapter 4. Customer-focused clinical care and PHOs both require this. The doctor is, and will be, the patient's agent in many things. He or she can be a better agent when the medical voice is part of the system's governance.

6. Back both the clinical and the economic program with resources—people, information, leadership, and dollars—and allow time for thorough discussion, learning, and conflict resolution. The hospital's strategy and financial plan should explicitly recognize that these processes take both time and money.

In short, customer-focused care and introduction of PHOs have much synergism. Steps 4–6 can be particularly effective in making the institution a more attractive place for doctors, nurses, and others to work. Economic reorganization becomes easier, not more difficult.

Ten Steps to Customer-Focused Clinical Care

1. Take leadership

Both management and physician leaders need to be knowledgeable about quality improvement. They cannot delegate this task. As leaders become increasingly knowledgeable, they need to understand and crystallize their conception of specific quality problems facing the institution. They need to relate the success of the organization to solving these quality problems. They need to discuss how much poor quality costs the organization in terms of wasted resources, lost customers, and the lowered reputation of the organization. As part of leadership, senior managers and physicians need to increase their involvement in quality issues. They need to participate in setting the quality improvement goals. If the organization has developed a quality steering committee, leaders need to actively participate in this group.

2. Develop a culture of customer focus

Leaders need to constantly put forward customer viewpoints, their needs, and concerns. By listening to customers and encouraging employees to understand customer needs at every opportunity, management can develop a culture of customer focus. When new process improvement teams are formed, they should be encouraged to identify customer needs and concerns. As process improvements are implemented, evaluations must include customer feedback data.

3. Involve physicians

Leaders need to constantly develop means by which more and more physicians are involved in the clinical improvement process. Physicians must feel that they are in charge of the process improvement activities in their own specialty and that they would benefit from the improvements made. Physicians must also understand how these process improvements will not only benefit the organization but also their patients.[42]

4. Communicate actively

Both management and physician leaders must actively communicate the aim of the improvement process: better care for patients and communities. They must constantly stress that it is not a witch hunt and that the objective is not cookbook medicine but development of shared learning among physicians practicing together. Meeting with physicians and developing a comfort level among them is critical to the success of clinical process improvement. Leadership must constantly stress the benefits to the patients, physicians, and the organization.

5. Increase training and education of physicians

Increased resources need to be put into physician education and training, by offering in-house courses and by sending physicians to selected external courses. Inviting physician leaders from other organizations to present successful process improvement initiatives in their own organizations and circulating articles that present clinical improvements made at other institutions will raise awareness among the physicians.

6. Set priorities

Every medical delivery organization has hundreds of clinical processes. It is the leaders' task to focus the energies of the organization on a few selected organizationwide clinical process improvement initiatives. When selecting clinical processes, consider the volume or number of cases and the clinical leadership in the area. In the early stages, selecting processes in areas where there are physician champions will accelerate the process. Also selecting processes for improvement where the cost of poor quality can be easily documented will help everyone to focus on the improvement effort. At Intermountain Health Care, senior management prioritized three clinical conditions to be developed into care process models in 1993. These conditions were chosen by an analysis of clinical importance as measured by volume of cases, risk of death, cost, and internal variance of cost for care. Intermountain picked coronary artery bypass grafts (CABGs) for process improvement at the four tertiary care hospitals. Hip arthroplasty was selected for the secondary hospital focus, and community-acquired pneumonia was picked for the smaller hospitals.

7. **Provide technical assistance**

Physicians are very busy people. Serving on clinical process improvement teams is extremely time-consuming. Management needs to find ways to reduce this time demand while at the same time keeping the physicians actively participating in the process improvement. Providing management analysts who can assist in documenting current processes, collecting data, interviewing customers, and meeting with individual physician team members to update them on the progress of the team will ensure that teams make progress while at the same time physicians will feel involved and in control of the process improvement.

8. **Encourage benchmarking**

Management should encourage clinical process improvement teams to learn from other organizations who have worked on process improvements in a given area. Sufficient literature now exists that presents clinical process improvement team efforts in many other institutions. By contacting these other institutions and exchanging ideas, a clinical process improvement team can accelerate its own improvement. Many formal organizations have also made clinical process improvement their priority. These include the Group Practice Improvement Network (GPIN), an organization of 58 group practices that have developed a shared learning network to implement CQI in their organizations. Similar efforts have been initiated by the Quality Management Network (QMN), with 35 hospitals and health care organizations as members. Both of these organizations have been sponsored by the Institute for Healthcare Improvement (IHI), led by Don Berwick, M.D.

9. **Look for ways to recognize accomplishments**

As clinical improvement teams achieve results, the members of the team need to be recognized. Management needs to think of creative ways to recognize accomplishments including such activities as team presentations at board of trustee meetings, medical staff meetings, management meetings, and quality improvement conferences. Team accomplishments can be published in internal newsletters and medical staff publications. Both Henry Ford Health System and Intermountain Health Care clinical team results have been cited in *Wall Street Journal* articles.[43] Recognition creates champions who further the process improvement culture within the organization.

10. Develop an organizational quality report
Leadership should develop an organizational quality report that presents the quality results on key clinical processes. By sharing this report throughout the organization and by using the report to set priorities in resource allocation decisions, clinical process improvement will be further accelerated.

Notes

1. Berwick, D. M. 1989. "Continuous Improvement as an Ideal in Health Care." *New England Journal of Medicine* 320 (1): 53–56.
2. Gaucher, E. J., and R. J. Coffey. 1993. *Total Quality in Health Care.* San Francisco: Jossey-Bass.
3. Byrne, J. A. 1993. "The Horizontal Corporation: It's about Managing Across, Not Up and Down." *Business Week* (20 December): 76–81.
4. Ibid.
5. Ostroff, F., and D. Smith. "The Horizontal Organization." *The McKinsey Quarterly* (1): 148–68.
6. *Quality Letter for Healthcare Leaders.* 1993. "Improving Cardiac Care." 5 (9): 1–12.
7. Ibid.
8. *Joint Commission Journal on Quality Improvement.* 1993. "Defining Performance of Organizations." 19 (7): 215–21.
9. Rupp, L. B., and T. Doyle. 1993. "A Successful Physician-Led Multidisciplinary Approach to Process Improvement for Inpatient Chemotherapy." *Journal of the Society for Health Systems* 4 (1): 18–33.
10. Ibid.
11. Gitlow, H., S. Gitlow, A. Oppenheim, and R. Oppenheim. 1989. "Documenting and Defining a Process." Chapter 3 in *Tools and Methods for the Improvement of Quality*, 38–53. Homewood, IL: Irwin.
12. Scholtes, P. R. 1992. *The Team Handbook.* Madison, WI: Joiner Associates.
13. Ibid.
14. Moen, R. D., and T. N. Nolan. 1987. "Process Improvement." *Quality Progress* (September): 62–68.
15. Shewhart, W. A. 1931. *The Economic Control of Quality of Manufactured Products.* New York: VanNostrend. Reprinted by ASQC Quality Press, Milwaukee, WI, 1980.

16. Deming, W. E. 1993. *The New Economics for Industry, Government, Education.* Cambridge: Massachusetts Institute of Technology.
17. Batalden, P. B., and P. K. Stoltz. 1993. "A Framework for Continual Improvement of Health Care." *Joint Commission Journal on Quality Improvement* 19 (10): 424–52.
18. Berwick, D. M. 1992. "The Clinical Process and the Quality Process." *Quality Management in Health Care* 1 (1): 1–8.
19. Rupp and Doyle, "A Successful Physician-Led Multidisciplinary Approach."
20. Winslow, R. 1993. "Health-Care Providers Try Industrial Tactics to Reduce Their Costs." *Wall Street Journal* (3 November): A-1, A-5.
21. Nightingale, F. 1863. *Notes on a Hospital,* 3d ed. London: Longman, Roberts, and Green.
22. Codman, E. A. 1916. *A Study in Hospital Efficiency.* Reproduced by University Microfilms, Ann Arbor, MI, 1972.
23. Roberts, J. S., J. G. Coale, and R. R. Redman. 1987. "A History of the Joint Commission on Accreditation of Hospitals." *Journal of the American Medical Association* 258 (21 August): 936–40.
24. Merry, M. D. 1992. "The Evolution of Quality Assurance and an Overview of Total Quality Management." *The Physician Leaders Guide,* edited by J. T. Lord. Published by *The Quality Letter for Healthcare Leaders.* Rockville, MD: Bader and Associates.
25. Health Care Advisory Board. 1993. *Outcome Strategy: Measurement of Hospital Quality under Reform.* Washington, DC: Health Care Advisory Board.
26. Lohr, K. N. 1988. "Outcomes Measurement: Concepts and Questions." *Inquiry* (Spring): 37–50.
27. Health Care Advisory Board. 1993. *Line of Fire: The Coming Public Scrutiny of Hospital and Health System Quality.* Washington, DC: Health Care Advisory Board.
28. Wennberg, J. E. and A. G. Gittelsohn. 1982. "Variations in Medical Care among Small Areas." *Scientific American* 246: 120.
29. Brook, R. H., and K. N. Lohr. 1985. "Efficiency, Effectiveness, Variations, and Quality: Boundary Crossing Research." *Medical Care* 23: 710.
30. James, B. C. 1993. "Implementing Practice Guidelines through Clinical Quality Improvement." *Frontiers of Health Services Management* 10 (1): 3–37.
31. Institute of Medicine. *Annual Report.* Institute of Medicine, 1990.
32. Ball, J. R., and P. Bousxein. 1991. "Practice Guidelines Can Contribute to Better Healthcare." *Quality Letter for Health Care Leaders* 3: 13–15.
33. James, "Implementing Practice Guidelines."
34. Berwick, D. M. 1991. "Controlling Variation in Health Care: A Consultation from Walter Shewhart." *Medical Care* 29 (12): 1212–25.
35. Burbas, C., D. McLaughlin, and A. Schultz. 1993. "The Minnesota Clinical Comparison and Assessment Program: Bridging the Gap between Clinical

Practice Guidelines and Patient Care." *National Quality of Care Forum*. Chicago: Hospital Research and Educational Trust.

36. Eddy, D. M. 1990. "Designing a Practice Policy: Standards, Guidelines, and Options." *Journal of the American Medical Association* 263 (22): 3077–84.

37. Camp, R. C. 1989. *Benchmarking: The Search for Industry Best Practices that Lead to Superior Performance*. Milwaukee, WI: ASQC Press.

38. Corrigan, J. M., and D. M. Nielsen. 1993. "Toward the Development of Uniform Reporting Standards for Managed Care Organizations: HEDIS Version 2.0." *Joint Commission Journal on Quality Improvement* 19 (12): 566–75.

39. Nerenz, D. R., B. M. Zajac, and H. S. Rosman. 1993. "Consortium Research on Indicators of System Performance (CRISP)." *Joint Commission Journal on Quality Improvement* 19 (12): 577–85.

40. O'Leary, D. S. 1993. "The Measurement Mandate: Report Card Is Coming." *Joint Commission Journal on Quality Improvement* 19 (11): 487–91.

41. Burbas, McLaughlin, and Schultz, "The Minnesota Clinical Comparison."

42. Wittrup, R. D., V. K. Sahney, and G. L. Warden. 1993. "Building a Culture of Participation in a Vertically Integrated Regional Health System." *The Quality Letter for Healthcare Leaders* 5 (8): 22–25.

43. Winslow, "Health-Care Providers Try."

4

Decision Processes for Success

Controlling the Decision Infrastructure for CQI

Decision processes are the systems for setting goals, resolving priorities, identifying alternatives, building consensus, and appealing wrongs. Decision processes—who decides what, when, and how—define the organizational culture and determine its success. They are the method by which the various stakeholders (those groups whose contribution is essential for success, and who could therefore close the organization down) negotiate a mutually beneficial accommodation. Decision processes are the unique domain of managers; nobody else thinks about them much. As the market gets more demanding, hospital decision processes must deal with more difficult decisions—and better and faster.

Any firm or organization faces four kinds of decisions: mission/vision (what the business will be, and why), resource allocation (products, quality, method, volume, price, and profit), organizational design (decision procedures, communication, authority), and implementation (recruiting, selecting, and training personnel, plus specific, detailed procedures and technology). It must make these decisions continually and collaboratively among both worker and customer stakeholders, building new consensuses as needs, power relationships, and technologies change.[1]

Continuous quality improvement (CQI) in its most mature forms, with effective *hoshin* planning and extensive delegation to cross-functional teams, will reengineer the four decision processes. The easiest change to grasp is in mission and vision setting, where CQI gurus put heavy emphasis. One of the first results of CQI is a change in implementation, the use of cross-functional teams to specify procedures and technologies. The case study institutions are discovering that change spreads to worker selection issues; to the resource allocation processes for planning, operating budget, and capital budget; and finally to the organizational design as the teams become more independent and replace line managers.

This chapter describes how, as well as it can be seen today, mature health care organizations will make their critical decisions and organize their work in the twenty-first century. Our case study organizations are well along in the transition. Their current positions and directions illustrate what's happening. Their executives describe many of their decision processes in their own words below. They are saying it's not just a matter of training and motivation, it's also a matter of the processes the organization uses to make decisions.

Building New Decision Processes

Figure 4.1 shows the four classes of decisions expanded into the processes that are now necessary to remain in business. Organizations exist because they make and implement these decisions; they thrive when they do it well and fail when they do it poorly. The "overhead" costs of Henry Ford Health Services, Intermountain Health Care, and Walke-Parker Medical Center are justified only because of improvements in the ability to deliver service, and these improvements exist because decision processes are carried out well.

Mission and vision setting rest on environmental assessment and market analysis and include customer-oriented product specification. Resource allocation begins with long-range planning, which in turn defines operational procedures, budgeting, and capital budgeting. Implementation begins with personnel selection and continues with detailed procedures, training, performance evaluation, and rewards. Organization design establishes the formal structure of accountability and the roles and membership of standing and ad hoc committees. Policies for information access, conflict resolution, and performance evaluation support the design.

Real-life processes are iterative and less orderly than Figure 4.1, but each process evolves from left to right and is linked to the one above. One frequently views them as seamless, as in the case of a product like home care services, passing through the four processes repeatedly during its life cycle. But this view overlooks some important facts. The decision methods, the

Figure 4.1

A Classification of Decision Processes

Type	Level	
	Strategic	Programmatic
Mission/vision	Environmental assessment	Marketing plans
	Strategic plans	Specific joint ventures
Resource allocation	Services plan	Facilities plan Human resources plan
	Financial plan	Operating budget Capital budget
	Technology selection	Equipment selection
Implementation	Personnel selection	Individual credentialling, recruitment, and development
	Human resource policies	Incentive programs
	Process design	Patient care protocols Policies and procedures
Organizational	Accountability hierarchy	Information plan
	Management system	Participation in care teams Conflict resolution mechanism Appeals mechanism

kinds of information, and the interest of various stakeholders differ with the process. Most importantly, there are interconnections between the products; the budget for home care cannot be decided independent of that for the ICU. These interconnections are increasing as pressures for cost control mount.

Good decision processes under CQI must lead to decisions that have two characteristics. The first is *realism*, that is, the decisions which result must be economically viable and timely. The second is *alignment*, that is, the decisions must win widespread agreement and support among the organization members. Realism means the processes will result in a successful future for the enterprise. They will meet the test of the marketplace. Alignment means that they must be persuasive; that is, most members of the organization will believe that the processes are sound, the decisions are realistic, and they as individuals will have a successful future.

The consequences of lack of realism are obvious, but the consequences of lack of alignment are equally serious. Lack of alignment makes timely decisions difficult and encourages people to fight for their individual good at the expense of the whole. Firm alignment is necessary to keep good people loyal to the organization and to encourage the extra effort that CQI entails. Alignment involves both emotional acceptance of the goal and cognitive acceptance of the implementation. It is a critical feature of CQI because it is the psychological event that changes the nature of control from "enforced" to "internalized." Individuals are convinced the goal is valid, taught how to achieve it, and convinced they can succeed. As consequences of this transformation, failure to achieve expectations becomes a rare event, monitoring is greatly diminished in importance, and blame virtually disappears.

Mission/Vision Setting Processes

Mission/vision statements that are specific and complete are both more realistic and encourage greater alignment. A vague or incomplete mission lacks realism. It also reduces alignment. It provides no guidance to potential workers and physicians on the kinds of values the organization promotes, and therefore loses the opportunity to attract like-thinking people. But the rhetoric of the mission/vision is clearly less important than a record showing that real decisions reflect the underlying concepts and lead to real achievement. Evidence of achievement of the mission/vision is more important than the words. Intermountain Health Care's key words in its mission statement, "excellent service . . . integrity . . . employees . . . diverse needs . . . caring and noble . . . model health care system . . . financial strength" (see Figure 6.4), reflect an attitude that sounds good but might be hypocritical. A visit reveals the reality of the commitment, and makes Intermountain Health Care (IHC) attractive to talented people. Gary Pehrson, vice president of Professional Services at IHC, explains:

> When we started CQI, Brent [James] and I thought that if we could educate people, we could change the environment and the culture. That has remained our strong strategy, and we've done a lot of education. What we're now running into is that education doesn't always mean

environmental change, because there are systems of accountability that people can't always change. They bump up against those. If management continues to focus on productivity or standards or bottom line, that's where people will spend their time.

We started from the basis of quality assurance, but it branches into financial issues or strategic planning. We got Greg Poulsen interested, and sent him to some courses. He said he wanted to change some aspects of the Japanese *hoshin* planning model. We developed out of that a whole planning model that fits more with the CQI thing.

Surprisingly, even though the mission and vision are alignment-building statements, they are rarely set by widespread discussion and debate. They are set by the board, the CEO, and a small group of key executives. (Henry Ford Health System will bring its top management into its next-round revisions, but the basic ideas are already set.) The mission and vision are changed only rarely and are supported by the most global measures of performance. Rather than extensive polling of the customers or members of the organization, the board identifies a mission and a vision that reflects the beliefs of others. One might use focus groups to evaluate alternative wordings or even concepts, but our study institutions did not, as far as we could determine. Gail Warden, president and CEO at Henry Ford Health System (HFHS), describes their process:

We began mission and vision-setting with senior management of all the Ford activities (including its medical groups) and a "blank sheet of paper." The process of establishing the mission/vision initially involved only the board and senior management. It became clear that the mission must include commitments to (1) patient care of the highest quality, (2) education and research, and (3) managed care. A "Futures Committee" of the HFHS board developed a lengthy vision. This was shortened [to the statement in the case study (see Figure 8.3)] which we view as a summary of needs for the year 2000.

The second and third missions are potentially conflicting. We resolved the conflict by recognizing that our tertiary care reputation is important in our overall marketing, and that managed care forces an appropriate accountability on education and research. The board's opinion is clear and everybody understands it: in the end, education and research must be limited to what the customer can afford. This establishes criteria to judge the teaching and research budgets. It also establishes a principle that the most expensive medical care is not always the best, and encourages the medical faculty to implement it.

The revision now under way will incorporate "grass roots" participation. We will continue to refine the relation between the academic medical center and the managed care perspectives in the current revision.

It is understood in the case study organizations that the market is the ultimate judge of the mission/vision. The market will express collectively individual customer evaluations of the price and quality of health care, and the providers will interact with that expression. The mission/vision must be detailed enough and convincing enough to win the alignment of line managers, physician leaders, and trustees. Extensive environmental assessment and market analysis make the mission/vision realistic and convincing. The assessment has stimulated major changes in direction at all three sites. Walke-Parker changed the basic strategic direction from niche markets to managed care capability. HFHS has offered a new insurance product with a multiyear premium guarantee, in a unique partnership with Blue Cross/Blue Shield of Michigan and Mercy Health Services (another large system). IHC is investigating its medical staff relationships. At all three sites, these changes carry through to the operating and capital budget priorities.

Resource Allocation Processes

Resource allocation processes translate broad directions to specific commitments. They often overlap with strategic direction setting, sharing the environmental assessment and market analysis, and they take up a lot of time in most institutions. Resource allocation processes occur in three interlocking levels:

1. The vision is translated to specific services and a long-range financial plan.
2. Specific plans for facilities, human resources, and information are developed.
3. Plans are translated to annual operating and capital budgets.

In the theory of CQI, all three of these steps follow the principle of *hoshin* planning.

Hoshin *planning*

Hoshin planning strives to link all levels of resource allocation closely to customer needs. *Hoshin* means a core belief, an intellectual pole star or reference point. In CQI, the *hoshin* is customer needs. The best examples of *hoshin* planning go far beyond meeting immediate customer requests to anticipate and even implant ideas customers would never have thought of on their own. Examples abound in the high-tech Japanese companies, Sony's Walkman being one of the most dramatic. The *hoshin* planning concept involves a sophisticated interplay of market analysis, technology analysis, creativity, and role-playing, leading to breakthrough inventions and fundamental redesigns.

We in health care have a long way to go to reach true *hoshin* planning.[2] What is missing, so far, is creativity, role-playing, and breakthrough innovation on behalf of the customer.[3] Provider logic has traditionally driven our innovation. The results of research have often been sold to the customer with much greater enthusiasm than the data actually support: Cesarian sections, circumcisions, tonsillectomies, prostatectomies, and executive physicals are among the more glaring examples. In the process of selling the customer, we have stimulated a specious faith in diagnostic machinery, drugs, and surgery as the source of eternal youth, values that are philosophically questionable and economically untenable.

Planning services and financial requirements

Successful resource allocation processes use time as an ally. Each decision is addressed as far to the future as practical, allowing the participants to conduct full discussions, adjust to unpleasant realities, find innovative solutions, and convince themselves that the decisions are well based, necessary, and fair. The result is that the debate centers on abstract future scenarios rather than current realities.[4] The scenarios develop realism and alignment over time, as they are tested and retested and become familiar to the participants. Here's how Greg Poulsen, vice president, planning and research, describes IHC's upper-level resource allocation processes. Note the emphasis on alignment by repetition and broad participation:

> Our goal is to take a top-down process of vision and a bottom-up process of implementation. Our planning documents put together the long-term vision and an implementation plan for it [see Figure 4.2].
>
> VISTA is a broad conceptual document—lots and lots of graphs, something people can grasp the ideas from. The Management Committee [the four most senior executives of the corporation] and the Executive Management Committee [EMC, Management Committee plus seven additional vice presidents] meet annually to review and

refine it. The board reviews VISTA in the fall of each year. VISTA has statements like, "Managed care will be the predominate form of care in the future," followed by charts and graphs showing the actual managed care market share and projections into the future. We go on to say that our success will depend upon both our ability to provide care and our ability to market managed care products. Then we talk about how we need to modify our delivery system and how to develop the managed care products. We raise questions like areas where managed care products need to be expanded, and how we need to change our relation to physicians, our compensation structure, and so forth. Most of these topics began to appear in VISTA eight or nine years ago. Initially, they were not disputed, but they were sort of ignored. Now I don't think anybody would disagree.

Once the board has approved VISTA, we encourage the EMC to share it with their subordinates. The board, the EMC, most of the Corporate Management Committee [the EMC plus the next level of about 20 managers] and all their planners see VISTA in full. The broad concepts of VISTA go in our employee newsletters. We recognize that it will be in our competitor's portfolios. Some of the details are kept confidential.

In *hoshin* planning, both existing and proposed activities are modeled in business plans against market and price trends. Quality measures establish minimums for acceptable performance, and the costs of meeting those minimums are tested against market price realities. The long-range financial plan provides the acid test for the enterprise as a whole. The achievable cost trend will be plotted against an outsider-determined price trend. The difference must generate the capital the organization needs for survival. That set of services or products that passes the acid test becomes the services plan. Realism centers on the assumptions for the models. Benchmarking information on the performance of competitors and market leaders becomes essential to achieve realism. Gary Pehrson, vice president of Professional Services at IHC, explains:

Now between 40 and 60 percent of our goals are related to quality. For financial guidelines, we use a 30-year capital planning model, which is reviewed every year by the Finance Committee and the board. It tells us that we'll need X dollars to stay in business. One of the complaints from the line managers was, "The central office always sets

Figure 4.2

IHC Planning, Budgeting, and Goal-Setting Interaction

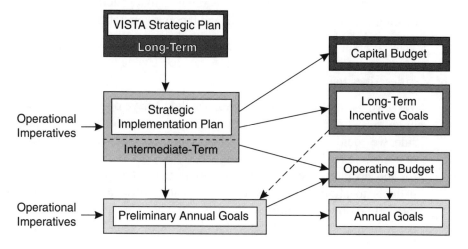

the targets without sufficient understanding." So the chief operating officer appointed two committees to look at the processes, and make sure we are getting the best thinking and more collective intelligence than just some finance people. The study got so complicated, we won't be able to implement it in 1994, but we'll get the report in time to implement in 1995. I think the report will emphasize more comprehensive measurement tools, looking more at satisfaction and quality measures, in addition to the bottom line.

At Henry Ford, Tom McNulty, senior vice president and chief financial officer, is a bit more graphic:

> We're committed to keeping this a financially strong institution, and we do it by paying ourselves first. We will maintain certain available debt capacity and certain financial ratios. The final budget and capital budget are approved by the finance committee in the light of its impact on borrowing power and cash flow.
>
> Our theory of financial management is a simple one. You have three sources of cash flow—operating margin, nonoperating income, and depreciation. Our theory is that depreciation should be used to replace facilities and equipment and to retire debt. Operating income

is used for expansion. If you don't set aside your nonoperating income, you are doomed to fail. If you don't have income for expansion, you will also fail. Nonoperating income is used to maintain the wealth of the corporation, by investment in instruments that generate income (including your own working capital, and income-generating expansions).

Walke-Parker's 25 percent reduction is a frightening goal, but at the time we visited, over half of it was in view. Joe Corrigan, chief financial officer, describes the situation:

> We have a ton of HMO contracts. If we didn't have our TQM methodology to get the cost down, both on the hospital side and the clinical side, we couldn't accept some of those contracts. We're on the strategy of accepting HMO rates, and using the TQM tools to make it profitable for the hospital. We've kept our cost per stay increases for similar patients to about 6 to 8 percent per year. We're in the process of ratcheting down, to drop our costs per case. We're trying to cut departmental costs by 25 percent and overhead costs by 50 percent.

Planning the specifics: Buildings, people, and information

Commitments that meet the test of financial planning are rolled out to specific plans for buildings, people, and information. Greg Poulsen explains that at Intermountain, this step is done for each regional cluster.

> The planning staffs of all of the divisions and my group pull together shorter-term (one to five years) strategic implementation plans [SIPs]. There is a planner assigned to every "cluster" plus a couple other areas with long-term responsibility, like our central laboratory, laundry, and purchasing units. The planners technically report to me. I think its more important that they report to the CEO of the cluster. In my view, planning isn't a staff function, it's a line function. Managers are the ones who really do the planning; planners are just the facilitators. If the planners do the planning, management won't put their heart and soul into it. If the planners facilitate, then things will go better. It'll be implemented with enthusiasm. The CEOs make the annual evaluation of the planners. The link between me and the cluster planners is service and data.
>
> VISTA should be precise on the concepts for what we need to do. The SIPs will take them to the specifics. We identify the key things that need to happen in the system. The VISTA concepts guide specific

SIPs and evaluate proposals like unit expansion and replacement. We aren't interested in large documents with lots of detail. Our goal for the SIPs is five pages for each operating entity and five pages on the system as a whole, so that someone could review the entire plan in about 30 minutes.

The SIPs are more a road map than a vision. It's a boring document. It's very mundane, but it outlines our physical building and our relationship building. It's multiyear. A lot of organizations would have what we have in our SIPs in their annual goals. Enough of what we're doing takes more than a year to do that you could get lost if you just focus on one year. It helps work out potential conflicts.

The process is similar at Henry Ford, as McNulty describes:

The units develop a "wish list" for the next three years. They say we need $100 million, prioritized, for the whole system. We then show the implications of that in terms of cash flow, operating income, and debt service ratios. The first iteration doesn't work. We go through successive iterations until we have agreed on the targets.

A hidden implication of customer-controlled prices and guideline-driven operations is that the human resources plan must be extended to physicians. It is already clear that primary care physicians will be in short supply and specialists will be in surplus. The implications of risk-sharing contracts focused on common provider entities or physician-hospital organizations, or simply physician groups, are that the organization must avoid overcommitting itself to providers who will soon be redundant. Pehrson notes:

We already see a problem with the distribution of primary and specialty physicians. We're working with McKinsey and Company to help us with this. Now with the changing marketplace, we want to develop the primary care network so it will feed the specialists. McKinsey is out interviewing specialist and primary doctors to help us make the right decision. The specialists have already realized that they need this desperately.

The case study institutions are clearly thinking in terms of long-term relationships with their physicians. A young specialist who affiliates with any of them is encouraged to think of a lifetime with the organization. The credibility of that offer depends on minimizing the number of physicians who become redundant, by avoiding excessive recruitment now, and encouraging prompt retirement, retraining, or refocus of practice among the older specialists.

A good *hoshin* process must include conflict resolution. Greg Poulsen describes the process at IHC:

> If the planners at the regional clusters hold tenaciously to an assumption that doesn't make sense to me, I'd call the cluster CEO and discuss it. In the end, the disagreement comes to the Management Committee when the SIP is presented. The Management Committee will make the decision. The EMC will hear it, too.
>
> Disputes are more frequent in capital proposals than in forecasting assumptions. Some of those have gone to the Management Committee, or one of its line executives. Even then, it tends to get to the EMC, where there are competing views. This happens with "border skirmishes" between clusters. The skirmishes are discussed at EMC. The final decision rests with the Management Committee.

Building capital and operating budgets

Both capital and operating budget guidelines are driven from the long-range financial plan. The capital budget limit establishes the funding available to support change. The annual productivity improvement or cost target provides an estimate of the changes necessary in operating budgets to meet price constraints. It becomes the survival threshold that the line managers must achieve. The guidelines should be forecast several years into the future, because major changes require longer lead times.

Greg Poulsen describes Intermountain's final planning step:

> The operating budget guidelines are set by the board, on recommendation of the Finance Committee. They will set the net profit and the rate increase. They approve the capital budget as a specific list, rather than a guideline, so that the Management Committee has flexibility to ask for what is necessary. If we value our jobs, we will present nothing to the board that is unnecessary, or that is not within the bottom line and rate increase guidelines.
>
> The guidelines are driven from a long-run capital planning model. The Finance Committee has reviewed the model and the assumptions. The Finance Committee's goal is to keep the bond rating. When we look at our history, we've always underestimated both the actual

revenue and the actual costs, but the model has kept us from investing too much.

The operating entities take over when the SIPs are approved, to set the preliminary annual goals. Demand is forecast by having the planners from the clusters sit down with our staff and go through the assumptions. We discuss issues like, "How aggressive will managed care be?" The local planners then modify those assumptions for their locale. We challenge those assumptions, not from an adversarial point of view, but in a collegial one.

Capital budgets are developed by clusters, rather than facilities. The local balancing between the facilities is handled locally. The proposals used to be judged principally on present value, but that's changing. It's much more difficult when you're building a network. Marketing issues are much more important. There are many more proposals each year than can be funded. The capital allocation is important. The cluster CEO gets his administrative council together, and says, "Let me tell you, friends. We have a list of $120 million here. We've been allocated $18 million. What should we do now? How can we cut by a factor of ten?" With the reality we face now, we increasingly say, "Look, folks, we only have this much to spend." If there were something absolutely critical, would we spring for more? Absolutely, but rather than our evaluating each project, we just say, "We don't have the money. You figure out what to do."

When somebody asks for something they want, but which isn't going to be funded, our people do two things. One is they blame. They say, "Corporate won't give us any more." The other is they use the arm around the shoulder: "In the managed care environment, we only have so much coming in. Anything we spend is going to come out of your compensation in the end." We leave that to the lowest unit— the chief of surgery for the operating rooms, for example. That's what he's paid for.

At Henry Ford, Gail Warden, president and CEO, said, "I met with the line managers today, to start the annual budget process. I told them to think in terms of CPI increases, this year and for the foreseeable future." Tom McNulty amplifies what happens:

Our system isn't perfect, but we have a process that is articulated in writing [abstracted in Figure 4.3]. We look at all the external activities and go through a series of specific reviews from different perspectives—market, government, etc. This year we took the proposed budget, and we did a SWOT [strengths, weaknesses, opportunities, threats] analysis in each division. We used this to identify "critical developments" to monitor for each unit. We picked six or seven things that will significantly influence the year's performance. They don't need to be quantitative; they can be milestones.

Quarterly reports include progress toward these items. This keeps reminding people what they agreed to—the increase in fee-for-service admissions, the increase in Health Alliance Plan admissions, reduced salary expenses, overtime expenses, agency personnel costs, staffing hours, and so on. What happens is that these feed the next year's budget. They become real facts in the next environmental assessment. We don't have to reconstruct; we're trying to build a continuum. It's made a much more open process, but at the same time made it more tolerable.

The capital budget tracks the strategic plan, and it drives the operating budget. We have a process of target setting. You've got capital demand leveraged against the staying power of the institution or corporate wealth. You've got new program development requirements and returns. You have to solve those simultaneously, as interdependent decisions. The target setting establishes the cost increase, the operating margin, and the capital budget guidelines.

We don't use a formal flexible budget. Flexible budgets are only useful when you have an operating system and individuals who are willing and able to make changes. We're not there yet. For example, if you have nurses sitting around the OR some afternoon because there is no surgery, you have to be willing to send them home. We're afraid to do that. We have to give our managers some kind of gain sharing to get them to do this.

You have to have the buy-in of the line managers to do this. They have to understand the financial relationships, and accept the board's policy on protecting the financial strength. You have to have good communication and information on an ongoing basis. The SWOT analysis and the "critical developments" do that for us. So do the forecasts. We already know our revenues for next year. They'll be up about 3.5 percent. An operating manager knows all this and knows what his margin has to be.

We've been averaging about 5 percent cost increases per year. We expect our operating units to be within one-tenth of one percent on costs and revenues. A large error is $1 million out of a $1 billion operation. Our operating margin is only one-half of one percent—$6 million out of $1.2 billion. We get surprises, but we have so far been able to adjust them.

Joe Horton, chief operating officer, Primary Children's Hospital, tells us how he responds to a similar process at IHC.

We've been one of the leaders in implementing the budget process, and I'm more of an advocate than most COOs in the system. We negotiate a productivity goal of expenses over revenue with the corporation. It's always an improvement over last year. We [a small committee of line officers and budget officers] figure out how we want to spread the goal to the departments.

Each department comes up with a one-time productivity goal. If they meet it, their work is done. The downside is they do not have the option of not meeting it. If a department head feels that they have had to do things that are unwise or destructive, they submit a separate memo documenting what those are. If their assistant administrator agrees, he or she can negotiate within his or her departments for relief, because the assistants have freedom within their totals. If necessary, they can appeal to me for a contingency fund we set up for the purpose. What's interesting is how few appeals there have been. On the front end, there was a lot of apprehension about the project. On the back end, though, only a handful of departments submit in writing.

We've also related productivity improvement to our mission and our rates, pointing out that our prices drive insurance premiums, which cause people to drop insurance and cut access for children. We've taken that message to our people. Last year we had no rate increase at all.

This was the first year for a flexible budget. Half the units in the corporation met their budget. There were a lot of problems, including too-tight targets, not enough tools, and the wrong incentives.

In the capital budget, we have two to four times the requests as we do funding. We invite the medical directors to a meeting to review the projects. We tell them up front, "You are all competing with one another. If the radiologists get a $1 million CAT scan, that's $1 million out of the pool. If you think it's not justified, or you know something that's not out on the table, now is the time to bring it up."

Figure 4.3

HFHS Operating Budget Process (abridged)

Time Period	Activity	Responsibility
June	Design customized Budget Index Model and formulate indices for Business Group.	Business Group representative in conjunction with the Corporate Budget staff
July 1–15	Review assumptions compiled for the Budget Index Models, 1992 Reforecasts, Environmental Assessment Document, and the models themselves. Define a total system Net Income requirement.	Corporate Budget Committee (CBC)
July 31	Present initial assumptions, reforecasts, and Environmental Assessment Document to HFHS Board of Trustees Finance Committee. Recommend a total system Net Income target.	HFHS Executive Mgt.
August	Review results of the Budget Index Models. Resolve differences between Budget Index Models and total system Net Income requirement. Set Net Income targets by Business Group.	CBC
Aug./Sept.	Review results of strategic planning retreat outcome and update issues for budget index model. Determine 1993 salary increases.	CBC
September	Negotiate and refine Net Income targets per Business Group.	CBC in conjunction with Group representative
Oct. 19	Present Preliminary Operating and Capital Budgets to HFHS Board of Trustees Finance Committee for review and recommendations.	HFHS Executive Mgt.
Nov. 9–13	Review recommended Capital Needs and final document for Board meeting.	CBC
Nov. 20–Dec. 7	Review and approve Operating Budgets by Board of Trustees of respective Business Groups.	CEO or President of Business Group
Dec. 15	Present proposed Final Operating and Capital Budgets to HFHS Board of Trustees Finance Committee.	HFHS Exec. Mgt.
	Review and Approval.	HFHS Board

The final decision is made after the meeting by a committee of the COO, medical director, director of nursing, and CFO, and our final list is circulated through the Medical Executive Committee. It's been a very different dynamic from what we did three years ago, which was essentially a radiologist coming and lobbying to death his assistant administrator. It's a different orientation.

An eight-person committee, four department heads plus directors of DP, bio-engineering, facilities, and finance, collectively evaluate projects under $20,000. The members rotate each year. They meet with every department head to go over their list. They prioritize the projects into A, B, and C. If we bought through the C level, we would be $500,000 ahead where we would have been with the old method. The rest of the requests were dropped by the department heads.

Joe Corrigan, chief financial officer at Walke-Parker talks about how the results of their budgeting process have changed with the environment:

The capital budget system [described at the end of Chapter 7] is now automatic. It's just engrained in what we do. Recently, our priorities have changed. Cost-based [as opposed to revenue-based] projects move much faster now. We used to approve 60 percent of our projects based on [their ability to generate] new revenue. Now it's 70 percent cost saving and replacement.

Charles Christiansen, CEO, adds:

We for years spent money trying to get open-heart surgery. We came to the conclusion that when we are putting the health system together, we can buy open-heart surgery from the lowest bidder. TQM has clearly shifted our views on "make versus buy." This hospital will have the things that we need to have to fulfill the community's image. We'll continue to do cancer research, and sports medicine, but in the context of cost control and managed care.

Gary Pehrson notes a similar change at IHC:

The capital budgeting priorities are changing. It's more sensitive to what we can and cannot afford. The COO has been meeting with the hospital managers. We will have about $200 million in requests, and we'll fund about $40 million. We literally can't afford to do more. People are looking at the request list in a different way, saying, "We can't afford two MRIs. We'll have to figure out how to share one."

We recently purchased some updated CT scanners. We told the people making the requests we could save $900,000 if we could standardize on one machine. That said a lot to the docs. In the recent past we've done much more of this.

Are the case study processes good models?

Our case study institutions are quite good at resource allocation processes. They distribute the environmental assessment broadly to guide the actual resource allocation decisions (especially IHC's VISTA process and document). Each project or process is expected to have clear and quantitative expectations on cost and quality. Budget development is taken seriously, and agreed-upon budgets are met. Henry Ford's level of sensitivity, one part in a thousand, is exemplary. IHC's troubles with its new flexible budget were clearly a source of pain and embarrassment. Whether they are due to overly ambitious goals or the need for better processes, the record is likely to improve dramatically. Walke-Parker's ability to reposition itself as a markedly less expensive provider is risky with CQI. Without CQI, it would have been almost impossible.

The case study processes have begun the transition from a provider *hoshin* to a customer *hoshin*. They establish the validity of the customers' viewpoint. They invest heavily in measuring it. All three have very sophisticated customer assessment programs. They have alignment on three landmark premises at a level of conviction beyond debate. The premises and their process implications, shown in Figure 4.4, are conditions of membership in the case study organizations.

The case study institutions have resolved debates over the rules. Despite the strong tradition of community service at both Henry Ford and Intermountain, it is taken for granted that the strategic plan will shape the budget, the budget will be met, productivity will be improved, and many capital requests will be denied. The "mission versus margin" debate has been resolved: "We will make our margin in order to fulfill our mission." There are many hospitals and medical staffs who have not yet reached those conclusions, and some who doubt their wisdom. In fact, the premises strip bare an important euphemism of the "quality movement": it is about quality only if you define the term to include economic productivity.

IHC and Walke-Parker have both begun to move beyond the traditional budgeting process. In these organizations, cross-disciplinary clinical teams have become critical to meeting the financial and quality goals. At Walke-Parker, three teams are the vehicles for meeting the cost reduction. What

Figure 4.4

Resource Allocation Premises of the Case Study Institutions

Premise	Process Implication
1. Economic constraints on medical care are inevitable.	1. Corporate survival will dictate budget guidelines.
2. Continuous improvement in quality *and productivity* is the only realistic response to economic constraints.	2. The guidelines will require continuous productivity improvement in the operating budget.
3. Specific services can be justified only on grounds of long-run cost-effectiveness as judged by the customers and measured by their willingness to pay the price.	3. Capital and new program proposals will undergo competitive review made more intensive by a strong bias for liquidity. (In other words, each proposal will be a tough sell.)

the teams decide will strongly influence operating and capital budgets. At IHC, the effort of many care process model teams has been to reduce costs to or below Medicare payment levels, eliminating the need to cost shift. While the tie to the operating budget is not as explicit, the line managers and the physicians understand it.

Clinical guidelines or patient care protocols are the future in resource allocation. As they become more common, they will be compared by insurance carriers and buyers. National consensus will emerge on what survival rates, customer satisfaction, and price ought to be. Provider institutions will copy the methods as well as the measures, and the methods will establish the details of resource allocation. Clinical guidelines will specify the number of hours of nursing care and therapy, the drugs and appliances to be used, and the location and duration of care. These decisions will drive the facilities and human resource plans—the number of beds, operating rooms, and physical therapists, for example—and the operating and capital budgets.

In short, *hoshin* resource allocation processes are real, rather than ideal. The leaders of CQI health care institutions have two pressing tasks—the moral obligation to avoid unrealistic assumptions and the practical one of maintaining alignment. Our case study leaders seem to have done well on both. Their processes contain a number of safeguards to insure realism, and alignment appears high. The workforces of all three institutions appear to be convinced of the validity of the approach.

Implementation Processes

IHC people told us several times: "We share the theory with anyone, including our competitors. We plan to beat them on the implementation." Mission/vision and resource allocation decisions establish what the organization intends to do, but implementation decision processes determine whether it gets done and how well. Processes to recruit good people (including physicians), select among them, and provide training to maintain and expand skills are becoming more formal. These processes are also subject to the tests of realism and alignment, and they can be continuously improved.

A realistic process for personnel selection and development is one that offers better employment and security than its competitors in the labor marketplace. It is convincing if current employees agree that the record is good. All three places have invested in ongoing surveys of employee and physician satisfaction. All three organizations anticipate extensive cross-training of both professional and technical clinical support personnel. The processes are not far beyond the talking stage at present. They are developing files of employee skills. They have approached workforce reduction gingerly, and made efforts to avoid layoffs.

Henry Ford has significantly revised the incentives for both doctors and employees over the past several years. The emerging incentives emphasize corporate as well as unit goals. Joe Horton notes that IHC is examining its formal incentive structure:

> One of the corporate QI teams is looking at the budget process. We're seeking a reward-based, department-initiated, target-setting process backed up with real accountability. We want to define up front how much of their pay increase is dependent on meeting the budget. Right now, pay increases are based on a list of 25 process items. Most people do well on 23 or more.

IHC's innovative use of pilot demonstrations are worth noting. They use "relief from the budget guidelines" as rewards in two major pilot projects. Joe Horton describes how one got started, and where it stands:

> We had a two-day CQI training program for all the pediatric ICU staff. We then empowered them by freeing them from the budget guidelines on cost, and allowing them to keep 20 percent of any documented

savings to spend on departmental needs, as defined by IRS rules. They reported to the Quality Council in June. They described seven or eight projects in detail and listed 22 in process. One was a project to evaluate intravenous versus naso-gastric [NG] feeding. The ICU staff had decided in favor of the less expensive NG feeding, and would have just implemented it. We have some physicians on the council who are grant-funded researchers who suggested a randomized trial for that and helped them design it. With the trial, we may get a published paper, and something that would help others.

We think they'll save $100,000 by the end of the year from all their projects. We will extend this empowerment model [gain sharing and relief from budget guidelines] as a reward. It won't be automatic. The group will have to be trained, and it will have to have shown some results.

Carol Bush describes a similar concept in nursing:

The philosophy we're adopting here is that the manager, the person in charge of any given unit should be in control. The [old] system put the staffing tool [acuity measurement and work standards] in control. We believe nursing managers can make better judgments than the tool. Our pilot project uses historic data acuity and staffing for the budget as in the past. The charge nurse knows the available dollars per patient and overall. She or he looks at actual care to real patients. She sets her own staffing for the shift, rather than setting acuity scores. We're saying, "We trust you. If you think you need more or less today, go ahead." We plot the actuals against the budget over time, and our experience to date is that they are very responsible. Costs are below what they would have been. We've been working with the managers on the pilot units to find more outcomes quality measures.

The incentive here is not monetary, despite some small monetary elements. It is empowerment and recognition, "You've done good work, and the reward is increased independence to do more." In order to make this work, alignment has to be high. The employees and physicians must believe that (1) IHC understands the market, (2) IHC has a reasonable plan to survive, (3) they can improve their performance, and (4) IHC will reward initiative to the extent it is able and better than its competitors. The fact that these pilots are in place and yielding positive results is as good evidence of IHC leadership as we can offer.

Customer-controlled prices, patient care protocols, and cross-training will have important implications for procedures and activities in hospitals. To get optimal patient outcomes, protocols will be increasingly precise on what, when, and how specific care processes occur. Line managers will commit their units to increasingly specific measures of cost and process quality. They will achieve these by using more uniform procedures. Henry Ford's automated nursing procedure manual is an example. No matter what procedure the doctor orders, the nurse has a complete, up-to-date, step-by-step procedure to follow. The implications go beyond uniformity; they include nurse self-confidence and empowerment of technical personnel. It is no longer necessary to say the process is right because a trained professional did it. Instead, the process is right because it followed the correct procedure. The latter statement allows the quality of the technician's work to exceed the professional's.

The implementation process must address conflict resolution and appeals mechanisms. It should also address decision-making styles, emphasizing fairness, empowerment, and candor. Styles include what subjects can be openly discussed, the acceptability of dissent, how performance will be judged, rewards, and rights and perquisites of individuals. These are incentive issues that may turn out to be the winning edge. A careful reading of IHC's record shows not one but four different philosophies about clinical protocols. All four have been allowed to proceed; the issue will be resolved empirically, not philosophically.

The actual incentives may even be too strong. The unarguable premises for resource allocation raise the specter of real harm from excessive fiscal conservatism or excessive zeal in implementation. Horton says, "The downside is they [the line managers] do not have the option of not meeting [their assigned budget target]." If necessary they can appeal in a formal written document to use the contingency fund. He adds, "What's interesting is how few appeals there have been. There was a lot of apprehension . . . though only a handful of departments submitted in writing."

Actions here speak louder than words. You would have to be pretty insensitive not to understand the message. Henry Ford replaced several senior managers because they seemed to have trouble keeping up with their budget targets. Warden says, "I'm looking for line managers who like the challenge of managing." Walke-Parker dropped several levels of line managers so they could keep up with their targets. One might argue that Horton's separate memo strategy is not enough to protect quality of care. (So far as we could tell, it was more than Henry Ford or Walke-Parker had.)

Systematic pressure for cost reduction will eventually cause some people to cut quality corners. Because not all aspects of quality are reliably measured, these shortcuts could result in disasters. Any number of historic tragedies (the *Challenger* space shuttle, for example) show the dangers. The fact that a few managers *did* submit in writing is reassuring.

Implementation decisions need to recognize this danger. There are several protections. Making quality an unarguable requirement iterated throughout the resource allocation process is one. Personal example by senior executives is another. Reward for actions protecting quality is a third. CQI concepts actually reduce the danger of exploitation by demanding objective assessment of quality, customer satisfaction, and worker satisfaction. The best financial models and budget practices address the danger of exploiting patients explicitly. Safety valves for people inadvertently under more pressure than they think they can bear are essential.

Organizational Processes

Organization is the assignment of tasks, accountability, and authority to individuals. It includes not only the traditional accountability hierarchy shown in the charts, but also the charge and membership of standing and ad hoc committees and the accountability assigned to the medical staff. Realistic organizational decisions are those that identify someone responsible for each task who knows when and how to do it, has the tools, and gets it done. Alignment in these decisions means that people are enthusiastic, or at least in agreement, about that accountability.

CQI and cost control are forcing a much more dynamic organizational process. Accountabilities are more specific, more flexible, and more variable. The annual budget, a dynamic response to customer needs, is rapidly replacing the traditional job description as the fundamental statement of accountability. Teams and task forces are taking over responsibilities that used to be reflected in the organization chart. Walke-Parker prefers not to use an organization chart at all. Peggy Hanford, chief operating officer and chief nursing officer, describes the teams at Walke-Parker:

> Each nursing unit has a manager. The three cross-functional teams are made up of the managers, plus a fourth team made up of the outside product line managers. There are two patient care teams, and a third for support services. We organized the patient care teams along lines of the most natural customer/supplier relationship (see Figure 4.5). The teams share services to many of the same patients and have a

lot of interaction. They began to look for elimination of rework and handoffs in these patient care processes.

The teams don't have budgets, but they have explicit goals. The teams will look at how is it we reengineer and redesign the jobs to reduce the costs, without hurting patient satisfaction. From the perspective of the traditional department head, they have a budget, their measures derived from the radar chart, and selected other measures they have picked for themselves. They have to make the reduction and work with the teams. Their fear is heightened right now. Some folks were totally immobilized for a week or so. They've begun to settle down now. The teams have begun to realize that some of the changes may mean, say, a reduction in physical therapists, or respiratory therapists. I think we will see some ebb and flow of the fear reaction as the process evolves, but the teams keep people on track. The teams together make the decisions, not outside the teams. They decide they have a person in PT who is redundant. They look at how they can find a new job for that person, but it may mean a relocation. It's pretty new at this point, but we've done some work on job redesign and retraining.

Three years ago the assistant directors were eliminated, and authority went straight to the nurse managers of the units. The managers themselves eliminated staff in their processes. For example, hiring new employees—we cut out all reviews for any position being refilled.

A great deal of the dynamic organizational process depends upon the two-way flow of information (about forecasts and needs from the top, about commitment and performance from below). As a result, organizational processes focus on the distribution of information, again emphasizing a two-way flow. Organizational decisions for a line manager are specific goals negotiated at the time of the budget that go far beyond the financial targets. Hanford's above statement, "traditional department heads . . . have a budget, their measures derived from the radar chart, and selected other measures they have picked for themselves," is only one example. Intermountain's Poulsen recognized that "40 to 60 percent of our goals are related to quality." Henry Ford's "critical developments," "six or seven things that will significantly influence the year's performance," is another approach. Teams and committees have charges that specify the subject, distribution, and form of the output, selected membership, and coaches and suggestions for information input.

Figure 4.5

Operations of QI Teams, Walke-Parker Medical Center, 1993

Patient Care Operations I	Patient Care Operations II	Support Services
Radiology (chair)	Pharmacy (chair)	Food service (chair)
2N Nursing	3W Nursing	Finance and accounting
6W Nursing	4W Nursing	Material management
Surgery	3E Nursing	Environmental services
ICU/CCU	7W Nursing	
Physical therapy	Gyn/2E Nursing	
Health information	Emergency room	
	Wound care	
	Laboratory	
	Obstetrics/IE	
	Cardio-Pulmonary	
	Social services	
	Options	

Charge to the teams:

Decrease the cost per unit of service
Increase the patient "brag about"

The organizational changes that are occurring include the following:

- Physicians participate more actively in decision processes, accept more accountability, and develop new organizational roles.
- Clinical teams influence clinical processes formerly controlled solely by individual practitioners.
- The teams cut across traditional accountability hierarchies.
- Work groups accept accountability with less supervision.
- As care moves from inpatient to outpatient venues, the direct supervision of some caregivers is decreased.

The full implications of these changes are still emerging. The most important is the need to extend formal organization to primary care physicians' offices. The requirements for cost and quality control give organizations

Figure 4.6A

Traditional Hospital-Physician Organization

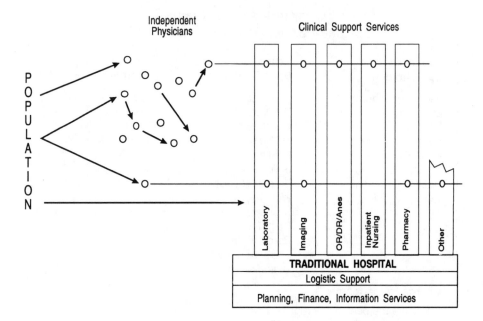

with specified accountability an advantage over loose affiliation of individuals or small groups. Organized primary care groups can achieve control by a variety of means, including member selection and education, formal incentives and risk sharing, improved relationships with suppliers, and clinical guidelines for care. The second implication is a restructuring of referral care, based on clinical guidelines and careful integration of the appropriate services. These two developments will profoundly affect clinical support services (CSS), from radiology to social service.

Both referral and primary providers will construct clinical guidelines around discrete clinical entities. The referral entities will be diagnosis and procedure oriented, like DRGs, while the primary entities must also include symptomatic and preventive care. (The ambulatory visit groups are an early version.) Primary care protocols will include criteria for referral or the use of services. The referral criteria are likely to be more stringent than the current system. Demand for CSS will be both price and quality sensitive, and will drop in many services. Lower prices will enforce a constant search for more efficient, more effective services. Quality demands will require uniformity of services and greater attention to customer satisfaction.

Figures 4.6A and B show these organizational implications. Up to 50 different clinical support services respond directly to independent physicians who order inpatient and outpatient services. They are the traditional departments shown as smokestacks on the right of Figure 4.6A. The seminal change is the insertion of explicit clinical guidelines, represented by diamonds in the patient flow lines, in response to the demand for more cost-effective care. As managed care spreads, the CSS will no longer be revenue centers. The clinical guidelines will establish the demand for CSS and the funds available for their operation. The changes in finance and control will affect both the formal accountability hierarchy represented by the table of organization and the collateral organization of cross-disciplinary task forces, committees, and work groups.[5] The "smokestacks" of the traditional hospital will be supplemented by the new disease- and procedure-oriented

Figure 4.6B

Emerging Health Care Organization

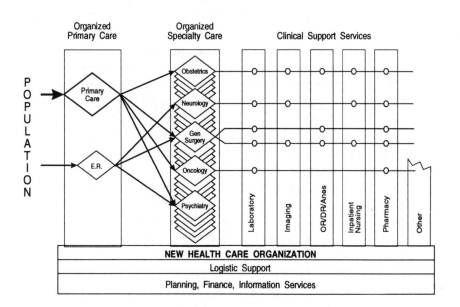

cross-disciplinary task forces. The formal organization of Figure 4.6B will incorporate direct accountability for the cross-disciplinary committees and the guideline-setting process as this trend continues.

Who gets to participate in the guideline setting, and where the information for it comes from, are critical organizational questions. Obviously, all providers will want to participate, and the task forces will be cross-disciplinary. CSS professionals will have a lot to contribute to guideline design and improvement in cost and quality, but the shift to clinically oriented approaches means sharing of power for these hospital line personnel. Their customers will be committees setting protocols, who will ask for patient satisfaction, strict adherence to procedures, outcomes quality standards, and minimum unit costs. Committees setting protocols will address both treatment paths of homogeneous patient groups and procedures that determine minute-by-minute actions within CSS.[6] Care plan decisions will drive the detailed expectations and budgets of units like laboratories, intensive care wards, and food service; that is, authority to set major operating parameters will pass from technical experts in clinical support services to permanent task forces oriented around specific clinical conditions, led by the medical specialists most familiar with the condition.

One implication of Figure 4.6B is closer affiliation within the medical staff and between the staff and the hospital, and the extension of the decision process and information system activities of the institution to serve physicians directly. Hospitals need to begin the development of effective physician-hospital organizations (PHOs) to facilitate this interaction. Using CQI principles, PHOs will offer substantial advantages to physicians practicing in a price-constrained environment, but a lengthy process of experimentation and development will be necessary. This is a process that is well under way at all the case study sites. Henry Ford, by virtue of its history, already has large employed medical groups, but it is working to extend organizational services to its fee-for-service physicians. Intermountain and Walke-Parker are actively studying how they can improve support to their physicians, who are largely fee-for-service.

Figure 4.6B does not show the final effect of the changes on the clinical support services. Presumably the final result will be a multidimensional hierarchy. The primary care providers as a group will have direct accountability for outcomes quality and capitation costs (including primary and referral services). Referral groups will be accountable for cost per episode or treatment and specific outcomes related to their services. Clinical support services will be accountable for process quality and costs per unit of service. All three classes will be accountable for patient satisfaction related to their services. Budget processes of the future will set financial, market, and quality targets for each group, using available total revenue as a guide. The institution as a whole will serve as an information and logistics resource, but also as a forum for the resolution of the most global expectations about the quality, quantity, and price of services.

In carrying out the future design, the main contributions of the Figure 4.6B organization will be

- Financial strength to bear risk and support capital expansion
- Marketing strength to compete in attracting satisfactory patient volumes
- Information collection and processing skills to support clinical protocol construction and continuous quality improvement.
- Conflict resolution skills to sustain a cordial environment and insure equity for individual members.

The future, like today, will reward organizations that are not afraid to address fundamental questions, that encourage and use a broad range of inputs, and that have robust mechanisms for appeals and conflict resolution.

The Infrastructure of Good Decision Processes

Some subtleties of the decision processes at these leading institutions go well beyond the outline in Figure 4.1. A health care organization could copy all of IHC's elegant processes and fail miserably to make them work. The most likely reason would be misunderstandings of role—who participates in each of the decisions and how they participate. Those questions—patterns for delegating authority for decisions and styles of participation—are more complex than they look. In the customer-oriented environment of CQI and cost control, they require more attention than they have received in the past.

The case study institutions are working through these problems by trial and error, by emphasizing CQI principles, and by relying on the sensitivity of their people. Rarely do the issues surface explicitly, but they are being addressed nonetheless. Progress begins with recognition of the mutual nature of stakeholder rights. It includes establishing new dynamic rules for delegating decisions. It is supported by deliberate implementation steps that encourage constructive adaptation to the new roles and authorities.

Recognizing Mutual Stakeholder Rights

We are in an environment where all stakeholders have opinions and expect their opinions to receive serious attention. Most of us grew up in a different environment, where traditional treaties assigned authority for decisions and rigidly divided the organization turf among the stakeholders. The doctor knew best, the nurse was his handmaiden, and the patient followed orders rather than participating in care. Trustees felt they handled the business matters, and often thought of themselves as beholden to the institution, rather than the constituencies it serves. Managers thought of themselves as the third leg of a wobbly three-legged stool with the physicians and the trustees.

Ideas like these fail both realism and alignment tests. Few will regret their passing; now they sound sexist and even absurd. Today's world requires a much more democratic and dynamic structure of decision-making authority, as Gary Pehrson notes:

> Demand in Intermountain is shifting out of the hospital business and into the outpatient and managed care market. We need liaisons with two important bodies. One is the business community. The other is physicians. Because of the demand, we're going to have to be more selective in our medical staffs. We'll have to build a real partnership with the doctors, on the basis of management decision making, true decision making, and rewards. We have a task force with the physicians, and they've begun to catch the spirit of this, in part because of the solid data and in part because of the efforts of Brent James. In part also because of the marketplace. The far-thinking doctors are really engaged. They recognize that when we can offer best value, we can sell that to the customers.

The shift means that people from a variety of backgrounds must learn to share decisions they once considered their professional prerogatives, and also that they must learn to make decisions outside their professional areas. People will have both cognitive and emotional difficulties with the transition. At a cognitive level, training can overcome ignorance of outsiders' values and lack of technical knowledge. A broader fact base in the presentation of each decision will help people reach beyond their field. Specific rather than general education will help people meet the cognitive requirement. We will teach people how to choose between TPA and streptokinase, not how to be cardiologists and health economists. This expanded cognitive requirement is a major force in the growth of information systems, discussed in the next chapter.

CQI's focus on a shared vision and emphasis on coaching and leadership helps the emotional adjustment to new roles and authority. Revising the mission and vision starts a process of reeducation because it focuses all stakeholders' attention on what the organization in fact is—the best device available to the stakeholders to achieve common goals. It is done annually partially to reinforce everybody's adjustment to new ways. The initial years particularly require leadership skills, patience, and sensitivity from health care managers. Beyond revisiting the vision, it is important to reinforce the new style with examples and cases showing its advantages; that is, the decision system must advertise its successes. So the first clinical protocols are easy ones where most people agree improvement is possible. The capital and operating budget programs evolve over several years as people become comfortable with the accountability involved. Pilots test next steps, provide visible examples, and develop coaches. At each step, victories are deliberately identified and celebrated.

The case study institutions demonstrate all of these points. Cognitively, they advertise their mission and vision at every opportunity. They have sound information systems now and ambitious programs for expansion. They put heavy emphasis on the CQI philosophy of objectivity and analysis. They provide helpful coaching to people making decisions. They approach the emotional aspects of relearning with considerable attention to giving people time to learn, letting them pick their participation rather than enforcing it, and tolerating contrary viewpoints and mistakes. But all of this is in a framework of the inevitability of customer focus. The term becomes a code word or euphemism for the required changes in attitude.

Dynamic Accountable Delegation for Decisions

New rules must replace the old turf domains for delegating decisions. The realism criterion demands continuous improvement of both cost and quality. The alignment criterion must assure all stakeholders that their individual interests will not be subverted by decisions beyond their immediate surveillance. The processes to meet these criteria must integrate complex patient and customer values with extensive technical knowledge from a wide span of professions. The integration should be complete, timely, and efficient. A missing or misstated stakeholder or technical viewpoint may lead to failure. Decisions should be prompt, if only to clear the field for the next problem; stakeholder gridlock will be fatal. Finally, the decisions should be efficient, optimizing the scarce time of the decision makers.

Dynamic accountable delegation is emerging to meet these criteria. "Dynamic" means that the topics are selected by the central governance structure according to stakeholder needs related to the topic itself, rather than unvarying treaties. There are no sacred cows or private domains. "Accountable" protects the right to have one's view heard if necessary. Each stakeholder understands that he or she has a reliable mechanism to a fair hearing on any question, at his or her discretion. Such a mechanism rarely existed under the old treaties. "Delegation" assigns decisions to the people most important to their implementation. Within accountability limits, delegation is complete. The boundaries of an acceptable decision are established in advance, and decisions within the boundaries are accepted without debate. The decisions are not micromanaged by meddling or ritualistic reviews. Pehrson notes that it won't be easy to change all the attitudes involved:

> Our organizational restructuring meets great resistance from the territorial imperatives of each specialty. My bias is that we let the marketplace drive the effort, rather than try to drive people into something that is foreign to them. They'll understand it better if we deal with the efforts through multidisciplinary teams. For example, management shouldn't ask for new standards of respiratory care using nursing instead of RT personnel. We should let work teams develop those decisions, as the need for them develops.

Dynamic accountability does not rule out using committees to negotiate specific conflicts, or giving direct representation to a minority position, such as placing physicians on governing boards. The best existing model of accountable delegation is the credentialling system, where decisions about individual physicians are made by physicians professionally competent to do so, but the criteria, process, and result are subject to review by a governing board representing a much broader constituency. At the same time, it allows a reversibility the old rules never had. A specific decision or a class of decisions can always be reviewed if some stakeholders feel aggrieved enough about the question. In practice, a very small fraction of the delegated decisions are challenged—much smaller than the number of old-rule decisions made by committee A, reviewed by committee B, passed on the board to be debated again, and frequently ping-ponged around several times in the process—because the delegates understand that it is in their interest to make the right to review moot by accommodating the needs of other stakeholders in the initial decision.

Under accountable delegation as the case study organizations do it, the governing board sets the mission and vision. Doctors and employees buy into the mission by signing on. Broad participation, understanding, and acceptance are essential. Beyond this, the more abstract, global, or central the decision, generally the upper left of Figure 4.1, the greater the need for direct outsider participation. Trustees evaluate mergers, acquisitions, and other external alliances. Internally, they focus on the scope of services, long-range financial plan, and budget guidelines. These decisions provide landmarks for insider delegation of the balance of the resource allocation and implementation decisions.

The larger the contribution of clinical knowledge to the solution, generally the right-hand portions of Figure 4.1, the more authority to propose solutions is delegated to the inside stakeholders. Most budget detail, care plan, and implementation decisions are delegated to insiders held accountable to the mission/vision and overall cost constraints. Cross-functional teams are also accountable delegation. In the case of clinical protocols, the delegation is actually from individual physicians to the team. It involves admitting the realism of customer input.

Our case studies are well advanced on accountable delegation. There are clear assignments for almost all the recurring decisions of Figure 4.1, and patterns for ad hoc issues. Their governing boards have focused almost exclusively on strategic direction setting, and executive-level activities have evolved to incorporate both attention to the delegation process and handling of appeals. Note particularly the role of the IHC and Henry Ford boards in the resource allocation processes. Almost all the dispute resolution is passed down the organization. Once the budget guidelines have been set, the board role is minimal.

Implementing the Decision System

Management is the accountable delegate for the organizational decisions of Figure 4.1. Management's attention is properly on the decision processes and their implementation, rather than the decisions themselves. It designs the processes and suggests the rules for accountable delegation in accordance with the stakeholder demands and the criteria of realism and alignment. Conversely, managers are generally not the delegates for the rest of Figure 4.1, the mission/vision, resource allocation, and implementation decisions.

There are four parts to effective implementation. First, the rules must have recognized authorities. Decision-making rules tend to be easy to forget and even easier to attack when the decision itself is not what the stakeholder hoped for. Conflicts about the rules can disable the entire continuous improvement program. The bylaws for the board and medical staff usually identify the major authorities.

Second, the alignment criterion requires that debates about the decision-making system itself must also have identified appeals bodies. These can be either line officers or specific standing committees: IHC tends to emphasize executives; Henry Ford, committees. Walke-Parker is small enough that there isn't much difference, but people clearly know where to turn. Any stakeholder who feels aggrieved enough must be able to request a review of the relevant delegation in addition to an appeal of a specific decision. If either appeal generates a majority for change, change can occur. If not, the individual can accept the decision or leave the organization. The decision system can do no more than provide an avenue for prompt and fair hearing, but it must do that much. The board and its major committees will be important as the final appeals bodies.

Third, the rules are enforced by appointing and charging committees, setting agendas, keeping minutes, training people to follow procedures, and supplying information and coaches. Managers in all parts of the organization must know what the relevant bylaws and procedures say, or how to find out. A beginning doctor, worker, or trustee is not expected to memorize the decision-making rules, but rather to know and trust someone who does. Knowing or finding the answer is properly the role of every first-line supervisor and medical division chief. Training these people in decision making is an obvious step, already incorporated in CQI.

Fourth, the decision system must be enforced. Even a few flagrant departures can destroy it. Exceptions to the rules and special pleadings beyond the appeals process must be strongly and promptly resisted. Enforcement means that behavior is redirected according to the rules. Punishment is not involved. Except in the rare case of deliberately destructive behavior, the individuals are simply shown that following procedures is the effective path.

Henry Ford Health System, Intermountain Health Care, and Walke-Parker Medical Center are very different cultures. If you were transported from one to another, you would feel the difference as soon as you started to talk to somebody. In none of them would you find people arguing over how to decide things. Just as the missions and visions are agreed upon, so are the processes for resource allocation, clinical guidelines, and organization. People expect to go to meetings to get things done. When they get there, the tools are in place—the agenda is set, the chair enforces it, the information is at hand, and the members commit to action. That is what implementation is all about. Gary Pehrson, perhaps unintentionally, expressed it in a few graphic words:

> It's not tolerated around here to be a poop. It's a combination of the board, Scott Parker's own attitude, and—even though we're not part of the church—to some extent the belief of the Mormon people that you should get along. It's not accepted to fight. That doesn't mean we don't have disagreements, but we try to handle them constructively.

Notes

1. Simon, H. 1976. *Administrative Behavior: A Study of Decision Making Processes in Administrative Organizations*, 3d ed. New York: Free Press.
2. See *Quality Management in Health Care*, 1 (Summer 1993), which is devoted to strategic quality planning and includes articles based on five different health care systems.
3. Demers, D. M. 1993. "Implementing Hoshin Planning at the Vermont Medical Center." *Quality Management in Health Care* 1 (Summer): 64–72. See especially p. 69, on which Demers offers no evidence that VMC has achieved breakthrough innovation to date.
4. Hatcher, M. E., and C. Connelly. 1988. "A Case Mix Simulation Decisions Support System Model for Negotiating Hospital Rates." *Journal of Medical Systems* 12 (6): 341–63. See also, Hatcher, M. E., and N. Rao. 1988. "A Simulation Based Decision Support System for a Health Promotion Center." *Journal of Medical Systems* 12 (1): 11–29.
5. Griffith, J. R. 1992. *The Well-Managed Community Hospital*, 2d ed. Chapter 4, pp. 106–39. Ann Arbor, MI: Health Administration Press.
6. Rosenstein, A. H. 1991. "Health Economics and Resource Management: A Model for Hospital Efficiency." *Hospital & Health Services Administration* 36 (3): 313–30.

5

Managing the Information Explosion

Information as the Linchpin of the Surviving Organization

No one "flies an airplane" anymore. Instead, pilots file flight plans stating destinations, departure and arrival times, altitudes, air speeds, and precise routes; they monitor progress against the plan and state performance facts in the flight log. In a quiet but rapid revolution, the same has happened with health care. No one "treats a patient" anymore. Instead, the care provider documents a diagnosis, plans a specific treatment, and indicates an expected outcome. Like the flight plan and log, this process has become routine and increasingly quantitative. Diseases and treatments are precisely coded. Quantitative laboratory data supports almost every treatment plan. Imaging is used frequently, and it is now often digitalized. Drugs have proliferated, and with increased power and specificity, dosages have become critical. The database that results has become an intrinsic requirement of practice for the individual patient's care and for monitoring the components of care across patient groups. The concept of "continuous improvement" is one of commitment to learning from variations between plan and actual.

To carry the analogy one step further, no one "runs a hospital" anymore. Instead, you treat specific numbers and kinds of patients in a variety of settings at specific costs and quality levels, and according to an advance plan. The database goes far beyond aggregating the individual care data and is an intrinsic requirement of practice for the manager, as it is for the pilot and the doctor. The manipulation of quantitative data has become the core technology for institutional survival in the twenty-first century.

Partly, this is because the technology is there to do it, but there are three reasons coming from health care itself. First, the information network defines the formal organizational hierarchy of obligations. Authority and accountability are defined by agreements about performance. Line managers and quality improvement teams alike accept responsibility for achieving improved levels of performance that are increasingly defined in precise quantitative terms. A head nurse is no longer "in charge of a floor." He or she is now accountable for a budget, certain staffing levels, certain outcomes and process quality scores, compliance to clinical paths or protocols, and certain levels of physician and worker satisfaction; that is to say, the head nurse's job is defined by expectations and performance measures more clearly than by the traditional job description. Similarly, a quality improvement team identifies a problem measured in several performance dimensions, commits itself to improvements in certain of those dimensions, and celebrates its results based on actual change in performance measures. The team, like the head nurse, the doctor, and the flier, defines its success by the information itself.

Second, the information resource supports effective operation, especially under CQI. The search for productivity improvement will succeed only when it is backed by reliable information. The range of information needed to support the search is vast. It includes sound market analysis and forecasting to properly size each activity to realistic demand, competitor analysis to develop benchmarks on price and quality, and internal data to support design and improvement of processes. CQI puts a high premium on delivering this information effectively to quality improvement teams at the point of service. The better an institution processes information and uses it to support the search for productivity, the better its performance will be.

Third, information defines the tenuous agreements between stakeholders that permit the enterprise itself to exist. Health care organizations, like all collaborative endeavors, exist because they fulfill goals of their participants or customers that cannot conveniently be filled some other way. Satisfaction of stakeholders' needs is essential for the organization to continue. The negotiations and the agreements that result between stakeholders are the essence of the governance function (see Chapter 4). They have become increasingly precise and quantitative—the institution will have such and such revenue; so many physicians will be available and they will earn so much; such and such levels of quality will be achieved. Quantitative information permits more effective governance function in *hoshin* planning, budget setting, and clinical performance evaluation. The results of stakeholder negotiations determine the acceptable ranges for the performance of the components of the organization. They define the survival goals for the organization, and they serve as the coordinating force that integrates all the caregivers, managers, and improvement teams.

The Case Study Institutions' Information Strategies

All three of the case study institutions recognized the importance of information some time ago. They have evolved complex plans for the use of information and implemented significant parts of their plans. Here is a brief summary of where each stands.

Walke-Parker Medical Center

Walke-Parker is relatively small. They don't waste time and money on overhead. They pride themselves on responding quickly to a difficult market. And they brag that they *don't* have a sophisticated information system.

There's a lot more sophistication at Walke-Parker than meets the eye. Consider this:

1. The monitoring and planning activities at Walke-Parker are driven by an elaborate hierarchy of information (see Chapter 7). Sixteen measures form the *hoshin* compass points. They have a major effect on what Walke-Parker will do next year, because Christiansen and his crew will change the operation to achieve acceptable scores on those measures. Twenty-four subsidiary measures are identified because they are statistically associated with the 16. Four hundred more measures are available to carry the rollout another step, to meet the needs of any specific work group or team.

2. The measures deliberately cover several dimensions. Their "radar chart" (see Figure 7.5) identifies four, with Walke-Parker's own labels, but you can think in terms of marketing, cost, finance, and quality.

3. The 440 measures are not fully automated, but they are understood to be reliable and valid numbers with specific definitions. This reliability and specificity never happens by accident; it represents a lot of work by the Walke-Parker people.

4. Walke-Parker has begun work on clinical paths. These "flight plans" for medical care set in motion a series of events that will eventually carry Walke-Parker to where Intermountain Health Center and Henry Ford Health System are going. The parent firm knows this, and will probably develop the clinical information systems to support it.

Intermountain Health Care

As Gary Pehrson, vice president of Professional Services at Intermountain Health Care (IHC) says, "The Management Committee is absolutely committed to information systems as essential." Brent James, director of the Institute for Health Care Delivery Research (IHCDR), adds, "Information systems are a business strategy for IHC, and they are awfully good." Intermountain has invested tens of millions of dollars over 25 years in the HELP clinical information system and will invest $40 million more as it rolls out to all the sites. It maintains competitive versions of the standard business office systems. It developed a nursing management system several years ago. It has an elaborate customer and employee satisfaction survey system. The IHCDR, two "medical informaticists" (physicians with training in medical information needs), an epidemiologist and several management engineers provide an exceptional data analysis capability. The IHCDR has three critical functions:

1. It educates IHC managers and physicians in CQI.
2. It stimulates care process model (patient care protocols) development.
3. It provides measurement tools like Horn's Computerized Severity Index (CSI).

IHC has an unmistakable, hard-headed focus on market performance, but it is deliberately balanced by other measures. For example:

1. The patient care protocols and clinical data reporting are oriented toward a clear quality goal as well as a cost goal. The goal is to get better clinical results, but also to get cost per case equal to Medicare payment levels. There are no excuses about "cost shifting."
2. Each site has rigorous goals for productivity and for a satisfactory margin (viewed as a dividend to the community) within the revenue made available by the market. The goals are not easy to make (half failed in 1993), and there is obvious tension about them.

3. There is strong emphasis on patient and family satisfaction, with carefully constructed and administered measures. This emphasis befits an organization with such a large market share that it could easily become lax and unresponsive.

4. Physician and employee satisfaction are carefully monitored, and their needs are met. The corporation accepts responsibility for recruiting, training, retaining, and retraining its workforce. Like customer satisfaction, this commitment is essential to maintaining effectiveness in a near-monopoly environment.

Figure 5.1 shows the relative importance of this expenditure in the IHC budgets. It excludes the information system for the health plan.

Henry Ford Health System

The plan at Henry Ford calls for rapid expansion of information services, emphasizing clinical expectations, improved costing, and concurrent control of care through an on-line care system. Henry Ford leadership feels the organization is strong on goal-setting information and short on actual performance data. Still, Al Sinisi, chief information officer, says:

> We have the conventional transaction systems on-line. They use software and hardware which are several years old, but they are as good as anybody's. The budget and monthly performance data are also on-line, and accessible to most responsibility center managers.

Figure 5.1

Planned Information Expenditures at IHC

Information Expenditure	Amount per Year	Percent of Total Operations
IHCDR	$ 700,000	0.1
Other analysis staff*	500,000	0.1
IS operations	17,000,000	2.2
Expanding clinical IS	8,000,000	1.0
Other IS investments	Contribution from joint venture on HELP system	Variable

*Informaticists, epidemiologists, and management engineers. Excludes planning staff.

We have E-mail for most managers. We're piloting teleconferencing. We have two help desks. One is for anything, and the other is for PCs. The calls are reviewed daily; any that aren't answered are assigned for completion. We try to stay away from developing new PC applications; we don't have the staff for it. If you ask for certain data, we have people who will find the data, retrieve it, and help you plan your analysis. We have preferred vendors for PC training. We have standard configurations of PC hardware and software, which we support with price and service contracts. If you stay within the configuration, your installation goes like that!

A Ford line manager such as a clinic director or a hospital department head can count on the following:

1. Direct access to significant amounts of individual patient data.
2. Conventional cost and revenue data compared to budget and automated for building future budgets.
3. Data on customer satisfaction and human resources from the several surveys routinely maintained by the HMO and the major delivery units.
4. Reports, commentary, and benchmarks on the "balanced scorecard" measures developed by his or her unit. (These include the six or seven "critical developments" described in Chapter 8.)
5. High-quality staff assistance for pursuing CQI projects, preparing the future budget, developing capital requests, and other innovative activities.
6. Steady improvement and an information system that remains equal to the best in the state.

Clinical Information Systems at the Case Study Institutions

Clinical information systems (CIS) provide on-line medical record data to physicians treating individual patients. Early versions included order entry and results reporting; the vision is of a fully electronic medical record accessible for patient care during treatment and for analysis afterwards. CIS are emerging rapidly, and both Intermountain and Henry Ford plan major investments in their development. Larry Grandia, the Intermountain chief information officer (CIO), says:

IHC views the computerized medical [or patient] record [CPR] as the goal for all patient records within the decade. As a key component to our CPR strategy, the HELP system supports clinical decision making and can link different types, sites, and episodes of care. At LDS Hospital, approximately 50 percent of the patient record is already stored in the HELP system. The development of the CPR is an ongoing process, however, and is an evolving goal rather than a specific outcome.

And, he adds, the effort is beginning to pay off:

Some of the documented successes IHC has experienced using the HELP System include

- Reduction in adverse drug events through automated alerts— $400,000 in annual savings
- Reduction in postoperative wound infection rates through automated reminders to administer preoperative antibiotics— $800,000 in annual savings
- Improved survival rate for patients with adult respiratory disease syndrome using standardized treatment protocols—from 10 percent to 45 percent
- Support for clinical CQI studies, including uncomplicated transurethral prostatectomies studies leading to reduced variation in clinical care
- Improved access to the presentation of data for physicians, including physician-specific rounds reports.[1]

Brent James adds:

The HELP system captures virtually all orders and results, and supports nurse charting. It supports a true expert system. IHC will install it in every medium to large facility within a few years. The hospitals will pay the costs of installation and maintenance in their operating budgets. The data from HELP are archived to form a research base. IHC uses two M.D. informatics specialists and a staff to teach people how to find and use the data.

The information goals for the next few years are the HELP rollout, using HELP and other systems to support horizontal integration of IHC, and developing an effective central data repository. Another long-term goal is an ambulatory care system.

The Ford system has taken a different approach. Al Sinisi, CIO, says:

Right now, our Medical Information Management System [MIMS] has radiology and lab reports. Pharmacy data, operating notes, discharge summaries, pulmonary and EKG results are available now. The big return for the doctor is on the results side, and that's where we try to focus. Order entry comes next; we're now in the process of installing it. In nursing, the "Excellcare" system operates independently. Over 2,000 care plan elements are accessible to the nurse planning care for the individual patient, and the individual care plans are summarized automatically to estimate unit staffing needs and annual budgets.

Our overall strategy relates to the patient: a clinical data system that is totally seamless, integrated, and makes no distinction between inpatient or outpatient. No matter where he or she is in HFHS, the practitioner can access the data in the way the practitioner wants it.

Tom McNulty, senior vice president and chief financial officer, talks about a "neural network" where a physician can get integrated sound-image-data communication on-line through the MIMS:

The "neural" system, which is the most ambitious plan the MIMS planning group is likely to request, will cost $90 million to $120 million over five years, or an increase in total expenditures of 1.5 percent to 2 percent per year.

The message here is of CIS as a strategic weapon of the organization. Before CQI, boards and executives looked at information systems as productivity improvement devices, and often sought specific efficiency gains as justification for investments. Henry Ford and Intermountain are not thinking that way. They are thinking about CIS as something a health care organization cannot do without, like laboratory and x-ray. They envision three layers of justification for the CIS:

1. Doctors and clinical personnel will use the CIS for most orders, results, and notes, speeding entry and vastly improving accuracy.

2. Case-specific data can be accessed and aggregated for study by function (e.g., drug usage), by site (e.g., outpatient), by disease (e.g., pediatric asthma), by insurance plan (e.g., Medicaid), and by individual physician. These data will provide the major analytic resource for CQI teams, who will use them to develop improved procedures or protocols.

3. Procedures and protocols can be built into the CIS, permitting clinical personnel to depart from them where necessary, but reducing the variance in care.

As Larry Grandia indicates, large benefits in both cost and quality are likely.

Smaller health care providers will not be able to make investments of the magnitude Intermountain and Henry Ford contemplate, but they won't have to. Earnie Lester, director of Managed Care at Walke-Parker remarks:

> We are working on a new clinical information system to support our primary care network. We looked at all the existing systems and picked one still under development. It will have information on each patient's history, physical, diagnostic test reports, and therapy and use advanced database techniques for retrieval. It does scheduling and office management functions. It will support remote consultation, transferring detailed clinical data via telephone. It's a relatively inexpensive system.

Most health care institutions will follow the Walke-Parker model. The technology developed at sites like HFHS and IHC will be made commercially available soon after it is demonstrated; Intermountain Health Care has already licensed the HELP system to 3M for marketing. Subsequent installations will be substantially cheaper. The lesson for most of us is that development will come piecemeal. It is not necessary to pioneer CIS, but it will be essential to keep up with commercially available developments.

Coaching with Information

What wisdom can be transferred from the cases to others? First, and most important, these institutions have a firm understanding of the role of data—what it is and how to use it in CQI. Second, they have used that understanding to improve their measurement systems to make the next step in continuous improvement easy for the line managers and the quality improvement teams, whatever the next step is. Third, they have tailored their systems to meet clinical needs, recognizing that any "reform" of health care must change actual care delivery.

The Role of Data in CQI

Obviously, strategic use of information involves large numbers and varied kinds of data that must be classified and organized. Below is a taxonomy based on dimension, type, and level that provides a checklist for planning information needs. The three case study organizations have substantially followed the taxonomy, although they sometimes omit parts and they frequently regroup the measures as they think convenient. Many of the omissions are mentioned in future plans.

Dimensions of performance measurement

Any activity or process in a hospital or clinic can be described and quantified in six major dimensions of performance, as shown in Figure 5.2.[2] Although a clinical activity is shown, the dimensions apply as well to support services and manufacturing functions. The specific measures for each dimension differ by application. Each of the six dimensions is managed in some sense. Demand is deliberately stimulated, diminished, and scheduled based on clinical needs; costs are kept to a budget; needs of doctors and other personnel are met; charges are posted and revenue is collected; and output and quality are maximized within demand and resource constraints. Each measurement dimension is backed by an information system, and measures for all six dimensions are used to improve performance.

Six is the safe minimum number of dimensions. Some people expand the number of dimensions (usually by elevating a component of the six,

---

Figure 5.2

Dimensions of Health Care Measures

Input Oriented	Output Oriented
Demand	**Outputs**
Patient management	Treatments
Clinical management	Productivity
Logistic management	
Cost/Resources	**Quality**
Costs	Clinical outcomes
Physical counts	Patient satisfaction
Resource condition	Procedural quality
Human Resources	**Revenue**
Worker/Physician	Profit
Satisfaction	Implicit price
Supply	

such as worker satisfaction, or outcomes quality) or use different labels and different groupings. Any specific application should have quantitative measures for all six dimensions. Quantified measures tend to draw attention from unmeasured or implicit ones. The unmeasured dimensions can become accidents waiting to happen. Two of the six dimensions, cost and output, are routine components of traditional budgets. The other four are evolving rapidly as part of the reengineering process.

Direct measurement of worker and physician satisfaction recognizes that the success of the organization and its working units depends upon a competent, satisfied worker group. Continued CQI progress is impossible if workers are marginally trained or dissatisfied with working conditions. Satisfaction is measured with surveys, measures of recruitment success, and absenteeism, turnover, and grievance statistics.

Quality measurement is developing rapidly. Patient satisfaction is surveyed using stratified random sampling of inpatient and outpatient populations (Ford and Intermountain are both considering universal sampling of important groups) and nationally available standardized questionnaires. Valid outcomes measures are expanding rapidly at a disease-specific level. They frequently require sophisticated severity adjustments or narrow case specification, as shown in the Intermountain measures of acute myocardial infarction and major joint replacement, Chapter 6. Global outcomes measures have not fared well. Global mortality statistics have not proven stable; readmissions do not appear to be valid;[3] measures of functional recovery do not aggregate over the variety of conditions and procedures. Process quality measures continue to be important. The measures are specific to the activity at hand, and the number and scope of measures are expanding. Intermountain's AMI study, for example, uses time to get an EKG diagnosis as an important component of the care.

Contribution is an increasingly difficult concept, as payment moves from individual fees to global payment like DRGs and finally to capitation. Its function in the measurement system is to relate the performance of the specific operating unit to economic requirements imposed by the external market. Under traditional fee-for-service, the revenue opportunity, less agreed-upon contributions to overhead (non–revenue-generating units) and to profit (capital needs), established the maximum operating cost of the unit. This is not to say the unit had to make a profit, but simply that the unprofitable unit had to be treated as an exception, and justified under other criteria. Its losses, of course, became part to the overhead burden of other units. Under a completely capitated system, the organization as a whole is the only revenue center. The test of the economic requirement changes—the organization must now operate all its component units at a total cost consistent with the overall needs. Most institutions will operate under capitation and various kinds of global payments for the foreseeable future. The result is that there will be three tests of contribution which any unit must meet simultaneously:

1. *Fee-for-service*: Unit costs less than unit price less agreed-upon overhead and profit contribution
2. *Global payment*: Costs per episode less than agreed-upon share of global payment
3. *Capitation*: Total costs less than agreed-upon share of total revenues

The traditional method rewarded increased volume; it led to lower unit costs and higher profits. The global and capitation payments have the opposite effect. As they begin to dominate the unit's activity, cost control efforts must move to reducing demand and making the department smaller.

Demand also presents special problems in itself. Under traditional fee-for-service, the logistics of demand are managed—for example, patients and internal customers are served within maximum time limits and simultaneous efforts are made to balance work loads and avoid idle periods. Deliberate promotional efforts are often made to keep the total level of demand high. Under global prices, unnecessary services must be identified and eliminated, but certain services are identified for 100 percent compliance goals. For instance, efforts might be made to eliminate redundant chest x-rays for pneumonia patients and to assure prompt chest x-rays for all patients going to surgery. Under capitation, demand management is extended even further. Patient behavior modification is used to diminish some elements of demand and encourage others, depending upon the clinical ramifications. For example, smoking cessation programs will be used to reduce smoking-related diseases and telephone advisory service will be used to eliminate unnecessary emergency visits, but simultaneously, prenatal care and immunizations will be promoted.

Types of information

The airplane pilot uses three types of information: *expectations*, that is her or his flight plan; *performance*, that is the flight log; and *reference*, that is maps, benchmarks, and other information that help determine the expectation and solve problems that arise. CQI assumes we also will use all three types.

The essence of control under CQI is expectations. The organization empowers people in quality improvement teams (QITs). The teams redesign processes and set new expectations. Clinical QITs frame these redesigned processes as care protocols. It is important to conclude the teams' work with new expectations for all six dimensions. These then become elements to factor into budgets, and benchmarks for the actual change in performance. Team performance can also be assessed on the six dimensions.

The focus on expectations, rather than performance, is a central CQI philosophy, building in control rather than enforcing it. Accomplishment of expectations, the satisfaction of the job well done, is the major reward. The teams use both reference and performance information to set expectations. Expectations drive performance, and performance plus reference drive expectations, in a circular manner. It is the reference information, what other people are doing and how, and what the market demands, that keeps this circle near the limits of currently feasible performance. Without reference measures, expectations and performance will decline, and the CQI process will become unstable.

Reference information services are relatively new in electronic format. They supply data that are external to the institution by definition:

- Epidemiologic data, such as the anticipated incidence of major diseases and conditions, functional status measures, and survival measures
- Risk data, such as smoking, drinking, immunization, and disease-prevention habits
- Utilization data, such as hospitalizations and procedure rates
- Competitor data, such as scope of services, unit costs, and health insurance premiums
- Comparison data, such as the performance of similar units in other geographic locations, useful for benchmarking.

In a cost control environment, these data are essential to the strategic level decision processes. They indicate what the priorities and opportunities are from the customer perspective of CQI, not only in the mission and vision, but down into the individual processes like mammogram waiting times and prenatal care expectations.

Levels of performance measurement

The six dimensions of the Figure 5.2 model apply to any level of the traditional organization, from individual activity units like pharmacy service or emergency physician care, to the strategic activities of the institution as a whole. At the higher levels, most cost, human resource, output, and quality measures are aggregated from the values for the individual activities; the aggregation rules may get quite complex, but they are spelled out in standard accounting, financial, and statistical procedures. The introduction of quality improvement teams, and the movement to hold the clinical teams accountable for episode-specific results, present special complexities.

The traditional method of organizing individual activities is an accountability hierarchy reflected in the conventional organization chart and cost-accounting reporting aggregates. The hierarchy remains useful to match professional skills (the labs under the pathologist, for example) and to control resources, or inputs to the activities. However, it does not match clinical processes or outcomes. Many different activities make up a clinical episode. As suggested by Figure 5.3, few activities serve only one kind of patient, and almost no patients require only one activity.

Thus, the information system must be capable of organizing data both ways, from the responsibility centers (the vertical elements of the new organizational structure shown in Figure 4.6B) to the clinical task forces (the horizontals), and back again. Outcomes control is achieved by cross-disciplinary clinical teams. Activity control is achieved by the traditional accountability hierarchy. Neither is likely to disappear. As a result, the six dimensions and three types of data must be reportable for traditional aggregates like "all clinical laboratory" and "all diagnostic services," and for all episodes of care, like "coronary artery bypass surgery"

Figure 5.3

Competing Needs for Information Organization

Inputs Organized by Hierarchy	Outputs Organized by Kind of Patient
Laboratory	Orthopedics
Radiology	Hip fracture
Operating room	Hip replacement
Recovery room	Knee repair
Inpatient nursing	Knee replacement
Physical therapy	Leg fracture

and "outpatient diabetic care." This duality is a major justification for automation because of the number and variety of important reporting combinations.

All three of the leaders already have systems for reporting data both ways. Joe Corrigan, chief financial officer at Walke-Parker, describes a commercially available system for clinical cost allocations:

> We support our clinical teams with case-specific data from the Ernst and Young "Claims Management System." We supply a lot of information—total charges, charge per day, charge by kind of service. Costs are based on a cost-to-charge ratio. We're installing a true RVU-based cost reporting system early next year, and we routinely report quality data. The data are continued after the teams finish their work to monitor what actually happened. We set up the reports the team requested on an automatic basis in our quarterly printouts. It used to be there weren't many things that were right around the borderline on a go/no go decision. Now people pay much less, you've got more stuff in the gray area. The systems are not cheap, but by the time you wait to see what data you'll need, it's too late.

Both Henry Ford and Intermountain want to go beyond this by improving the accuracy of the clinically oriented reports. Tom McNulty, HFHS senior vice president and chief financial officer, wants to improve cost allocation accuracy and accessibility, making it possible to estimate profit or loss on an individual patient during his or her care.

> We are developing an RCU system [relative cost unit system] for care which will provide unit cost for either actual patient ledgers or clinical paths. Then any proposed path can be costed, and actual care can be concurrently costed, compared to protocol, and compared to revenue. The system will enter inpatient alpha testing in 1993.
>
> The RCU system will use groups of similar items within a cost center (e.g., similar lab tests or similarly handled pharmaceuticals) to reduce calculation volumes. Items within each group will be assigned relative value units based on studies of relative cost. We'll estimate the unit cost for groups of similar items using the 80/20 rule and this formula:

$$\text{unit cost of group average} = \text{direct labor}$$
$$+ \text{ direct supplies}$$
$$+ \text{ other direct costs}$$

> \+ departmental overhead
> \+ depreciation and capital cost
> \+ allocated space cost
> \+ corporate overhead

The last four cost entries are largely fixed costs; the allocation will be based upon anticipated or budgeted volumes. So the cost center accountability is translated to a unit cost based on a standard volume, eliminating any incentive to increase volumes in the center.

The patient ledger items, multiplied by an estimated unit cost, summed by individual patient within an identified episode of care, becomes the referent for clinically oriented cost reports. The clinical summary can be prepared instantaneously from an automated billing record. Costs can be compared "to date" against the protocol, empirical averages, or anticipated revenue. The physician managing the case can be accountable for the cost. For both the cost center manager and the physician, the actual control will be built in through expectations (protocols or budgets), consistent with the CQI philosophy.

Susan Horn, Ph.D., senior scientist at Intermountain's IHCDR, notes an important problem in comparing patients or aggregating patient data. Diagnosis or procedure alone is often not enough to remove acuity differences between patients. She has developed a severity index to make patient groups more homogeneous.

> The Computerized Severity Index has been reprogrammed on DOS as a totally relational database. You can retrieve the data supporting the index very quickly. That data is captured from HELP and downloaded to the database. It's useful for specific studies, like the partial prothrombin time study, and for nursing staffing evaluation, and for adjusting quality and cost measurements.

Improving a Measurement System

All three of our case study institutions have strong information systems covering most dimensions, a clear focus on expectations and references, and competitive capability in dual reporting. They are rapidly expanding their coverage of the dimensions, adding explicit measures for quality and worker satisfaction and increasing the frequency of patient satisfaction surveying. They are developing archives to make performance data retrieval easier, expanding their reference data sets and making them more accessible, and supporting more sophisticated analysis. The number of clinical protocols is expanding rapidly at both Henry Ford and Intermountain. While QITs do not universally conclude with six dimensions of new expectations, the importance of these numbers is now understood and the batting average is improving. All three have ambitious plans for further improvement. These plans balance four different areas: activity measures, corporate vision measures, expectations, and analysis.

Improving measures for individual activities

The first improvement possibility for most health care organizations lies in expanding coverage of the six dimensions of Figure 5.2. Automated systems have allowed demand data to be distinguished from output (fulfilled demand) and separately captured. Understanding demand opens opportunities for demand management through marketing, scheduling, and prospective appropriateness review. Traditional hospital budget systems now quantify the cost and output dimensions and use revenue as an estimate of contribution. They are being refined by increasing the number of cost centers and the detail of functional accounts, so that estimates of direct costs are reliable and overhead allocations can be analyzed in depth. Fixed and variable costs are being identified, permitting better understanding of the relationship between price, cost, and demand. New measures of both procedural and outcomes quality have been implemented. Henry Ford is a member of a group striving for externally reportable quality measures, including disease prevention and health promotion demand measures and a broad range of cost and quality measures.[4] Satisfaction surveys for physicians, workers, and all kinds of customers are routine.

The case study organizations do not seek perfect measures in their expansion of measurement. Their criteria are much more pragmatic, even expedient. They recognize the opportunity for continuous improvement of the measures themselves. Do we understand it? Might it mislead? Is there anything else we could get at that's better? Should we try it and see how it works out? Should we make this a stop-gap, and try to do better next year?

External demands for cost control will require improvement in the specificity of all dimensions. Both fixed and variable cost estimates are essential to the make-or-buy decisions implicit in *hoshin* planning, to track the implications of demand changes, and to evaluate new procedures designed by cross-disciplinary task forces. Henry Ford's RCU project is a major effort toward this need. Similarly, more frequent surveys and larger samples of satisfaction and process quality data are necessary to support

Figure 5.4

Plan for Information Improvement at IHC

CQI Measurement—Current and Future

Recipient			Freq	Customer Service		Clinical Quality	Finance
IHC	Cluster	Hosp					

CURRENT

	Nonmedical Outcomes	Satisfaction	Medical Outcomes	Cost per Case
	• Inpatient admissions • Outpatient registrations • Average inpatient age • Average length of stay • Case mix index	• Perceptions of overall hospital quality • Perceptions of hospital staff • Perceptions of clinical process and outcomes	• Mortality • Infection rates • Repeats & returns to OR • Adverse drug reactions	• Net operating income • Controllable expense variance • Charge per case (CMI-adj) • Medicare charge per case

FUTURE

	Process	Satisfaction/Expectation	Medical Outcomes	Cost per Case
	• Patient delays & waiting times • Forms per patient • Person-hours per STAT (efficiency) • Number of processes analyzed	• Referral & hold rates (MDs/clinics) • Employee retention & turnover rates • Satisfaction by dept & specialization • Expectation profiles & patterns	• Injuries • Severity indices • Functional status • Cure rates • Complication rates • Readmits • Long-term clinical outcomes	• Uniform cost per case (adjusted for severity) • Uncompensated care • Cost per day of stay • Volumes

Source: Intermountain Health Care System.

more specific applications. Outcomes quality data require acuity scales and refinements of the diagnosis and treatment categories to identify extraneous factors. Worker and physician satisfaction will be more critical as more is asked of the workers. All three of the case studies are moving in these directions. IHC has an explicit plan for information improvement, outlined in Figure 5.4.

Continuous improvement in data quality is particularly important. The stresses of change will lead to repeated attacks on the data themselves. Confidence in the data—perceived reliability—will be as important as real reliability. Any measures used outside a single unit or activity should be subject to common definition, collected according to established procedures, and centrally archived. The data should be audited as often as feasible. Using audits to establish accuracy of critical data is often viewed as "keeping people honest," but it has another function, encouraging trust in the numbers.

Data quality is a particular problem in larger systems because so many people are involved in entering data. Grandia at Intermountain and Sinisi at Henry Ford both set rigorous standards because they know that even slight differences in definition will lead to irreconcilable differences when the numbers are compared. These differences cause a loss of conviction— people no longer believe they can rely on the numbers. Sinisi says:

> Data from the transaction systems are thoroughly audited and filed in the "Repository," which uses different hardware from the clinical system to keep clinical response times satisfactory. Major measures of demand, output, cost, revenue, and human resources are in the Repository. Data are stored with definitions in a form accessible by a user with "Windows" or "Apple" technology.
>
> There are a lot of departmental-based systems. Those can be housed to the department. If the data are shared in the Repository, then those systems must meet higher standards. We have one ADT system, so anyone who wants ADT data has to meet central standards. If you use the communications network, you have to meet central standards.

Measuring and guiding the corporate vision

Integrating the activity measures toward a common goal is essential, but it seems to get overlooked in many organizations. The CQI failure cases often seem to be reports of improvement teams that did not work hard enough on the core business issues. They rearranged the deck chairs while the ship sank. They celebrated small gains without doing the *hoshin* planning to identify and achieve the big ones. Protection against this danger comes from managing the levels of information—having a clear mission, developing measures that are clearly related to mission achievement, using references appropriately, and relating the CQI effort to those measures in an explicit annual planning review.

Both IHC and the Ford system have clear, community-based, vertically integrated missions and visions. Walke-Parker's vision, to become the best facility in Southern City, may lead it in a very different direction. The community-based vision puts much heavier emphasis on core measures for the vision itself, and on the use of reference measures to assess overall corporate performance and stimulate *hoshin* planning.

The core measures are guiding beacons that make clear what the improvement task is. They deal with the same six dimensions as the activity measures, but they relate directly to market forces. They say what cost, profit, and quality will meet customer requirements, and what demand and output will be. Even if the connection between the activity unit or a clinical cross-functional team and the core measures is unclear (it usually is), the direction for improvement is clear, and some sense emerges about how much change is needed. This central focus is essential in a rapidly changing market.

Our case studies are very good at this. Walke-Parker's elegant pyramid of measures ties everything to the 16-dimension radar chart (see Figure 7.5). Ford has its "balanced scorecards" up to the corporate board level (see Figure 8.12). IHC has a new quality report for their board, discussed by Gary Pehrson:

> We presented our Quality Measurement Team report to the Professional Standards Committee of the board in June. We've worked out the kinds of measures that should be presented to them routinely [see Figure 5.5]. They approved the draft and we'll begin reporting in September. It's a measurement tool we thought would focus everybody in a more business base, and not just FTEs or bottom line or one of those things. The bottom line's important, but there are a whole host of things that affect that bottom line that we haven't looked at, and I want to look at those in a comprehensive fashion. The theory is we will focus everybody from the middle managers all the way to the top on the same indicators.

Figure 5.5

Proposed Board Quality Assessment Report, IHC

1992	1Q'92	2Q'92	3Q'92	4Q'92	Yr Mean
Measures of Clinical Outcomes					
1. Surgical Wound Infection Rate					
2. Severe Drug Reactions		0.004%	0.003%	0.005%	0.004%
3. Returns to Surgery		0.63%	0.69%	0.47%	0.60%
4. Mortality (exclude NBs, ER, DOA)	0.99%	0.95%	0.58%	1.11%	0.91%
5. C-section Rate	16.65%	17.02%	16.26%	17.24%	16.79%
6. PRO Quality Denials		2.19%	1.72%	2.16%	2.02%
7. Readmissions within 30 Days		2.19%	1.72%	2.16%	2.02%
Future 8. Severity Level (CSI)					
9. Functional Status					
10. Deep Vein Thrombosis					
Measures of Patient Satisfaction					
Patient Perception of: 11. Severe Quality—on a scale of 5					4.24
12. Clinical Quality—on a scale of 3					2.84
Measures of Financial Outcomes					
13. Net Operating Income (000s)	$16,824	$13,008	$6,295	$2,885	$9,753
14. Charge/Case (adjusted for case mix and rate increases)	$4,527	$4,495	$4,567	$4,556	$4,536
System Demographics					
15. Inpatient Admissions	26,968	26,308	25,312	24,662	25,813
16. Outpatient Revenues (000s)	$82,957	$86,579	$87,651	$89,406	$86,648
17. Average Length of Stay	4.46	4.26	4.19	4.28	4.30
18. Case Mix Index	1.280	1.265	1.249	1.305	1.275

Source: Intermountain Health Care System.

Reference measures are critical to evaluating the core measures. Identifying realistic standards of excellence will be essential. A "zero defect" approach will not succeed in a cost-constrained environment. Success will lie in identifying gains that can be made within available funds. The broader the search for opportunities and the more rigorous the benchmarking, the more likely the organization is to succeed.

Focusing on expectations

Continuous improvement is in the expectations; it is in the flight plan before it is in the flight log. It is in the "Plan" of the Shewhart "Plan, Do, Check, Act" cycle before it is in the "Act." There are three basic types of expectations in health care organizations. *Procedures* describe how each activity of each task is to be performed. *Clinical protocols* state the usual care plan for similar cases. The *budget* states the anticipated values of the six dimensions for organizational or clinical aggregates. CQI in the case study institutions is a multiyear, expectation-oriented, information-guided, core-measure-driven process. It works like this:

1. Financial planning identifies revenue expectations and goals for profit levels. At the level of the institution as a whole, these approaches are still essential.

2. Environmental assessment and reference data identify benchmarks and lead to a new set of core measure goals—satisfactory overall future performance on the other five dimensions, quality, demand, output, human resources, and cost dimensions.

3. The goals are translated to the annual budget guidelines for all six dimensions. The guidelines are promulgated both to the traditional activity managers and the quality improvement teams. They must meet the guidelines by improvements in processes and clinical protocols.

4. The managers and clinical teams redesign additional processes and clinical protocols to achieve improvements indicated by the future needs.

5. The improved processes are used to set the unit and clinical team expectations that meet next year's more rigorous core measure goals.

This approach works only because the redesign effort is directed at the future, not the present. The annual budget guidelines are no surprises for the operating managers. They are within reach because of redesign activities already under way. Today's redesign activities will support the forthcoming budget, not the current one. It is critical that each year's budget be achievable. Repeated failures to achieve budget actually destroy CQI. They pull the efforts from redesign to patching up and catching up. They regress from building in control to enforcing control.

Our case study organizations are not perfect at this, but they are doing better. HFHS reports close conformity to budget in recent years. Walke-Parker, after some difficulty, expects to achieve its ambitious goal of 25 percent reduction in unit costs. IHC has a high failure rate at the operating facility level, but this may relate to the ambitiousness of the goals and their move to flexible budgeting in 1993.

Supporting expanded analysis

Information is numbers, and most people are at least a little bit afraid of numbers. If your plan calls for responsiveness to clinical workers, and they are afraid of numbers, you may never get where you have to go. How do you resolve this dilemma? All three organizations are broadly seeded with people who make numbers their business. Beyond the usual accountants, the larger institutions have tiers of expert advice available. There are statisticians, management engineers, epidemiologists, software/hardware consultants, and experts in clinical protocol design. Bill Schramm, vice president of Management Services, describes some of HFHS's services:

> Several staff functions are centralized under the senior vice president for Planning, Vin Sahney. Environmental assessment has about one and a half FTE, throughout the year, and is supplemented by an outside contract and personnel in the units. A CQI manager tracks task forces and provides CQI educational support. Management Services also provides support to the units. Our services are billed to users at $50 per hour, with an initial evaluation provided without charge. Demand for Management Services is twice what we can service. We encourage units to go ahead on their own, refine their ideas, and return, or hire outside consultants. The initial consult can involve several dozen hours. We also access the databases for clients, and suggest the best analytic methodologies to use. This accounts for about 10 percent of my staff's time.

IHC adds an expert in experimental design (Horn), and several informaticists. The point is to make these people helpful, which means available, trained in the right tools, and trained in human relations and teaching skills.

Walke-Parker can draw on Corporate resources, but Joe Corrigan, CFO, explains:

> We have two data analysts. One supports cost analysis and budget preparation and works in the Finance Department. The other works for the clinical teams and reports to the medical director. We don't pay a lot of attention to the reporting relationships.

A full program of analytic support begins with CQI facilitators and basic CQI training. There are three reasons to teach the basic CQI course to large numbers of managers, physicians, and workers. First, it helps empower them. Second, it gives them tools to understand their problems. Third, it teaches them how to use numbers, and not be afraid of them.

Having the data is one thing, and using it effectively is something else. The seven analytic tools of CQI are taught to large numbers of workers. These tools are easy to use, and using them develops an appreciation for analysis as a concept. But they are beginners' tools, and more sophisticated techniques are soon necessary in the complex health care environment; the elaborate and rigorous processes for data analysis, severity adjustment, and formal experimentation at IHC are the best example. Surviving institutions will develop an analytic support system that will become more powerful as the years go by.

The needs suggest that smaller institutions should copy Walke-Parker, creating a development general staff that would be responsible for information services, planning and marketing support, analytic assistance, and training (in analytic statistics, cost accounting, quality control, surveying, forecasting, methods improvement, and experimental design). Its job would be to assist others in setting expectations, from the mission to the most detailed productivity and quality standards.

Developing Clinical Expectations

The people who use and pay for health care are demanding control of cost and quality at the global level of capitation or health insurance premium. Their demands will be met principally by systematic continuous improvement of clinical quality focusing on improved clinical expectations. Paralleling the dual reporting system shown in Figure 5.3, there will be two types of clinical expectations:

1. Clinical care protocols developed by cross-disciplinary teams outlining agreement on treatment of recurring problems and diseases,

organized by diagnostic or treatment code, will be used to specify the anticipated cost and quality of care for each disease entity. They will specify directly the demand for specific procedures. For example, the cardiac surgery protocols will specify presurgical testing, postsurgical monitoring, and rehabilitation service requirements.

2. Clinical procedure expectations developed by support services like nursing and radiology, outlining the content of identifiable services, will be used to specify anticipated process quality, some intermediate outcomes such as functional status, and unit costs.

As health systems replace hospitals, a complete, integrated, dual system of control will emerge.

1. Cross-disciplinary teams will manage clinical care protocols.
   - They will need complete information systems of six dimensions and three types, and codes aggregating disease, treatment, and symptom.
   - Implementation will take several years. It will begin with the most clearly defined care episodes and progress to the least: common inpatient surgeries, outpatient surgeries, obstetrical episodes, and medical episodes.
   - The focus on cost per episode of care will lead to requirements for fixed and variable costing by episode, and formal budgets and cost accountability for cross-disciplinary teams.
   - Outcomes quality measurement will be an essential marketing tool. There will be demand for expansion and refinement of measures to reflect both global and episode-specific outcomes.
   - Pressures to refine episode definitions and remove variability from cost and quality will require new clinical aggregates analogous to DRGs, but appropriate to capitated outpatient care, and severity refinements such as IHC's Computerized Severity Index and others.
2. Cross-disciplinary teams and primary care physicians will become the customers for support services. They will seek
   - low unit costs,
   - high process quality, and
   - ways to reduce the demand for support services.
3. Line managers of support services will use unit cost, rather than total cost, in budgeting. They will

- benchmark unit costs against outside suppliers,
- seek to discontinue services with insufficient demand,
- strenuously resist overhead allocations,
- use lower-skilled employees and patient self-care, and
- improve scheduling, time per patient, and amenities.

4. Line managers will offer evidence of consistent high-quality performance. They will use procedural expectations to maintain
   - procedural quality scores and
   - timeliness, patient satisfaction, and uniformity of service.
5. Line managers will seek to validate their services by showing
   - relationships between support services and the outcomes measures achieved at the episode level and
   - relationships between outcomes and the procedural quality of support services.

Making Information a Strategic Weapon

All three of the case study institutions are making information services part of their strategic weaponry. Information does not replace the other elements of strategy, like planning, financing, and control of performance. It improves each, and it makes the whole greater than the sum of the parts. Developing information as a weapon requires a significant capital commitment. It also requires the corporation's willingness to take risks about itself; the investment in systems will only pay off if it is backed by a commitment to use the data and a corporate structure that emphasizes continuous improvement. Three elements seem to improve the odds that the information strategy will pay off: an information vision, an information services plan (or more accurately planning process), and a mechanism for continuous improvement of the value of information.

An Information Vision

You need a vision for information itself. It should state a commitment to information as a strategic weapon and indicate a willingness to undertake information expenditures that are not justified by forecasts of specific savings, but that offer reasonable promise of general future improvement. If you seek specific savings, you will spend too little. The major investments HFHS and Intermountain are planning will never have specific justification.

They take too long, affect too many people, and too many outside events will occur while they are being installed.

On the other hand, your vision should avoid excess spending. It should say, "We're going to take risks to spend enough on information, but we won't take foolish risks." As Larry Grandia, the CIO at Intermountain, says, there should always be tempting projects left unfunded.

The vision for both Henry Ford and Intermountain is clinical—the core of their future information systems will be an electronic medical record, a transaction system supporting most clinical decisions and incorporating clinical protocols of all kinds. They are probably right in their vision, but HCA may be right in its strategy, too. If it is planning a multimillion dollar investment to provide an automated medical record, it has not announced that yet. Should it? Should even smaller systems make the kinds of investments necessary to develop clinical transaction systems? Probably not yet. The price of the technology will fall once a few more giants have completed development. Clinical transaction systems should be in your vision, but not in your plan until the price is reasonable.

An Information Services Plan

The vision is implemented over several years, so a plan is necessary to keep track of the parts and progress. An effective planning process is more important than a plan document. Both Henry Ford and Intermountain talk more about process than document. Here are their own descriptions of how these organizations plan. Larry Grandia, vice president for Information Systems, Intermountain Health Care:

> There is no dedicated computer capital allocation, but beginning in 1986, IHC committed to a program of approximately $40 million per five years. The commitment is reviewed annually and continues. We anticipate no more than modest growth in that level. It was approximately the value that had been invested per year prior to 1986. We've been running under that number, because it's taken longer to develop and gain support than we anticipated. The expenditure includes all telecommunications, which saved $1 million annually in telephone charges. We use the same network to send computer data.
>
> We've been very prudent in the hardware platforms we adopted, and we developed all of our own financial systems in the early eighties. We sold the financial systems to GTE and recouped the vast majority of our investment. We started developing the HELP system years ago.

The HELP system is supported by a joint venture with 3M, which underwrites some development and maintenance costs.

There are two reasons I think are most important to our success. First, we had McKinsey and Company do a companywide study. One of the recommendations was that we should create an information systems committee of the corporate board of trustees. We did that in 1986. That allowed us to make sure information gets reviewed at the very top strategic level. It doesn't get mingled with other stuff and lost in minutia. This allows the board committee members to query us on what we're doing, and help us fit it into corporate strategy. This process unites top management and the board. If we believe information is a critical resource, like capital and human resources, why is it that we have board committees for them, and not for information?

Second, we merged our traditional hospital information services with medical informatics—the academic, medically oriented application of information to medicine. Our informaticists are part of the department at the University of Utah. These people have tremendous information systems capabilities. They relate very closely to our clinical community.

We have a corporationwide strategic planning committee that includes our CEOs of major hospitals and senior VPs from the corporation. They help me refine the vision. The real message of the vision is enterprisewide integration. Linking the information so that wherever the information is needed—hospitals, offices, corporate—it's available to them.

The first step was a strong business/financial system. The second step was a communications network. We have over 3,000 people on E-mail now. The third is close coupling with the health insurance plan. The last phase is a focus on clinical activities. We've done a pretty good job on staffing ratios, inventory controls, reducing A/R, and so forth. We believe the area of greatest opportunity is the variability in consumption of resources and outcomes of clinical procedures. So we have automated pharmacy and radiology and laboratory, those infrastructure things, to get to the payoff clinical applications like infectious disease/antibiotic therapy. With the capture of this clinically rich data, our researchers and clinical leaders can use it to determine the most appropriate way to get the physicians and nurses to coalesce around practice patterns. Then we can structure the ordering process for individual patients. We think one of the greatest opportunities for reducing costs is reducing unnecessary orders. One of the key steps is in getting the clinical systems automated and creating the electronic medical record.

I would say that on balance IHC is conservative, but we're making appropriate progress. If we had more money, could we move more quickly? I think the answer is yes, but the challenge is not spending on technology. It's how you're organized to adopt and absorb that technology. There's only so much change you can impose. It takes a while for doctors and nurses to become comfortable. I believe you are better off pacing implementation as time goes on, and then taking advantage of changes to improve productivity in hardware or software. If I had my druthers, I'd have us spend a little more, but I don't think a lot more.

Grandia says his formal plan is a little out-of-date and in some disarray, but he says, "That's not important." What is important is the annual review process. Putting this at the board committee level demonstrates a commitment to the information vision. It also brings outsider perspectives to bear. Note that the board concerns itself only with the broadest planning strategies for the corporation, (the VISTA level, not the SIPs of Chapter 4). Its committees are designed to delve one level deeper in information and finance.

Henry Ford is striving for the same thing with a dual-committee approach. Al Sinisi, chief information officer, describes the ongoing planning and budgeting:

We have an Information Steering Committee of physicians and senior managers that helps develop the budget and plan. Membership has shifted toward the second level of major units over the years. Anybody who wants an information system larger than a PC must prepare a proposal for review, even if they have independent financing. The committee also has $2.2 million to use for routine developments and upgrades.

We have a three-year planning document which is based on the institution's strategy. We create an information strategy, a long-range information systems plan, with five components: applications, technology, data, client needs, and management control. Our overall strategy relates to the patient; a clinical data system that is totally seamless, integrated, and makes no distinction between inpatient or outpatient.

No matter where he or she is in HFHS, the practitioner can access the data in the way the practitioner wants it.

Tom McNulty, senior vice president and chief financial officer, describes how Ford will overlay a special planning committee for a major information services investment:

We need to develop a new information services plan. I'm going to follow some rules I learned years ago.

1. Start with a "philosophical approach" which emphasizes the overall purpose of information services, user support, in a pragmatic context:

   The general consensus [from a survey by an outside consultant] . . . is that we need an overall strategic plan. . . . From a practical point of view, constructing one is not a simple task. The technology available today provides the necessary platform for most of the expressed needs. The availability of neural networks [integrated voice-image-video communication] is not simple, but can be developed. The use of artificial intelligence . . . is still a vision in the minds of many, practical in the hands of a few, and not widely acceptable to the economics for a solid platform that would stand the challenge of time.

   The vision . . . is to place the need to know within practical reach of each and every authorized requester; a rapid single access process [will be the] . . . hallmark of the system."

2. Carefully select a task force that balances user requests with knowledgeable technical resource people.

   I'm forming a "policy group" of eight members, overlapping the Information Steering Committee but not identical to it. I'll chair the group personally. Five members are physician representatives, and the remaining two are the top line officers for the provider business group and the insurance business group. Personnel from Information Services, the Information Steering Committee, and Research and Education are designated to support the group.

   I want to use an outside facilitator to arrange sessions to obtain input toward the vision statement: We need to talk to the three management committees, [Senior Operating Team, Senior Physician Team, Senior Support Team] some [medical department] chairmen, HAP [Health Alliance Plan, the Ford HMO] executive group, Information Steering Committee, and a selected group of others. That would give us the awareness we need."

3. Let the policy group develop the vision, a series of policies for the future and a plan for monitoring and implementation.

The policies and plan are circulated to all other units of the organization for review and comment, but there is strict control on expansion of the policies. It comes from two sources: the financial limits for operations and capital, and the technical limits imposed by current realities.

The neural system, which is the most ambitious plan the group is likely to request, will cost $90 million to $120 million over five years, or an increase in expenditures of 1.5 percent to 2 percent per year. It will not be easy to get this money in the financial management process even though I designed the process. The policy group will keep the lid on. Somebody who comes in with some willy-nilly star wars idea that adds a half million dollars to the total just won't stand a chance. In fact, the policy group's most central decision will be how far to go toward the neural system.

4. Develop "champions" and ownership of the components of the plan. Negotiate the potential turf disputes so that people have ownership of significant parts in a context of an integrated whole.

For instance, instead of sitting around arguing about how membership files work, you might assign them to HAP Information Service to do systemwide. You could get the Ford Service to operate the MIMS activity systemwide.

Champions become sources of truth for a given outcome. . . . You can then get people cooperating because they have their own ownership and they keep maintaining their territorial prerogatives. Creating a source of truth, what you really do is you empower people to have a good sense of feeling about themselves and their accomplishments so they are identified as an individual and not just a small cog.

5. Do the implementation with a second team, putting the original task force in the position of monitoring progress.

You develop the goals at a "pro forma" level, and you double check it with both users and technical experts, piece by piece by piece. You go out and get some people with good judgment and you put them in a room and you show them the plan. You say to them,

"Don't tell me what you don't like, because I can change that. Tell me what's wrong with it. Does the philosophy work? Does it have an engine, and a transmission, and can it take you where you want to go? You don't put one line of code on paper; you don't sign any vendor contracts until you've done this.

You then code it *without* change, and you call that iteration 1.0 and you put it in place. Once you've got 1.0 running, you can take a look at the problems and start to fix them. The biggest mistake that's made in system design today is that people don't design the system and install it. You go along when people ask for this variant and that, because they are easy to do and you don't foresee the system implications. All of a sudden you have this huge cost to fix everything.

The process of planning for smaller institutions need not differ from these models. The cross-discipline planning teams, the board level oversight, and the multiyear commitment of capital funds all flow from the decision to use information as a strategic weapon. The teams will be smaller, and the financial limitations will be tighter. The decisions will focus on commercially available services that have been developed and tested elsewhere. Joe Corrigan, chief financial officer at Walke-Parker, explains:

The information strategy is developed corporately. The Field Operations Activity Committee [at the parent corporation] now does the planning. It's trying to meet our needs, whether by purchase or development.

Information systems costs are kept low because of the support from corporate. It's probably between 2 and 3 percent. We buy a lot of data from corporate and other sources for benchmarking—comparative data with other institutions. We also get the corporate customer satisfaction survey from corporate. Corporate is looking toward a system that relates costs to clinical paths, so we can deliver current cost reports to the physician. We'll go to things like the automated medical record when the cost of the investment is justified. We're exploring budgeting by DRG or product line. We do some of this on PCs. We have a variety of scheduling systems and departmental management systems on PCs.

Budgeting Information Services

The budget of a well-run information service will include cost limits based on the overall financial needs of the institution, just like any other operating unit. It will also have expectations for the other five dimensions in Figure 5.3. "Customer" satisfaction will be user satisfaction. Outcomes quality will address completeness, response timeliness, and reliability and validity of information. Process quality will include audits of compliance with key procedures, rework rates, and backlogs. If the vision is to be competitive, a comparison to services offered by peer institutions may be useful, even though it is difficult to quantify. Demand and output will be measured and explicitly forecast. Productivity measures and expectations will be used at both departmental (cost per service unit) and clinical (cost per episode) levels.

Only revenue is problematic; under capitation and bundle payment it is difficult to attribute a specific revenue to information services. Estimates of benefits may take the place of revenue. Larry Grandia's analysis of HELP contributions (see p. 147) is an illustration.

How do you decide how much to spend on information services? Right now, the study sites appear to benchmark costs on peer institutions, expressed as a percent of total costs. For example, Tom McNulty says:

> Ford spends a relatively small percent of its annual budget on information services, but the level of decentralization is so high that it is difficult to estimate. The 1993 information services operating budget, $19 million, and equipment budget, $3 million, are directed toward the inpatient and outpatient delivery sites. Other units, particularly the Health Alliance Plan HMO, add $4 million. The corporation spends $26 million per year in operations, or about 2.2 percent of the total and $6 million in capital.
>
> Analytic support personnel costs are approximately $750,000 per year, in addition.

There are serious limitations to benchmarking on percent of total costs. There is nothing magic about what other people are doing. The total cost of using information is difficult to estimate, both in your institution and in others; for instance, decentralized processing makes it easy to overlook certain costs. As a result, the benchmark is quite crude. McNulty and Grandia both know other people spend "2 to 3 percent"—in their organizations that is a range of about $10 million. The benchmark doesn't even hint to McNulty whether he should spend another million next year, although he gets this level of precision in his other units (see p. 118).

In the reengineered institution, a better approach may be to assess cost in relation to information value, recognizing that the value of information lies solely in its use. Conceptually, if an increase in cost would yield a large improvement in effective use of information, it is justified. This approach encourages information services (IS) personnel to design their service to maximize the same goals as the information users, that is, patient care quality and cost control. When combined with user satisfaction scores, it means the following:

- The IS department and IS users will both look for information improvements that contribute to the same mission and goals.
- Proposals for improvement will be measured against their end contribution, in terms of the institutional vision and the core measures of success.
- The IS department will emphasize user acceptability and user analytic support. Effective use of information will become a CQI opportunity for IS staff.
- Success of new IS projects will be defined by user behavior. If the information generated is not used, the project is, at best, not yet finished.
- Any service which suffers declining user satisfaction will be a priority for redesign by internal CQI teams.
- Competitor analysis will focus on new or expanded services and their apparent value, rather than on costs.
- The ideal expenditure for information services will be determined by user needs. The optimum expenditure for IS is reached when the requests left unfunded would yield only small improvements in patient care quality and cost.

Conceptually, this approach makes the "percent of total expenses" benchmark irrelevant. It no longer matters to Ford what Intermountain spends for information services. What matters is strictly what Ford can gain from an increased expenditure. While none of the study sites articulated a policy like this, it may not be far from their minds. While all three were proud of being near the benchmark expenditure level, most of their conversation is about the value of information.

Peters and Waterman[5] identified the concept of "simultaneously loose/tight," meaning that the goals are firmly adhered to, but the implementation is open to experimentation, chance opportunity, and personal preference. It applies as well to information. All three sites are using worker/physician reaction as a guide to short-range planning and implementation. They are sensitive to people's ability to use data, as well as the objective evidence about the value of data. They do not force information systems or data down their members' throats; they constantly make data available and encourage its use. That may be the essence of their leadership position.

Notes

1. Grandia, L. 1993. "Intermountain Health Care: How a Regional Health Provider Is Using Information Technology to Meet Its Strategic Objectives." Paper presented at the Healthcare Information Executives Forum.
2. Griffith, J. R. 1992. *The Well-Managed Community Hospital*, 2d ed. Chapter 3, pp. 59–71. Ann Arbor, MI: Health Administration Press. See also Kaplan, R. S., and D. P. Norton, 1992. "The Balanced Scorecard—Measures that Drive Performance." *Harvard Business Review* 70 (January–February): 71–79.
3. Thomas, J. W., and J. J. Holloway. 1991. "Investigating Early Readmission as an Indicator for Quality of Care Studies." *Medical Care* 29 (4): 377–94.
4. Nerenz, D. R., and B. M. Zajac. 1991. *Indicators of Performance for Vertically Integrated Health Systems*. Detroit, MI: Henry Ford Health System Center for Health System Studies. See also, Goldfield, N. 1991. "Measurement and Management of Quality in Managed Care Organizations: Alive and Improving." *Quality Review Bulletin* 17 (11): 343–48.
5. Peters, T. J., and R. H. Waterman. 1982. *In Search of Excellence*. New York: Basic Books.

6

Intermountain Health Care Case Study

Intermountain Health Care (IHC) is a not-for-profit integrated regional health care system serving the Intermountain Region of Utah, Idaho, and Wyoming (see Figure 6.1).[1] The heart of the system is a network of 24 hospitals with 2,779 licensed beds and 18,500 FTE employees. IHC hospitals have provided close to 50 percent of the hospital care in Utah for almost two decades. Ten of the hospitals are urban, and 14 are rural, 12 with less than 50 beds. The two tertiary care facilities, LDS Hospital and Primary Children's Medical Center, are located in Salt Lake City.

Reflecting a strategic decision made in 1985, IHC offers a continuum of care ranging from acute inpatient hospital care to outpatient and home health care services. To this end, IHC operates a total of 81 units including 42 urban and rural clinics, 24 hospitals, 13 home health agencies, a medical equipment and supply division, and a home intravenous therapy division. The hospital complexes include 10 women's centers and 9 psychiatric and behavioral medicine units. The system also provides dialysis, ambulatory surgery, occupational health, urgent care, and blood donor centers, as well as inpatient and outpatient rehabilitation programs. Eighteen of the clinics and several of the home health care agencies focus on rural areas. IHC also operates an air ambulance and rescue service to provide emergency transport to and from the remotest parts of its service area.

Intermountain's managed care program, started in 1984, has grown to around 400,000 members today—over 50 percent of the persons in managed care in the region—and is growing about 10 percent per year. In 1991,

Figure 6.1

Hospitals in the IHC System

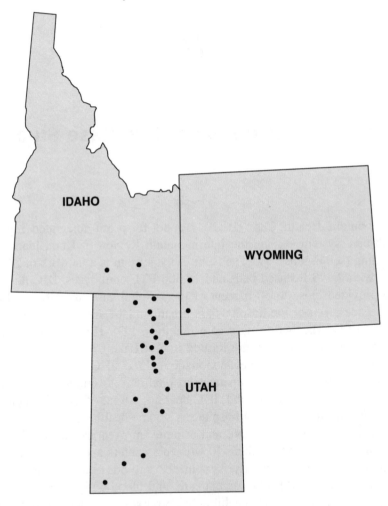

Utah ranked eleventh in the nation in HMO penetration; 60 to 70 percent of the population is in some form of privately insured managed care, and a large proportion of the remainder are covered by Medicare, Medicaid, or are uninsured. Key trends for IHC as a system are shown in Figures 6.2 and 6.3.

Figure 6.2

Operating Statistics for IHC

	1989	1990	1991	1992
Acute admissions				
Rural	21,115	21,125	21,983	25,610
Urban	79,799	80,506	80,522	78,011
Total	**100,914**	**101,631**	**102,505**	**103,621**
Deliveries				
Rural	3,556	3,940	3,956	5,096
Urban	18,229	17,449	17,143	16,759
Total	**21,785**	**21,389**	**21,099**	**21,855**
Inpatient surgeries				
Rural	7,255	7,201	7,587	9,285
Urban	27,831	29,009	28,461	33,653
Total	**35,086**	**36,210**	**36,048**	**42,938**
Ambulatory surgeries				
Rural	8,163	8,708	9,163	11,602
Urban	42,917	44,731	45,198	49,801
Total	**51,080**	**53,439**	**54,361**	**61,403**
Outpatient visits				
Rural	261,743	292,721	366,414	505,088
Urban	1,135,588	1,171,452	1,280,522	1,294,849
Total	**1,397,331**	**1,464,173**	**1,646,936**	**1,799,937**
Emergency room visits				
Rural	65,422	69,211	74,828	101,582
Urban	207,479	210,879	227,502	170,087
Total	**272,901**	**280,090**	**302,330**	**271,669**
Long-term care admissions				
Rural	368	365	503	686
Urban	1,503	1,665	1,963	1,941
Total	**1,871**	**2,030**	**2,466**	**2,627**
Home health care visits				
Rural	40,681	69,791	61,193	106,033
Urban	123,361	227,405	324,580	167,962
Total	**164,042**	**297,196**	**385,773**	**273,995**

Notes: 1989, 1990, 1991: Urban and rural designations reflect IHC administrative regions. 1992: Urban and rural designations reflect U.S. Census Bureau Metropolitan Statistical Areas, not IHC administrative regions.

Sources: Intermountain Health Care Annual Reports, 1991 and 1992.

Figure 6.3

Key Financial Trends for IHC
($ in thousands)

	1990	1991	1992
Revenues			
Inpatient services	$601,784	$656,219	$ 686,413
Outpatient services	239,244	280,586	328,642
Gross operating revenue	$841,028	$936,805	$1,015,055
Uncompensated care, community services & contractual discounts	(180,711)	(214,985)	(243,803)
Net operating revenue	$660,317	$721,820	$771,252
Nonoperating revenue	92,616	141,985	180,574
Total revenue	$752,933	$863,554	$951,826
Expenses			
Salaries & benefits	$383,606	$425,370	$474,816
Other	326,897	396,394	425,058
Total expenses	$710,503	$821,764	$902,874
Operating margin	−7.6%	−13.9%	−17.1%
Net margin	5.6%	4.8%	5.1%
Comparative margins			
Utah hospital average	3.0%	5.2%	5.0%
Idaho hospital average	7.2%	8.6%	8.5%
Wyoming hospital average	.2%	2.9%	.9%
U.S. hospital average	3.8%	4.3%	4.6%

Sources: Intermountain Health Care Annual Reports, 1991 and 1992. Comparative margins from *The Universal Health Care Almanac*, Phoenix, AZ: Silver and Cherner, 1993 and 1994.

Organization Structure and Leadership

IHC is governed by a board of trustees composed primarily of prominent Intermountain Region citizens. Five physicians (representing IHC, the Great Basin Physicians Corporation, and private attending physicians) serve on the board. Each hospital or hospital group—19 in total—has its own governing board composed of representatives of the local communities and their medical staffs. Local boards act in an advisory capacity. The president of IHC reports to the board of trustees; all subsidiary organizations report through him.

Approximately 1,600 physicians are affiliated with IHC. Of these, 1,500 are closely affiliated in the urban areas. About 150 are directly employed by IHC. For example, at McKay-Dee Hospital Center in Ogden, 25–30 physicians providing community-based primary care are employed through the hospital. Another 100 rural physicians are closely affiliated; about 70 percent are employed. The balance of physicians are in solo or group practice, largely fee-for-service. All physicians with active privileges at IHC hospitals are eligible to join the Great Basin Physicians Corporation (an entity legally independent from IHC). This group elects three representatives to the IHC board of trustees.

IHC's mission statement is presented in Figure 6.4. It reflects a strong commitment to health care as opposed to the operation of institutions, to the provision of care to persons in rural areas and to those in need regardless of ability to pay, and to the fiscal responsibility necessary to achieve its service goals. The stated mission has remained consistent over IHC's existence.

Unique Factors

IHC History and Culture

Intermountain Health Care was formed April 1, 1975, when leaders of the Church of Jesus Christ of Latter Day Saints (Mormon) divested the church's holdings of 15 hospitals. Church authorities appointed an independent board of trustees and, upon divestiture, turned all properties, assets, and liabilities of the hospitals over to it. This board then organized Intermountain Health Care, a not-for-profit corporation without ties to the church, to own and operate the 15 hospitals. In 1985, as part of IHC's major strategic planning effort, its goal of adding value to the community served was affirmed. Further, the IHC management team concluded that IHC should pay "dividends" like a for-profit entity, but that the dividends should be in the form of lower prices, better quality, and charitable service. The dividends should at least equal the taxes that would be paid if IHC were a for-profit entity, for it to meet its community obligation. The IHC management team was determined to have the same dividend accountability as a for-profit company. The result of this policy has been a strong emphasis on reducing costs. Further, the

---

Figure 6.4

The IHC Mission Statement

Our Mission

Excellence in the provision of health care services to communities in the Intermountain region.

Our Commitments

- **Excellent service** to our patients, customers, and physicians is our most important consideration.

- We will provide our services with **integrity.** Our actions will enhance our reputation and reflect the trust placed in us by those we serve.

- **Our employees are our most important resource.** We will attract exceptional individuals at all levels of the organization and provide fair compensation and opportunities for personal and professional growth. We recognize and reward employees who achieve excellence in their work.

- We are committed to **serving diverse needs** of the young and old, the rich and poor, and those living in urban and rural communities.

- We will reflect the **caring and noble** nature of our mission in all that we do. Our services must be high quality, cost-effective, and accessible, achieving a balance between community needs and available resources.

- It is our intent to be a **model health care system.** We will strive to be a national leader in nonprofit health care delivery.

- We will maintain the **financial strength** necessary to fulfill our mission.

---

needs of its patient population are sometimes defined in rather broad terms; for example, in an effort to meet the health needs of rural elderly patients, "coal and ash" services (stoking coal furnaces and removing the ash the next morning) are provided.

Utah

In the economic arena, Utah has generally performed well over the past ten years except for a regional downturn in 1986–87 that was due to declining oil prices, the completion of the Intermountain Power Project, and the temporary closures of Kennecott Copper and Geneva Steel. Utah ranked first or second in a number of measures of economic activity in 1992. This favorable performance is attributed to a more productive and diversified economy that emerged from the mid-decade downturn. Solid average growth is expected to continue, although Utah continues to be vulnerable to out-of-state and international economic conditions since much of the economy is based on the export of goods and services. Tourism and defense/aerospace continue to be important. Many of the rural counties in the Intermountain Region, especially those in Idaho and Wyoming, have deteriorating economic conditions.

The Utah population (1,723,000 in 1990) grew 16 percent between 1980 and 1990 and is expected to grow a similar amount between 1990 and 2000. Utah has by far the youngest population in the country, with a median age of 26.3 years (versus the national median age of 33.4 years). Total personal income per household in 1991 was 89 percent of the national average. Of Utah's population, 62 percent (1,200,000 people) live in the Salt Lake City–Ogden area.

Figure 6.5 presents information on admissions, hospital beds, occupancy rates, and number of physicians for Utah overall and the Salt Lake City MSA compared to national rates. Utah has been known for a number of years as a "low medical services use" area, at least partly explained by its age structure. Only 9 percent of Utah's population is over 65, and only 23 percent is over 45, compared to 13 percent and 32 percent nationally. Seventy-eight percent of community hospital beds in Utah are located in the Salt Lake City–Ogden area. The number of active physicians per 100,000 population is expected to decrease in all three of the Intermountain states between 1986 and 2000: Utah, down 13.9 percent; Wyoming, down 34.0 percent; Idaho, down 24.2 percent.

Hospitalization in Utah is also focused on the most critical care, especially at IHC. IHC hospitals have a case-mix rating 20 points higher than non-IHC hospitals in Utah, and 35 points higher than the national average. Overall, however, they report a slightly lower length of stay than the state average and 15–20 percent lower charges by DRG category than non-IHC hospitals in the state.

In 1989, the average rate of professional liability insurance per bed in Utah was $1,700, compared with $4,600 in Michigan and $1,600 in Southern State.

Figure 6.5

Community Hospital Demographics, Utah vs. United States, 1991

	Admissions (per 1,000 Population)	Hospital Beds (per 1,000 Population)	Occupancy (percent)	Physicians (per 100,000 Population)
Utah	101	2.5	58.3	169
Salt Lake City/Ogden	109	2.7	61.8	211
U.S.	123	3.7	66.1	198

	Revenue (per Patient Day)	Expense (per Patient Day)	Expense as % Revenue
Utah	$1,367.65	$1,296.72	94.8%
U.S.	$1,054.67	$1,009.71	95.7%

Sources: *The Universal Health Care Almanac*, Phoenix, AZ: Silver and Cherner, 1993. AMA, *Physician Characteristics and Distribution in the United States*, Chicago: AMA, 1992.
Note: Physician data is 1990.

Origins of CQI: Quality Evolution, Not Revolution

IHC's commitment to adding value to communities served through lower prices and better quality is reflected in the Quality, Utilization, and Efficiency (QUE) studies that originated with the Departments of Quality Assurance and Finance in the mid-1980s. QUE studies were an effort to match information on clinical care delivered for specific diagnostic categories with the costs associated with this care. The Medicare DRG payment for these diagnostic categories was of particular concern; in 1986, the IHC board set a goal to develop a methodology for comparative DRG cost analysis. The long-term objective was to provide low-cost patient care without sacrificing quality.

The QUE model separated hospital contributions from physicians' contributions to clinical care. The aim of the QUE studies was to compare and contrast physicians (in terms of resource utilization) and hospitals (in terms of efficiency), with the goal of identifying and eliminating inappropriate variation in utilization and efficiency. To do this, the study needed to start with a group of patients who were as alike as possible in terms of diagnosis, acuity (severity of illness), complexity (presence and severity of comorbidities), and expected outcomes (complications and medical results) so that variations in these factors were not the source of variation found in the study.[2]

Brent James, M.D., joined IHC's Department of Medical Affairs in the mid-1980s. He became quite interested in the QUE studies and became a participant in the research. His expertise in computers, statistics, and medical research complemented that of the staff already working on them. The QUE researchers at that time were not happy with the methodology that they were using. They felt that it required too many patients and too great an expenditure of resources to obtain results that allowed them to make statistical inferences about treatments. They were, therefore, searching for an alternative study methodology. With this in mind, James studied the work of Avedis Donabedian on quality of care and, at the suggestion of Paul Batalden, that of W. Edwards Deming on quality in general. He also attended one of Deming's continuous quality improvement (CQI) workshops. He brought what he learned back to IHC. More and more it appeared that the methodology used for CQI could meet their study design needs. At this time there was no particular interest in CQI as a management philosophy.

In late 1988, several staff members began to plot a strategy to extend the use of this methodology within IHC in order to produce faster clinical study results. Brent James, Gary Pehrson (then interim director for the Department of Medical Affairs), and Douglas Fonnesbeck (then administrator of Cottonwood Hospital) drew up a "hit list" of people that they needed to convince (mostly those with day-to-day operations responsibilities), prioritized the list, then started at the top and "ganged up on" them one at a time with the data collected from completed studies. Quality management staff, both corporate level and the heads of the departments at the larger hospitals, were their first targets to talk through what increased use of the quality improvement (QI) methodology would mean operationally. From there they branched out to the others.

They convinced IHC leadership that total quality management (TQM) had a lot of merit. In 1989, Pehrson (by then a member of the corporate executive team) was charged with assessing the potential of CQI for IHC and for determining what cultural changes would be necessary for it to succeed. A retreat on quality improvement was held for all of the people on the hit list. The retreat group drafted a quality mission statement and formed a Quality Council. Soon after that the Quality Council decided that a common language and a common understanding were needed in order to talk about quality improvement issues within the system. James volunteered to put together a course, which later evolved into the Facilitator Workshop Series, the core training effort of the current quality improvement initiative.

The Quality Council requested and was given the opportunity to present the program for the 1990 spring management retreat for IHC's top 200 managers. They did a first-pass rollout arguing for quality as a primary business strategy. During 1990, as part of a reorganization, Pehrson became vice president for Professional Services. The Institute for Health Care Delivery Research (conceived by James and Pehrson) was formed with its own budget as part of a strategic approach to legitimate quality efforts. James became its executive director. The institute had four goals:

1. To recommend strategic priorities regarding health care delivery and clinical research based on community needs
2. To provide data, statistical analysis, and coordination to internal and external health care delivery and research efforts that advanced IHC strategic objectives and were approved by the institute's board
3. To provide research and technical support for the IHC TQM strategy
4. To seek external collaboration and funding to achieve the above objectives with the approval of the institute's board of directors for specific projects.

The institute's board of directors, comprised of senior managers, was designed to ensure both a degree of independence and integration with the rest of IHC's activities.

In 1991, IHC management formally adopted TQM as its primary business strategy for dealing with the changing environment. By that time, IHC had had several years of good experience with quality improvement methodologically, and there was a large cadre of people who agreed that it made sense. Senior management had never cheer-led the effort nor mandated it. Those supporting it had convinced their colleagues on the basis of the internal clinically focused studies. Thus, IHC's quality effort was both uniquely clinical and uniquely collegial.

After official adoption of TQM, the Executive Management Council (approximately the top 20 managers) was designated the Quality Council. Fairly quickly it became obvious that this group was excellent for policy decisions but not as good for operational decisions for implementing the quality effort. They reorganized, keeping the Quality Council for policy decisions and adding a Core Quality Group (Pehrson, James, Ann Ward, Carol Bush, and David L. Larsen) to guide the day-to-day operational-ization. The Core Quality Group represents administration, medical staff, quality management, nursing, and planning, and it functions as a team to integrate the overall quality improvement efforts. A Physician Clinical Quality Group was added in 1991. This group has around 20 members—one representative from each medical staff organization as well as some corporate-level members (e.g., James). It started as a physician profiling group, but collectively the members decided that this was the wrong focus—they wanted to be involved with studies of cost and quality. In January 1993, they changed their emphasis and are now moving into the role of guiding James and the institute on research topics and related practical matters.

A Framework for Developing QI

The staff at the Institute for Health Care Delivery Research are responsible for developing and implementing the education and training efforts, includ-ing the basic Facilitator Workshop Series, an alumni conference, physician education and training, an advanced training program, conferences for per-sons outside of IHC, and QI support for non–health care organizations in the community. As noted earlier, the Facilitator Workshop Series grew out of a perceived grassroots need for a common QI language. James describes the education effort itself as a quality improvement project—in the early days, the workshop content and format changed fairly rapidly based on customer feedback.

Today, James and the institute staff continue to take primary respon-sibility for teaching these workshops, and spend about one-half of their time on them. The Facilitator Workshop Series trains trainers who will return to their own operating units to facilitate teams, provide general consultation regarding problem solving to their own local organizations, and teach—both through consulting with and facilitating teams, and by actually implementing local QI education programs. To attend the workshop series, people must be sent by their administrator. Administrators are asked to send people in small groups (2–4 at a time). Workshops are limited to 20–30 participants at a time. Participation by non-IHC people is also possible, on a space-available basis. A new series starts every two months.

The workshop series is nine days in length and broken into four segments to be attended about a month apart. The first segment (three days) presents QI theory and planning tools. The second segment (three days) comes one month later and focuses on measurement—computer skills, statistical process control, and the seven quality improvement tools. The third session (two days) focuses on team skills. The last session (one day) comes two to three months later and involves presentation of the completed QI project required for graduation. A certificate is awarded in a special presentation ceremony to all who graduate.

In addition to the workshops, the institute also makes materials (e.g., model curricula), a speaker's bureau, and a QI bookstore available to the operating units. The ultimate responsibility for educating employees rests with each operating unit. It is expected to tailor the education to its own needs and can use its own format. It also can make the decision not to do any QI education. James takes the position, "If I can't convince them that it is the right thing to do, then probably they shouldn't be doing it. We have enough data and it's picked up enough momentum within the system, that it's pretty much become moot."

Alumni conferences for graduates of the workshop series are held twice a year and feature a nationally prominent speaker. The overall focus is on assisting facilitators to handle roadblocks that they encounter. The planning for these conferences is based on a survey of the needs of the facilitators.

James personally presents quality improvement training to the various medical staffs. The introduction has usually been a medical staff leadership retreat presenting basic concepts in the context of clinical studies. James argues:

> The medical profession already has all the principles of quality control built-in—but called by different names. TQM/CQI's scientific component is at the foundation of American medical practice: Physicians commit to continually assess the treatment they apply to patients' diseases, and the medical outcomes they achieve, with an aim to improve treatment and outcome for future patients. Physicians also understand the importance of objective evidence when evaluating treatments and outcomes, and the use of the scientific method to systematically improve.

Therefore, he never calls it "quality improvement" when he starts with physicians, but "good medical practice, standard medicine, clinical research." Dr. James believes, "In many settings the terms 'TQM' and 'CQI' are now so strongly associated with their philosophical component that their methodological core is dimly recognized and poorly implemented, if at all."

There have always been some physicians who have wanted to learn more about CQI than what was presented in medical staff meetings, and they participated in the institute's regular facilitator workshops. However, since the medical staff retreats, requests for more training have increased. At these retreats, James presents clinical studies and tells the doctors that this is nothing new:

> It makes all the pieces of the puzzle fit together for you as a physician. And, it gives you a few useful tools that you didn't have before such as SPC [statistical process control] or the quality planning tools. These are relatively trivial compared to the core ideas that physicians already have.

James has had the experience more than once of being asked to make a one-hour presentation to a medical staff meeting of private practice physicians and of running over by three hours because they didn't want to stop. He is convinced that

> A physician is needed to lead with physicians. The issue is trust and credibility when you are starting. Now we have quite a number of physicians who have come through the training and are champions. It's been an evolution based on methodology and results. It was not a philosophical rollout [to the physicians]. [However] in order to not just stay a bunch of good methodologists, philosophy is critical to become a truly full-quality organization. The management philosophy creates an environment in which the scientific methodology that lies at the heart of TQM/CQI can flourish.

In turn, James urged his managerial colleagues to "think about this as a clinician, as a patient. We are not a bank. Our primary business is patient care." And they have agreed. As Pehrson stated:

> We are in the business of clinical medicine—and let's find out how we can improve that; let's not focus on the other kinds of things. We're finding out in the clinical studies—that's where the action really is; that's where the dollar savings really are; that's where we can really join physician partnerships in a more detailed way; that's what we will be able to sell in the health plans arena, managed care marketplace. It was a very logical thing for us [to start with the clinical aspect]. To me, it's illogical that others have started with admitting, billing

procedures. That's not to say that they're not good—and we've done some of that, too—but that doesn't focus on the base business of why we exist and who does the work. The clinicians do the work. We have forgotten in health care, to a great extent on the administrative side, that the physicians and nurses and the others are the ones who do the real work. We're the ones that ought to be there supporting it.

IHC modifies the way certain key QI principles are implemented— for example, physician involvement on teams. It has proven more efficient and effective for doctors to move in and out as the process goes on. They participate in the initial work on a diagnosis group, receive periodic reports on work in progress, and then become active when the analysis seems complete to review and respond to findings. The existing medical staff structure with its committees is used.

Many physicians have been stimulated by the retreats to pursue further CQI education. They participate in the facilitation workshops, but the most effective teaching tool for IHC physicians has turned out to be the advanced training program developed by Susan Horn, Ph.D. (senior scientist, IHC Institute for Health Care Delivery Research), and Brent James. This program runs twice a year as four monthly sessions of four days each. It is explicitly targeted at senior professionals from academic, business, or health care institutions who want to start a training program or a health services research program, or to implement a full-blown quality improvement clinical rollout. Forty people participate in each series. Because IHC sees implementation of QI as a means of survival in a managed care environment, it pays program costs, although physicians volunteer their time. This program focuses on health economics and quality—arguing that quality drives cost. It includes the material covered in the Facilitator Workshop Series but also allots 2–2½ days to presentations by prominent health care services researchers (e.g., David Eddy, Stephen Shortell, John Williamson), who are given a half day to a day to present their research.

CQI at a Single IHC Site

For several years, Primary Children's Medical Center followed an essentially "trickle down" evolutionary approach to quality improvement implementation. Key managers had taken the regular Facilitator Workshop Series, but there had not been extensive physician exposure, partly because the clinical studies had not focused on children's medical diagnoses. Until very recently, the medical center's medical director had been skeptical about CQI. Rather than push CQI on clinicians, Primary Children's administration elected to take some time to cultivate a credible champion for the quality improvement process. Recently such a person has come to the fore— Michael Dean, the medical director of the pediatric ICU, who is also the chair of the Medical Staff Quality Assurance Committee and considered a rigorous thinker. Primary Children's Medical Center now appears to be in a position to do something that it hasn't been able to before.

After going through the institute's workshops, the medical and nursing directors of the pediatric ICU came to Joe Horton (at that time chief operating officer, now chief executive officer, Primary Children's Medical Center) and said, "We'd like to really go after this in an intensive way. Are you willing to support it? If you are, these are the kinds of elements we'd want you to build into it, that would energize us to do it."

The ICU team requested assistance in identifying measures to relate changes in outcomes quality to team activities. They were especially interested in building in mechanisms for tracking financial savings in a manner that would allow cost savings that showed up elsewhere (e.g., pharmacy) to be credited to their efforts. Their interest in tracking cost savings related to their second request: They wanted a commitment that 20 percent of any documented savings through CQI efforts of their people would go back into a department fund to be used for more CQI efforts or for other training opportunities that aren't normally available through the operating budget. Third, the ICU team wanted to "go whole hog and not have anything that forces us into a defensive position where we have to regulate savings to stash some away for the next year."

Primary Children's administration agreed to these requests. They exempted the ICU from the usual productivity improvement pressures for 1994. They agreed to pay for CQI training and to participate with the team. In early 1993, Horton, along with the director of nursing, the CFO, members of the Medical Staff Quality Assurance Committee, and 34 other managers and clinicians from Primary Children's (most from the ICU) attended a special two-day training session presented by the institute. He feels that they have now brought on a key group of their physicians who are involved in the traditional quality effort of the hospital and are in a position to make the transition from the "bad apple" approach to a CQI approach. Primary Children's is "on the brink of developing the kind of core commitment and consensus around this that you have to have before anything dramatic happens."

The pediatric ICU now has prioritized 17 teams based on suggestions from staff members regarding where they think breakthroughs and improvements can be made. Horton will be on one, the director of nursing on another, and the CFO on a third. The three representatives of administration

Figure 6.6

Uncomplicated Cholecystectomy
Quality, Utilization, and Efficiency Study of IHC

Study Population: 708 cases of DRG 197 (total cholecystectomy without common duct exploration, age greater than 69 and/or comorbidities/complications) and DRG 198 (same but age less than 70) that passed a review verifying ICD diagnoses of cholelithiasis or other disorders of the gallbladder. All treated at one of four IHC hospitals during calendar 1986. All cases with major unrelated secondary procedures, gallbladder disease secondary to other disease, or lacking critical medical or financial information were excluded. 219 cases attended by physicians with insufficient case load to meet the study inclusion criteria or having serious pretreatment comorbidity or post-treatment complications were included in the analyses of outcome, comorbidities, and complications (i.e., quality), but were not included in the final utilization and efficiency analyses because they did not represent comparable, uncomplicated cholecystectomies.

74% were women with mean age 46.0 years. Mean age men, 55.3 years. Women were 1.5 times as likely to be classified as obese on the CDC Body Mass Index.

All four hospitals served comparable urban populations within a limited geographic area along Utah's Wasatch front. All offered a similar range of general surgical services. One serves as a teaching institution for a general surgical postgraduate training program so medical students, interns, and residents may have been involved with cases there. The remaining hospitals were staffed exclusively with independent, community-based general surgeons. All surgeons treated other general surgical illnesses in addition to cholecystitis. There were no significant differences among the hospitals in terms of the total number of cholecystectomies performed as compared to bed size, overall number of surgeons as compared to bed size, the percentage of surgeons who were board certified or board eligible, or the number of surgeons who were dropped due to lack of sufficient cases for analysis.

Selected Findings:

1. There is a difference in the average cost of performing an uncomplicated cholecystectomy among hospitals (see Figure 6.6A).
2. There is a wide variation in the average cost of performing an uncomplicated cholecystectomy among physicians (see Figure 6.6B).
3. There is a wide variation in the average length of stay among physicians (see Figure 6.6C).
4. There is a difference in average pharmacy cost per case among physicians (see Figure 6.6D).

Source: Baird, M. L., S. W. Busboom, B. Ingram, B. C. James, M.D., S. W. Lewis, M.D., D. S. Thompson, A. Ward, and M. Weed, Technical Report No. 2, *Final Analysis of the IHC Uncomplicated Cholecystectomy Quality, Utilization, and Efficiency (QUE) Study*, Salt Lake City, UT: Intermountain Health Care, Inc., March 1988.

Continued

Figure 6.6   Continued

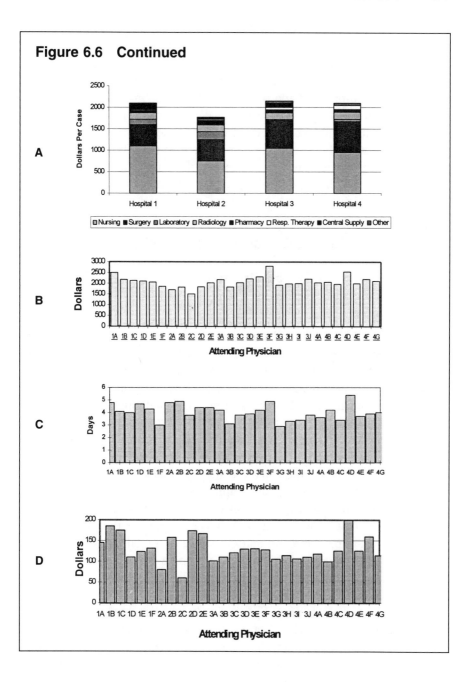

will also participate on a committee that will get quarterly reports from each team leader regarding the status of their team's activities and whether they need any additional assistance.

Horton sees this pilot as a test case that could support a leap from the traditional control-oriented approach to financial responsibility to one based more on CQI philosophy: "We trust you. We believe everybody does really want to do a good job. We believe in empowerment. We will help you to do the things we believe you will do." But it is an approach that would also "put some carrots out there in terms of reinforcing that 'something positive'—to keep the engine going and help you to get some of your people interested as well."

Putting Concepts into Practice

Research Informing Clinical Practice

Clinical studies

Over the years, IHC has fielded a number of studies oriented toward clinical practice improvement. Some have been focused on improving the extent to which specific standards are met (e.g., the surgical wound infection study and the adverse drug events study); others have been more focused on understanding a clinical process from the standpoint of outcomes in relation to what care is provided and how this care is provided (i.e., What units of care—for example, a single dose of a drug, one minute in a surgical suite, or one day on an acute nursing floor—are used in the treatment process and how efficiently are they produced?) The QUE studies on transurethral prostatectomy, uncomplicated cholecystectomy, uncomplicated total hip arthroplasty, permanent pacemaker implant, coronary artery bypass graft (CABG), and pneumonia are examples of the latter type of study. (See Figure 6.6 for a summary example of a QUE study on uncomplicated cholecystectomy.) While the above studies were initiated from the corporate office, other studies have been initiated at local facilities by local clinical providers.

In the past, findings from the studies have been shared with the participating clinicians. (Individual provider identifying information is blinded except to the specific provider.) The next steps—determination of whether to change practice patterns and if so, how—were left up to the individual provider. Follow-up has now been carried out for some period of time poststudy in each case. Decreases in variation have been noted, as have decreases in costs of providing the services. Figure 6.7 (an analysis of MEDPAR Medicare data) shows that for like DRG categories, charges started lower and increased more slowly within the IHC system than for non-IHC Utah facilities or U.S. facilities on average. Between 1986 and 1991, IHC experienced about an 8 percent increase in these categories, compared to a national increase of around 9 percent and a non-IHC Utah facility increase of close to 11 percent.

Quality does not appear to have been adversely affected. For the same time period, general physician ranking of IHC patient care quality increased (see Figure 6.8) as did patient satisfaction. Patient satisfaction was measured by a telephone survey of a 10 percent random sample of previously hospitalized patients. They were asked, "Would you return to this hospital if needed for further care?" and "Would you recommend this hospital to others?"[3]

These studies opened people's eyes regarding the amount of variation that existed and that could be addressed. However, IHC feels that even greater value (quality and cost) can be attained through management of key processes—and that this is critical based on the general situation in today's health care field. Therefore, next-generation studies are now under way. The original QUE studies were essentially point-in-time snapshots; the new studies are designed to be longitudinal and to involve providers from the local sites to a greater extent in the entire study process. An example of

Figure 6.7

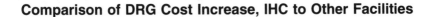

Comparison of DRG Cost Increase, IHC to Other Facilities

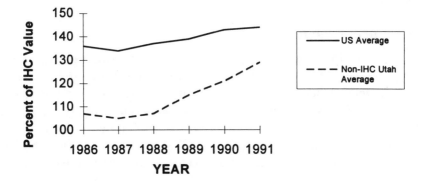

Figure 6.8

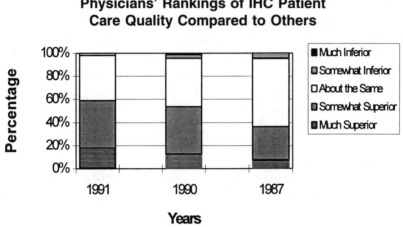

**Physicians' Rankings of IHC Patient
Care Quality Compared to Others**

such an evolving study (total hip arthroplasty) is presented at the end of this chapter.

Today, the institute tends to carry out the initial phases of clinical studies. The Department of Quality Management (QM) becomes more involved in spreading the results and processes from the studies throughout the system. For example, a manual data collection version of the postoperative wound infection study is now being piloted at McKay-Dee Hospital Center. QM is also working with Planning and Marketing to build patient satisfaction measures into ongoing studies of processes and outcomes in selected diagnoses as well as to include the tracking of functional status (for example, see the total hip arthroplasty study presented at the end of this chapter).

Care process models

All members of the Core Quality Group are involved with the local sites in the development of the multidisciplinary care process models (CPM). There are three general steps in the development of a CPM. First, a protocol is specified at the local level for a specific diagnostic category. Next, the CPM is implemented at the local level. The third step (critical to the process) involves standardization of the CPM across the system. The first and second steps have been under way since 1990. That year each facility was encouraged to develop three CPMs around clinical topics of their choice. (The authors identified at least 29 protocols apparently in local use.)

Since 1990, the topics have been chosen from those shown to have important consequences for the IHC system as a whole, as determined by a study of more than 850 major clinical processes that occur routinely in IHC hospitals. These processes were prioritized based on judgments of clinical significance, total case volume, cost per case, internal cost variability (an indicator for overall variation in practice patterns), and purchaser interest. The top 40 clinical conditions accounted for more than 70 percent of IHC's total patient volume and were chosen to be the focus for measurement and improvement efforts. Since what is important clinically varies depending on the size of the facility, the priorities for CPM development also vary with facility size. In 1993, adult tertiary care facilities will be focusing on CABGs, midrange hospitals (100–299 beds) on major joint replacement, and smaller rural hospitals on pneumonia. A multidisciplinary team develops the baseline CPM by "reducing to paper" how patients in a specific diagnostic category are handled as they go through their stay, producing a flow process chart driven by special clinical indicators or decision points. Now in the third year of implementation, this first step in the process of developing a CPM is becoming more standardized systemwide, with the objective of achieving quicker results.

In the second step, the baseline CPM is then used to manage the process of care for such patients at the facility that developed it. Each exception to the CPM is documented. The original group then reconvenes, looks at the variations from the original CPM, and evaluates it: "Was it off-target or is the variation unacceptable?"

In the third step of the process, the various local versions will be disseminated to all provider sites for review, discussion, and assistance to the corporate office in developing a system version. Ultimately, the goal is to gather variation information from everyone and to be able to say, "This is how we are doing in Intermountain Health Care."

Figure 6.9 is an early example of a CPM developed for step one and currently being implemented at one of IHC's hospitals. This version is a critical path model, driven by the day of stay rather than the more flexible clinical decision points. James prefers the latter, and current work emphasizes it. He feels that it is less arbitrary than the critical path method, is more acceptable to physicians, and yields higher quality. He notes that for many patients, and for parts of the care of almost all patients, it yields almost identical results.

Figure 6.9   Stroke Care Process Model

Time Frame	Day 1	Day 2	Day 3	Day 4	Day 5
Problems	**Interm. Goals**	**Interm. Goals**	**Interm. Goals**	**Interm. Goals**	**Interm. Goals**
1. Neuro Deficit 2. Knowledge Deficit 3. Immobility 4. Nutrition	1. Stable Neuro status 2. Pt. &/or family V/U room & unit routines 3. Pt. &/or family V/U restricted activity AROM & PROM 4. Prevent aspiration	1. Cont. 2. Pt. &/or family V/U neuro deficits 3. Pt. &/or family V/U PT/OT 4. Pt. &/or family V/U or diet	1. Cont. 2. Cont. 3. Cont. 4. Adequate nutrition	1. Cont. 2. Pt. &/or family D/U safety 3. Pt. &/or family D/U or therapy & appliances 4. Cont.	1. No further eval. 2. Cont. 3. Self care as much as possible 4. Cont.
1. Consults/Assessments/Indicators	Dr. H&P— Assessment to determine embolic or thrombolytic. Consider ECHO. Consider CRS. Consider Neuro & other consults. Nursing H&P v.s. q4° (Glasgow coma). All to consider swallow eval.	Cont. routine assessments. VS w/neuro's q4° if stable.	Cont. routine assessment. VS w/Neuro's q6° if stable. Assess need for home or Nrsg. Home appliances & follow-up.	Cont. routine assessments. VS q.i.d.	Cont. routine assessments. VS q.i.d.
2. Tests	CT of Brain Carotid—U.S. Doppler Chest X-Ray EKG Consider ECHO Consider MRI CBC w/Diff., MCP, PT, PTT, UA	Daily; Pt, PTT if indicated. Follow-up Day 1 lab abnormalities.	Consider repeat CT of head for Day 4—order is indicated. Follow-up Day 2 lab abnormalities.	CT of head if indicated (could be done as outpatient if necessary). Follow-up Day 3 lab abnormalities.	Follow-up Day 4 lab abnormalities.

3. Treatments	Medical problems—evaluated and treated. Assess managed deficits. Implement CRS recommendations.	I&O Cont. progressive treatment per CRS team.	I&O Cont. same progressive.	I&O Cont. same progressive.	I&O Cont. same progressive.
4. Meds/IV's	IV to maintain hydration. Medical therapy a necessity.	Maintain hydration. Cont. IV if necessary. Heplock if intake good. Cont. medical therapy as ordered.	Cont. same.	Cont. same. DC Heplock if still in place.	Cont. same.
5. Nutrition	NPO until initial assessment. Step 1 Dysphasia diet (no thin liquid).	Progressive diet per S.T. (Maintenance) and assistant as needed.	Cont. same.	Cont. same.	Cont. same.
6. Activity	PT or Nurse assisted.	Cont. w/Progressive activity per CRS team and Nrsg.	Cont. w/Progression.	Cont. w/Progression. Encouraging self care as much as possible.	Cont. w/Progression. Self care as much as possible.
7. PT & Family Education/Counseling	Orient to room, unit & routines. Review Meds. Family education regarding DX, tests, ancillary specialist, physician specialist, disposition options and course of care.	Cont. teaching. Coping w/changes and safety.	Reinforce teaching.	Reinforce teaching. Instruct PT &/or family on appliance, meds, diet, and follow-up.	Reinforce teaching. Discharge teaching on follow-up. Written instructions for meds., diet, follow-up, activity, appointments given.
8. Discharge Planning	Social Services Psych/Social assessment (Family & care giver assessment)	Cont.	Check w/attending physician re: discharge date & disposition	Written order for anticipated discharge in AM.	Discharge w/Home Health notified or transportation to SNF.

Carol Bush, R.N. (assistant vice president, Nursing Services) talked about the initial development process for what became IHC's care processt model. She described the approach as "tailored to our environment, our corporation, our beliefs, to where we were." Top management identified the need to guide patients through the process of illness as efficiently as possible as important. "It was up to the rest of us to determine how that looked." As they considered what their approach to monitoring patient progress through the system would look like, representatives from across the IHC system visited other health care providers throughout the United States and Canada. As they talked with others, one of the things that came through loud and clear was, "Make sure physicians are involved when you do this." Bush further notes:

> We kind of overcorrected for this, and nursing may not have been as involved as they should have been. Now we've gotten to implementation and the reality of the world is, if something is going to work, nursing has to be involved because nurses are the ones that can make most things work or not work. So now we are saying, "We've got to bring nursing up to speed with where we are on some of the stuff."

The HELP computer information system

Developed over the past 20 years at Intermountain's LDS Hospital, Health Evaluation through Logical Processing (HELP) is the clinical heart of the IHC information system. It is a computerized medical record that contains an integrated patient database drawn from many sources, including pharmacy, surgery, laboratory, radiology, respiratory therapy, blood bank, as well as nurses' notes and, in some ICU cases, physicians' notes. At LDS Hospital, HELP brings this information to bedside terminals. Clinicians can also access the information through personal computers and modems in their offices and homes. The assembled information is checked against LDS clinician-determined protocols and logic. When care decisions or patient conditions fall outside its predetermined bounds, the system issues alerts to the clinical staff (for example, see Figure 6.10). It has the ability to exchange information with other computer systems in order to use their specialized capabilities (for example, a commercial laboratory information system, a financial computing system, and commercial statistical programs).

HELP has assisted LDS clinicians to reduce postsurgical infection rates, medication errors, adverse drug reactions, respiratory therapy–related infections, and length of stay. It has promoted discussions generally among

Figure 6.10

LDS Study Utilizing HELP
to Improve Infection Control

Objective: To detect output failures (deep wound infections) and relate their occurrence to the process of care.

Method: Baseline data collected on all elective surgical cases admitted from June to November 1985 at LDS Hospital that received antibiotic prophylaxis. Timing of administration of antibiotic recorded as "premature" (>2 hours before surgical incision time), "optimal" (within 2 hours before incision time), or "late" (after incision time). Cases identified and monitored through HELP Hospital Information System, a complete electronic medical record system developed at LDS Hospital. *Intervention:* Starting in January 1986, HELP programmed to automatically evaluate new elective surgery patients and insert a reminder regarding the 2-hour "optimal" time period in the patient's electronic medical record. Copy of reminder also posted on patient's chart. Prospective monitoring of all elective surgical cases again carried out from June–November 1986 under new reminder system.

Findings: 4,484 cases monitored (2,098 in 1985; 2,386 in 1986). No change in % patients receiving antibiotics. Significant increase in % patients receiving prophylaxis during "optimal" time (40% in 1985 to 58% in 1986, $p < 0.0001$). Significant decline in deep post-operative wound infections (1.8% in 1985 to 0.9% in 1986, $p < 0.03$). Decrease in number of infections from 32 expected in 6-month period to 16 actual = over $400,000 per year savings in fixed costs to hospital, insurers, and patients ($13,000 to $15,000 average cost to treat each). Also, decreased potential liability for hospital and attending physicians and decreased potential permanent disability or death for patients.

Current Infection Control Capabilities of HELP: Daily monitoring and automatic identification of new hospital-acquired infections as well as reportable diseases, infections at sterile body sites, and unusual antibiotic resistance. Infection control personnel are also notified when a patient is at high risk of hospital-acquired infection.

Source: Larsen, R. A., R. S. Evans, J. P. Burke, S. L. Pestotnik, R. M. Gardner, and D. C. Classen, "Improved Perioperative Antibiotic Use and Reduced Surgical Wound Infections through Use of Computer Decision Analysis," *Infection Control and Hospital Epidemiology* 10 (1989): 316–20.

physicians regarding clinical processes and how to improve them. Larry Grandia, vice president of Information Systems, noted, "If we share objective, timely and reliable clinical data, we've found that clinicians openly receive it, debate it among themselves, and are very willing to alter the way they do things, as long as we can demonstrate that patient care is being improved."[4]

The HELP computer information system plays an important supporting role in the studies carried out within IHC. It is anticipated to play an even larger role as it is extended to link the hospitals throughout the IHC system. Currently, LDS Hospital in Salt Lake City is the only facility to fully implement HELP. McKay-Dee Hospital Center has been a second-generation pilot for five years; however, the clinical components are not yet up and running. Primary Children's Medical Center is expected to be brought on in 1993.

Computerized Severity Index

One of the institute's current projects is the expansion of Susan Horn's inpatient Computerized Severity Index (CSI) to include nursing as well as medical aspects, thus making it a multidisciplinary evaluation of severity of illness.[5] CSI is expected to form a foundation for the institute's clinical practice improvement (CPI) studies. Study protocols for appropriate care can be put together based on the detailed patient signs and symptoms criteria found in the CSI. It is also a building block in the development of a nursing acuity system for predicting the amount of nursing care a patient requires. Teams of nurses (specialists in the relevant areas, e.g., cardiology, oncology, OB/GYN) from across the system are putting together standards for nursing care for each of the 800 CSI diagnostic categories. The standards will be developed for each of four aspects of patient nursing care: physiological, behavioral (psychosocial factors, compliance, and communication difficulties), medication monitoring, and postprocedure care (e.g., postintubation care). At LDS Hospital (and at other sites as they go on-line), HELP will create a nursing care plan for each patient from the information that it has about each patient and the nursing care standards developed for each CSI category. With a standardized set of expectations for the care of a patient at a specific level of acuity and the requirement that exceptions be documented and explained, it will be possible over time to test whether certain approaches lead to better outcomes for the patient.

Decreasing variation

This approach of first decreasing the variation in related processes is being used in the institute's current study on pressure sores. First, agreement had to be reached on how each of the problems faced by patients at risk for pressure sores would be addressed. In this case, expected care is standardized within categories derived from a patient's functional level (e.g., mobility, nutrition). Once the care of patients within a category is standardized, then studies can be done that vary certain aspects to see if better outcomes are attained. For example, the literature in the area and IHC staff agree that specialty beds do not appear to help prevent the sores. Since the goal is to provide the best patient outcome for the least necessary cost, use of specialty beds will not be included in the initial protocol for prevention. However, plans allow for a randomized clinical trial after the original care processes have been standardized to test whether specialty beds do make a difference.

Brent James makes the point that

> It is arguably more important that health care be delivered consistently (without inappropriate variation) to groups of comparable patients than that such health care be "right," as judged by the opinions of individual practitioners. For when care is delivered consistently, systematic techniques can be applied that lead to optimal care. But when treatments are not delivered in a consistent manner it is impossible to systematically improve. In fact, if a particular treatment is not delivered to a well-defined group of comparable patients in a consistent fashion, it is impossible even to measure accurately the outcomes that the treatment achieves. For that reason both the random clinical trial approach and QI methods attempt to eliminate variation in the treatment process. This is necessary to allow practitioners to draw valid statistical inferences from their patient care experiences."[6]

The methodological component of TQM/CQI can be seen as creating a clinical laboratory from the everyday practice setting. It combines practice guidelines and outcomes management into a system designed to generate valid statistical inferences about the operational, day-to-day elements of the process of clinical care. It uses consensus and feedback on process to eliminate inappropriate treatment variation for well-defined groups of comparable patients. It tracks outcomes and feeds the resulting information back to practitioners so that they can objectively evaluate the effects of treatment consensus.

Results

IHC has a 16-year history of quality assurance and 6 years of clinical research and improvement consistent with, but predating, their formal CQI commitment. What difference has it made? Such questions are hard to answer, but the evidence is promising. As noted earlier, costs are increasing less rapidly within IHC than in non-IHC facilities on the average. In addition, patient satisfaction is very high, and physician ranking of quality is increasing. When talking about these findings, Greg Poulsen (vice president of Planning) observed:

When we thought about it, there was a correlation between our effort and the outcome. Small cogs in big wheels could feel, "We've made a real difference!" We can feel like we have really done something for the community. Maybe there are externalities here that are not apparent, but whatever, it has been a big boost to the culture of CQI and practice improvement.

QI methodology is being used effectively in both research studies and in day-to-day process improvement within the Intermountain system. It is a tool that is helping them to attain their goals in the area of patient care. As Ann Ward described it:

IHC is trying to make quality the focus of what we do, so it is not a "buzzword of the day" kind of thing. Since IHC's inception, quality has been in its mission statement. It's something we just feel—QI is the next step. There may be another next step; we just don't know yet what it is.

Administrative Support of Clinical Base Business

IHC is unique in that its implementation of QI methodology (as an underpinning for clinical research) preceded its commitment to TQM principles as a management philosophy. To this day, the emphasis on research to inform clinical practice continues. Now, however, this is supplemented by an administrative focus whose objective is to support the clinical "base business." This section presents an example of administrative implementation of QI concepts in support of the clinical focus at McKay-Dee Hospital Center in Ogden.

McKay-Dee is a 330-bed hospital with 1,600 FTEs providing comprehensive inpatient and outpatient services in Ogden, Utah. Thomas Hanrahan, CEO, describes the quality management process as reaching a turning point in 1992 after management and physician participation in several CQI workshops revealed a need to establish a foundation for the quality effort in their vision and values statement. From early to mid-1992, an intense educational effort took place. All employees went through a one-hour session where McKay-Dee's vision and values were described and dialogue about them was encouraged. A lot of emphasis was placed on everyone buying into a common vision and values—even though there was a risk of having to modify them during the course of the dialogue. These discussions set the stage for the ensuing emphasis in the quality management program and the planned structural changes. Figure 6.11 presents the vision and values statement generated by the discussions. Patient focus is the primary value: "the essence of everything we do." The other values are shown in relationship to it. The figure concludes with guiding principles that follow from the stated vision and values.

Hanrahan describes the statement of vision and values as "nothing particularly innovative there, except it was an expression of the community—of what we believe in. We made a commitment here that not the physician, not the company, not the community-at-large but that the patient would become the focus of everything we did and why we did it." They feel that they have received enthusiastic support from corporate for their consensus approach.

Hanrahan's advice to other hospitals interested in quality improvement is, "Get to the clinical aspect as fast as you can. Don't neglect this while you focus on the nonclinical." They, however, are trying to take it yet another step. McKay-Dee has a "continued and relentless focus on trying to document and improve our processes and our outcomes on the clinical side"—for example, the use of care process models. They term it, "doing the right things." Hanrahan notes, however, that it is also important that "we do the right things in the right way." The search for the "right way" (carried out in the light of their consensus-generated vision and values) has led them to initiate redesign of the care delivery network within the hospital.

The goal of this work redesign project is to convert the entire hospital to a patient-focused model of care delivery—to decentralize services to the patient at the bedside unit and to delegate knowledge and authority for patient care to the lowest possible level. The project is expected to both enhance the quality of patient care and to reduce the operating costs of the overall organization through reducing the number of FTEs required to deliver the same care. It is also expected that the development of self-directed work teams on the units will reduce the number of administrators needed.

Sustaining the Organization's Quality Awareness

There are a number of ways in which the awareness of quality is promoted and sustained within the IHC system. Certainly the ongoing education and training workshops with certificates of completion and the alumni conferences discussed earlier extend such awareness. Brent James's presentations of clinical research results to medical staffs also keep quality improvement in people's minds. Further, Gary Pehrson notes a sense of great personal

Figure 6.11

McKay-Dee Hospital Center
Vision, Values, and Guiding Principles

Vision: To be the leader in patient focused care.

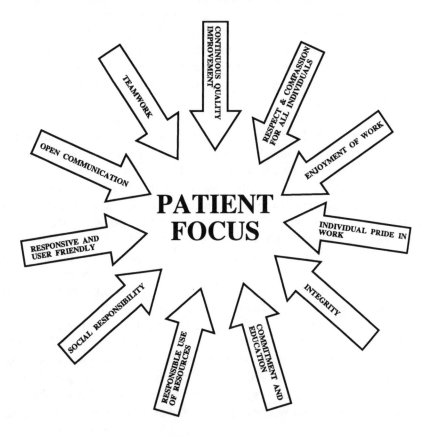

Guiding Principles
- Patients are the focus of everything we do.
- Quality comes first.
- Continuous improvement is essential to success.
- Employee involvement is vital.
- Integrity is never compromised.

support from Scott Parker (president) and the Management Committee: "Whatever I need to do in terms of quality, they say, 'Let's put them on the goals and we will start integrating across the line.'"

Quality goals have been integrated with the strategic planning process for three years now—for example, key goals are outlined in quality break-through goals. And, in fact, the value of clinical and service quality forms the core of the Intermountain Health Care Vista (strategic planning process) along with community access and lowest possible cost (see Figure 6.12). The budget planning process is also somewhat integrated into the Vista process. In 1992, two quality teams were reviewing the budget processes with the intent of increasing the integration by the 1994 planning cycle.

There is no systemwide scheme for the recognition of the contributions of various staff to the quality effort. However, Gary Hart (vice president, Human Resources) feels that there is a lot of recognition going on, but

Figure 6.12

An Evolving IHC Strategy

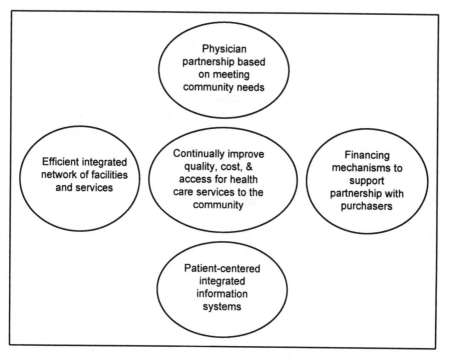

on a hospital-specific basis. For example, McKay-Dee Hospital Center has a number of methods for recognizing quality improvement contributions from employees. There is a permanent Quality Hall of Fame with changing storyboard exhibits, recognition awards, and sections on teams and customer focus. They also have an Annual Quality Celebration under a tent with a band and food, where accomplishments of teams are recognized and the "team of the year" is announced. Most recently, an employee recognition program has been revamped to focus specifically on contributions to quality improvement.

Under this recognition program (the Employee Involvement Plan), each department or cross-functional team is given credit for the total number or "value" of quality-related ideas that are generated and implemented by that team. Upon achievement of specified totals, the teams are recognized by a bronze, silver, or gold award. Individual team members receive pins and a designated amount of money goes to the appropriate department to be used for a celebration event or to purchase an item for the department.[7] A plaque is presented to all departments achieving the gold status. The "most valuable team" for the previous year is announced at the Annual Quality Celebration.

A protocol outlines the procedure: Ideas from individual teams are certified by a "service line" quality idea certifier (QIC). All certified ideas are then communicated to the hospital Quality Management Council for reporting and tracking purposes. All ideas that claim a financial impact are to be certified by the liaison from the Finance Department to the relevant department. Examples of certification criteria include the following: improves quality, improves productivity, decreases cost, improves patient satisfaction, improves customer needs, improves customer satisfaction, and increases safety/improves risk management. Figure 6.13 shows a sample idea submission form.

Importance of Underlying Culture

At IHC, virtually everyone interviewed mentioned the importance of that organization's culture on quality improvement. They identified four elements as particularly important: having a long-standing focus on clinical quality, being a mission-driven organization, having a consensus management orientation with a CEO who does not need to control everything, having a measurement orientation. Another element, an internal environment that empowers employees in their work, became apparent during the discussions of the other cultural aspects. Here's how they see these elements.

Figure 6.13

Sample Idea Submission Form for
the Employee Involvement Plan

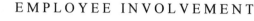

EMPLOYEE INVOLVEMENT

Quality Through Ideas * You Make the Difference!

Sample Idea Submission Form

Date: _____ Team Name: _____
Department Represented by Team: _____

Team Representative: _____
Idea Title _____
Department Affected: _____

Brief description of idea: _____
_____
_____
_____

Implementation Date: _____
How was it implemented? _____
_____
_____
_____
_____

What are the benefits of the idea? _____
_____
_____
_____
_____

If the idea has a financial impact, please project an approximate annual savings or gain. (This financial impact must be confirmed by the team's Financial Liaison from the Accounting Department.) _____

Team Financial Liaison _____

Please attach any supporting documentation.

For QIC Team Use Only
Log Number: _____
QIC Team OK: _____
Date Approved: _____
After entering data on the LAN System, keep
this copy for your records

Cecil Samuelson, M.D., (a 20-year resident of Salt Lake City and until 2½ years ago, dean and the vice president for Health Sciences at the University of Utah Medical School) describes clinical quality as "always important at IHC. This has been clear since 1975." He also compliments "senior management before his time" for having "the willingness and enthusiasm to bring on people like Brent James and giving them not only a sandbox to play in but the resources to play with." He calls this completely consistent with the quality movement, but it wasn't thought of as embarking on a program based on the principles of Deming or Juran at that time.

Pehrson points out that excellence in quality was one of the five major strategic directions specified in the 1985 strategic plan. Two administrators for operating units also echo this concern with quality in regard to their facilities. Hanrahan talked about the "RIGHT" teams initially formed at McKay-Dee Hospital Center around 1988—multidisciplinary teams that study specified clinical processes. Joe Horton (Primary Children's Medical Center) depicts his facility as one with a very strong mission-oriented culture, where the QI movement has not been a revolution because "we've always had objectives around quality improvement. The only thing that changed is we've introduced a different way of approaching that with some different tools."

Samuelson, James, and Gary Poulsen (vice president, Planning and Research) emphasized the sense of corporate responsibility to the community: driving a bottom line sufficient to meet responsibility to the community, having a charitable mission, and adding value to communities served.

Pehrson and James emphasized the importance of team playing and consensus building at IHC, but also the freedom to do one's job within the scope of one's responsibilities. The style and culture of IHC is characterized as solid and methodical with a very strong strategic plan. Samuelson lauds IHC for its early commitment to developing data systems—especially those that assist practitioners in handling patient data. It's been very important in the development of the organization's culture of "measuring everything that we do, to try to do better" and the related "infrastructure that allowed us to attract a Brent James" who was interested in clinical research. It also has attracted other people interested in "doing academic things in a nonacademic setting that you can't do in a traditional academic setting"—for example, Samuelson and Horn.

So while IHC's quality improvement effort has not actually been "led" by senior management, an environment had been developed that attracted a catalyst (James) and provided support to the elements necessary to grow a quality initiative into itself. James himself says that

> The lack of initial push from top management was the best thing
> that happened to us—because we focused on methodology. We got

provable results. I'm not too wedded to the philosophy. I don't think anyone is. The attitude is, "If it works, do it." And that's what quality improvement really is for us. That approach has worked very well for us. It hasn't led to the schisms that you might worry about. But I think that is due to the culture of IHC. We tend to be strongly mission driven—and our mission is a charitable mission. Quality improvement fits very tightly with that.

Special Focus: Studies on Total Hip Arthroplasty

QUE Study

In 1988, a QUE study was carried out at six IHC hospitals to assess and compare efficiency (hospital related) and utilization (physician related) on total hip arthroplasty (DRG 209). As in the cholecystectomy study in Figure 6.6, eligibility criteria were used to form a cohort of 252 comparable patients in terms of presenting disease, comorbidities, complications, and short-term medical outcomes. Many process and outcome factors were tracked, including number of physical therapy sessions, cases walking 100 feet, number of laboratory and radiology procedures, length of stay, total cost, cost of prosthesis, and type of prosthesis. Figure 6.14 presents some examples of findings from this study. The findings were shared with the clinicians involved (orthopedists, nurses, physical therapists, anyone involved in the care of these patients). Physician-specific information was identified by blinded code; surgeons were given a unique code so that each could recognize his or her own practice measurement within the group. The researchers did not make any determinations of what was "best care." That was left up to the clinicians to determine. As an outgrowth of the study, ongoing monitors of long-term outcomes on these patients were instituted at the six hospitals that do hip replacement. Although average length of stay declined, as did the variation within the group as a whole, the system continued to lose money on this DRG category. These results led IHC to the longitudinal-type study being carried out today by the Department of Quality Management.

Current Quality Management Study

The objectives of the current study are to (1) identify "inputs" that significantly affect the "outputs," (2) identify significant variation in practice

Figure 6.14

Selected Findings from QUE Study, Total Hip Arthroplasty

A. Recovery to Physical Therapy Start to Discharge

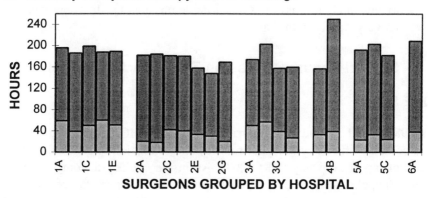

B. Average Prosthesis Cost

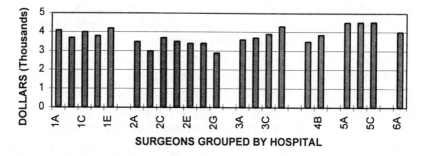

patterns among hospitals and physicians, and (3) reflect trends over time. In February 1993, Quality Management staff were about 18 months into the project. Patients complete a health status evaluation (the John Ware SF-36) presurgery, 6 months postsurgery after the postdischarge therapies are completed, and at 18 months postsurgery. Cost, type of prosthesis, and patient satisfaction are also measured. The six hospitals are compared to see who is doing what and if that correlates with patient satisfaction or health status outcomes.

Some preliminary analyses have been carried out on sample populations. To date, men show greater change in mobility at six-month follow-up than do women. The "very satisfied" group of patients had a shorter

Figure 6.15

Preliminary Findings of Quality Management Study on DRG 209 (Total Hip Replacement)

Objective 1: Identification of inputs that impact outputs

Dependent Variable 1 (DV1): change in pain from presurgery to six months postdischarge (as measured by John Ware SF-36).

Dependent Variable 2 (DV2): change in patient mobility from presurgery to six months postdischarge (per Ware SF-36).

No statistically significant impact on dependent variables 1 or 2 from patient age, length of stay, cost of prosthesis, or hospital.

Predictors	Change in Pain (DV1)	Change in Mobility (DV2)
Degree of pain prior to surgery	$-.63$ ($p = .0002$)	n.s.
R^2	.15	
Mobility before surgery	n.s.	$-.75$ ($p < .0001$)
R^2		.37
Gender	n.s.	-2.13 ($p = .0238$)
R^2		.04
Number of cases	88	86

Dependent Variable 3 (DV3): patient satisfaction.

Analysis of Variance
No statistically significant impact on patient satisfaction between very satisfied and less than very satisfied for patient age, mobility prior, level of pain before surgery or at 6 months, or cost of prosthesis.

Predictors	Very Satisfied	< Very Satisfied	p	Cases
Length of stay	5.26	5.98	.0103	209
6-Month mobility	24.50	19.80	.0050	47
Sufficient info. from surgeon	4.91	4.74	.0276	212

Continued

Figure 6.15   Continued

Objective 2: Variation in practice patterns

Analysis of Variance
A *p* value less than .05 was used to identify statistically significant differences in practice patterns. The following were not statistically significant: patient age, gender, level of pain before surgery or at 6 months, level of mobility at 6 months, change in pain or mobility from presurgery to 6 months, or variation in patient satisfaction. Level of mobility before surgery was significant ($p = .05$), as was variation in length of stay ($p < .0001$) and variation in prosthesis cost ($p < .0001$).

There was no significant difference physician to physician on presurgical mobility. Significance of other differences is shown in the following figure.

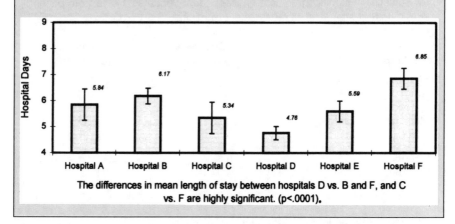

The differences in mean length of stay between hospitals D vs. B and F, and C vs. F are highly significant. (p<.0001).

length of stay, greater mobility at six-month follow-up, and were more satisfied with information received from their surgeons before surgery than were other patients. There were statistically significant differences between hospitals on patient level of mobility before surgery, length of stay (see Figure 6.15), and cost of prosthesis. Significant differences between surgeons occurred for length of stay and prosthesis cost.

The multidimensional picture of total hip replacement (e.g., functional outcomes, pain, satisfaction, length of stay, cost) is fed back to the multidisciplinary orthopedic teams at each hospital. As in the earlier study, any practice-related changes are clinical practitioner decisions. However, this time the multidisciplinary teams at each of the study hospitals are also developing CPMs addressing the care process for total hip replacement, starting with the initial contact to the physician's office and continuing through the postsurgical follow-up phase. Outcomes continue to be monitored on a comparative basis and shared across the system. In addition, discussions are occurring to identify what other information related to hip replacement would be useful.

Notes

1. The Salt Lake City Market Area covers parts of three states. The two hospitals in Wyoming fall easily into this area; the two in Idaho are only slightly outside it and are easily accessible by major highways.
2. For more information on QUE studies, see James, B. C. 1989. *Quality Management for Health Care Delivery*. Chicago: Hospital Research and Educational Trust.
3. IHC is in the process of revising its method of determining patient satisfaction. It expects to go to a monthly "every patient" survey that will ask the following: "How well did we meet your needs?" "How well did we meet your clinical expectations? For example, if you expected pain to be reduced or eliminated, has it been?" This is part of the effort to track three major outcome measures that have been identified: cost/case, customer satisfaction, and clinical outcomes. The "every patient" survey is expected to allow more granularity on patient satisfaction and clinical outcomes and to allow comparisons to be made, for example, between Dr. X and Dr. Y or Hospital A and Hospital B. IHC is also now measuring cost per case on type-adjusted cases and tracking this on a monthly basis to see whether costs for specific types of cases are increasing or decreasing.
4. *Hospitals*. 1993. "HELP on the Way." (20 February): 32.
5. CSI is disease-specific and defines the severity of illness as the treatment complexity presented to medical personnel as a result of the extent and interaction of a patient's diseases. Treatment complexity refers to the difficulty in returning the patient to baseline health. For more information, see Horn, S. D., and R. A. Horn. 1986. *CSI: Computerized Severity Index, Its Uses and Applications*. Salt Lake City, UT: Intermountain Health Care.
6. James, B. C., S. D. Horn, and R. A. Stephenson. 1993. "Management by Fact: The Relationship of Quality Improvement to Outcomes Management, Practice Guidelines, and Randomized Clinical Trials." Unpublished ms.
7. Awards are based on the assumption that a 10-person unit will generate about five implemented ideas worth $5,000, which would earn a Bronze Award, paying $5.00 per employee. The Silver Award, paying $10.00 per employee, requires 12 ideas worth $12,500. The Gold Award, paying $15.00 per employee, requires 25 ideas worth $25,000.

7

Walke-Parker Medical Center
Case Study

Walke-Parker Medical Center (WPMC) is affiliated with a for-profit system. WPMC is comprised of a 294-bed acute care facility (Walke-Parker Hospital), MediServ (a group of 16 minor emergency and primary care clinics throughout Southern City), and two surgical centers located at the main campus in a prosperous area of Southern City.

Southern City is a very competitive health services arena with a number of strong hospitals that draw patients from the rural areas of Southern State, especially for specialty services. Located on a major north-south freeway, Walke-Parker Hospital follows this pattern—it serves its immediate neighborhood and it also draws patients from 50–60 miles away. About one-third of the hospital's admissions are related to pregnancy and newborns. The next most important inpatient DRGs are psychoses, heart failure and shock, hysterectomy, major joint procedures, and cerebrovascular disorders. Its cardiovascular and cardiac surgery services are a strong point. In 1991, Walke-Parker Hospital recorded 9,775 discharges, 12,000 emergency room visits, and 26,000 other outpatient visits. Inpatient services represent only 76 percent of Walke-Parker's operating revenues. Figure 7.1 presents recent financial trends for Walke-Parker Hospital.

In the past, Walke-Parker has actively developed niches in several areas based on strengths in its 300-member private practice medical staff. Two of these niches are the management of overall medical care needs

Figure 7.1

**Financial Trends for Walke-Parker Hospital
($ in thousands)**

Operating Performance		1991
Net revenue		$86,890
Operating payroll		$22,942
Total expenses		$78,614
Net gain		$8,276
Operating margin		9.5%
Average Margin	**1990**	**1991**
Southern state hospitals	6.1%	8.0%
U.S. hospitals	3.8%	4.3%

Sources: *AHA Guide to the Health Care Field,* Chicago: AMA, 1991, 1992; *The Universal Health Care Almanac,* Phoenix, AZ: Silver and Cherner, 1991.

of patients with intercurrent diabetes or mental health–related diagnoses—that is, focusing on the patient as a whole while taking these preexisting conditions into specific consideration. A third is laser surgery. However, the 1993 name change of the overall entity from Walke-Parker Hospital to Walke-Parker Medical Center reflects an evolution in strategic thinking. As Charles Christiansen, CEO and president of Walke-Parker Medical Center notes:

> Process thinking converted us from being a hospital to being a health system. We will continue to look at what business we are in based upon our knowledge of process as opposed to looking for niches in the marketplace, which is what we used to do. We are more inclined to look strategically at the way we evolve our organization. We are more inclined to look at it as a system or a set of interconnected processes.

This view of themselves as a system led to the decision during 1993 to buy a group of 16 primary care clinics.

Organization Structure and Leadership

Organization charts have been de-emphasized at WPMC. Although the traditional departments still exist, an emphasis on teams (as shown in Figure 7.2) replaces much of the authority of the traditional hierarchy. Teams can draw from any level of employee (there are essentially four levels—the CEO, senior managers, department managers, and regular staff); the key variable is who has critical knowledge of the process under study. The director of Quality Resources is one of the six senior managers.

The local board of trustees is appointed by the parent firm of WPMC. This board consists of nine members, including the CEO of the medical center, who serves as secretary-treasurer. The other eight members of the board are medical staff members or local business or community leaders. The board is responsible for the medical-administrative powers of the hospital, as directed through the CEO, and it acts as the principal sounding board for management initiatives. It has complete authority and responsibility for all medical, professional, and ethical activities of the hospital, including the granting of staff privileges. Other than these explicit duties, it serves in an advisory capacity.

Walke-Parker prides itself on a long-standing sensitivity to its physicians and their needs. To ensure that this awareness continues, an administrative representative is assigned to each of the medical staff departments.

Walke-Parker's mission statement has remained unchanged in its 20 years of existence. The vision, "to be the best-value Southern City health system by 1996 and to be recognized as such," was kept memorably simple. It was adopted in 1990 after some experimentation with a longer version. In 1988, department managers developed a quality definition:

> At Walke-Parker Hospital, achieving quality means adding value to all that we do through a commitment to the continuous improvement of services that meet the needs and expectations of our patients, physicians, payers, employees, and the community we serve.

Unique Factors

Corporate Support

Walke-Parker Medical Center is a member of one of the nation's largest hospital chains. The quality vision within the System was initiated by its

Figure 7.2

Process for Aligning Vision, Stategic Plan, Management, and Leadership

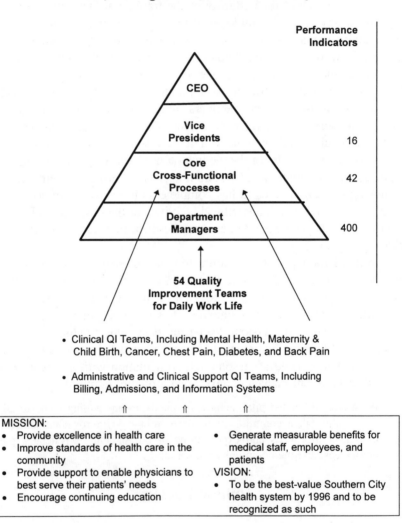

Source: Walke-Parker Medical Center.

CEO who was concerned about both increasing costs in the health care field and the potentially adverse effects that attempts to control these costs could have on the quality of care provided. In the mid-1980s, he hired a physician and give him the charge to create and champion a quality model for the System.

The culture of the System traditionally allows administrators a great deal of autonomy. Therefore, no hospital is required to participate in the quality improvement initiative. However, if a hospital does decide to participate, the CEO must first complete the training before other senior managers will be invited to attend. After those two levels have been trained, then the Corporate Office will conduct on-site training for middle managers. In addition, the facility's CEO is required to teach part of the on-site course. The CEO and senior managers also make up the hospital's Quality Improvement Council, which charters and monitors teams. (See Figure 7.3 for the road map of the process for System hospitals to follow.) Since 1987, Corporate Office has trained hundreds of hospital executives in the basics of quality improvement. Charles Christiansen, CEO of the then Walke-Parker Hospital, was one of the first executives to be trained.

Southern City

Southern City is the economic capital of the region, especially in the areas of transportation, wholesale trade, and professional services.[1] It has enjoyed decades of rapid, uninterrupted growth. The Southern City metropolitan area, and indeed the entire region, is expected to remain strong economically, although some effects from the nationwide recession have been felt recently. The population of Southern State increased 18.6 percent between 1980 and 1990 and is projected to increase another 22.8 percent by 2000. The Southern City metropolitan area population increased 32.5 percent between 1980 and 1990. Median age in the state was 31.6 years in 1990.

HMO enrollment has increased in Southern State in the last three years but still represents only 8.7 percent of the market. Public insurance covers 14.2 percent of the population insured, including 10.8 percent under Medicaid. In 1992, Walke-Parker reported the following breakdown of patients: managed care, 35 percent; Medicare, 18 percent; Medicaid, 5 percent; and commercial/other, 42 percent. Figure 7.4 presents health care information on admissions, hospital beds, occupancy rates, and physicians for the Southern City MSA, Southern State, and the United States. The number of physicians is expected to increase. In 1989, the average rate of

Figure 7.3

Hospitalwide Quality Improvement Road Map

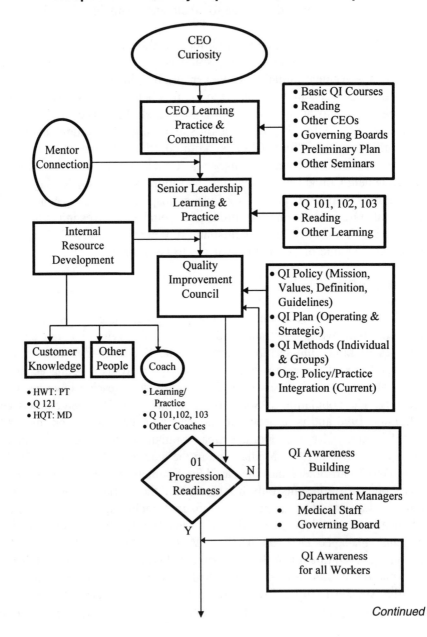

Continued

Figure 7.3   Continued

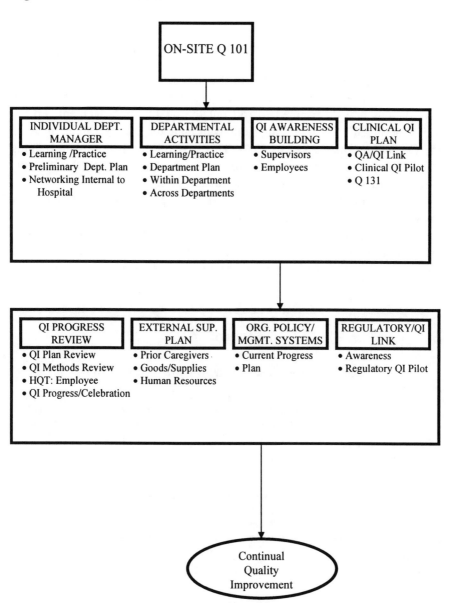

professional liability insurance per bed was $1,600 (similar to Utah's and about one-third of the Michigan rate).

Quality Management Awareness and Learning

Charles Christiansen participated in the first session of Q101 in February 1987. He was enthusiastic about the emphasis on customer needs and expectations and determined to roll out the quality improvement process at his facility. Five senior staff from Walke-Parker attended the courses in the Corporate Office early in 1988. This was followed by on-site training for department managers in June of that year. It was during this training that the hospital's quality statement was developed.

As part of the very heavy emphasis on employee education to quality improvement concepts the first year, Christiansen personally conducted orientation sessions for all employees. The goal of these sessions was to bring staff through the awareness phase of the learning curve—to make them aware of what quality improvement was, to relate quality improvement

Figure 7.4

Community Hospital Demographics, 1991

Area	Admissions (per 1,000 Population)	Hospital Beds (per 1,000 Population)	Occupancy (%)	Physicians (per 100,000 Population)
Southern City MSA	132	3.3	69.2	192
Southern State	132	4.0	64.7	162
U.S.	123	3.7	66.1	198

Community Hospitals	Community Hospitals Revenue (per Patient Day)	Community Hospitals Expense (per Patient Day)	Community Hospitals Profit Margin (%)
Southern State	$ 948.65	$ 872.83	8.0
U.S.	$1,054.67	$1,009.71	4.3

Sources: *The Universal Health Care Almanac*, Phoenix, AZ: Silver and Cherner, 1991; AMA, *Physician Characteristics and Distribution in the U.S.*, Chicago: AMA, 1992; *AHA Guide to the Health Care Field*, Chicago: AHA, 1991, 1992.

Note: Physician data is from 1990.

to Deming's Fourteen Points, to discuss QI's process orientation, and to make them aware that there are tools and techniques out there that can be helpful. The Corporate Quality Resource Group also conducted a course specifically for physicians in November.

Today, Walke-Parker offers two courses (Q101A and Q101B) based on content developed by the Quality Resource Group. These are taught in-house twice a year for all new managers, supervisors, and key personnel within departments. Vicki Dawson (director, Quality Resources) coordinates the courses, and all senior managers participate in the three- to four-hour segments (including CEO Christiansen). All new employees receive a two-and-a-half hour orientation to quality improvement. Department managers continue their education through a monthly leadership series, now a day in length.

As directed by the Corporate Office, WPMC's Quality Improvement Council (QIC) is composed of the CEO and senior managers. Initially, while the membership was identical to that of the hospital Operations Committee, the two groups held separate meetings. Eventually the agenda items became so intermingled that the two were merged into a weekly discussion of strategic and operational issues. By 1991, the annual strategic planning and quality improvement road-mapping processes were merged.

The QIC has primary responsibility for developing the annual quality improvement road map, chartering cross-functional QI teams, selecting facilitators and assuring that they are properly deployed and trained, and monitoring the progress of the QI teams, as well as for developing and implementing measurements for tracking QI results.

Over the five years of TQM implementation at WPMC, the role of the QIC and department managers has evolved away from "management by control" and toward more of a mentoring role. The approach asks, "How can I help you [the organization's employee] improve your processes?" rather than stating, "Here are your MBO objectives this year."

Quality Management Framework Development

A great deal of organizational introspection has taken place at Walke-Parker since Christiansen attended that first training session. Drawing on Peter Senge's "learning organization,"[2] participants in that first session were encouraged to ask questions such as the following:

- Why does your organization exist?
- What do you make?

- Based on what you make, how do you measure the degree to which you meet the needs and expectations of the customers of that product?
- Given what processes produce it, from the outputs and outcomes and measurements that exist, where are you in comparison to best practices?

The Radar Chart

Such questions guided Christiansen and his senior staff as they worked to develop a framework to transform their organization to one focused on quality improvement. The group began by identifying 16 measures in four areas: customer satisfaction, productivity, sales, and development. They then established benchmarks or goals for each measure. Actual performance is compared to the goal using a radar chart (see Figure 7.5).

The radar chart is used as a planning and operational tool in the search to achieve balance between areas. The inner circle represents acceptable minimum requirements for each indicator; the outer one, benchmark scores. In this format it is possible to see the big picture at a glance—Is something doing well at the expense of another area? The 16 target measures expand to 42 for senior managers and 400 for teams. Results are plotted on a regular basis. Christiansen notes:

> We respond faster than instantly to the slightest variation in efficiency or productivity and certain levels of clinical outcomes. That's probably true of any hospital. We aren't so rigid if we see an increase in length of time it takes to respond to complaints or a slip in the number of patients that answer Question 56 ["the care I received is so good I bragged about it . . ." from the discharged patient survey]. We're not going to react as rapidly. I hope we evolve to that point—that when we are close enough or in best value in those 16 indicators, that any slippage from being best value causes a sense of concern.

Christiansen outlines six sets of questions related to the radar chart that must be answered to achieve WPMC's vision of best value.

1. What are the best practices around the 16 measurements that we are tracking to show that we are on track? In other words, what do the outer points of the target diagram look like? Who has the best practices? How are we in relation to these practices?

Figure 7.5

Walke-Parker Medical Center: 1993 Targets

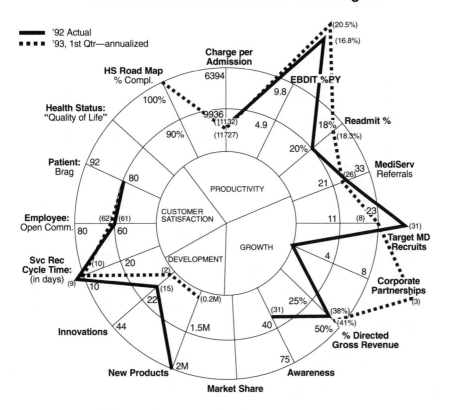

2. What are the high-leverage processes on which we can focus that will, in pareto-type thinking, drive us to best-value achievements?

3. What are the drivers that exist here that will help us achieve those best-value data points? What are the inhibitors that are holding us back?

4. What education and training needs to be offered here to capitalize on the drivers and to remove the inhibitors—or at least minimize their negative impact?

5. What does the measurement system [related to the targeted areas] look like? How is it structured?

6. What methods exist to celebrate when improvements are achieved?

Christiansen feels that this process for aligning vision, strategy, and performance can offer assistance to others in their pursuit of quality improvement.

The "Brag Abouts"

Some of the performance measures used at WPMC have been developed by the corporate office for use by all facilities participating in quality improvement. In addition, elements of an integrating framework are presented as part of the corporate-developed education and training program (e.g., Quality Improvement Council, coach, facilitators). How it gets specifically woven together at each operating entity is, as will be shown by various examples, up to that facility.

The Corporate Quality Resources Group developed the Hospital Quality Trends (HQT) surveys to elicit information from each of four important groups of customers (physicians, patients, employees, and payers) in order to assist System hospitals to improve their quality. The surveys used the phrase "brag about" in the summary question for each group because it represents a more difficult to achieve outcome than satisfaction with a service or situation. For example, patients were asked the extent to which they agreed that "The care I received at the hospital was so good that I have bragged about it to family and friends."

After receiving the results of the first surveys, the Quality Improvement Council at Walke-Parker developed a set of goals or indicators for their hospital based on features that were statistically significant in explaining what a particular customer group bragged about. These factors that contribute to a higher "brag about" score are identified in Figure 7.6. The QIC used the "brag about" terminology to emphasize its importance.

The 24 "brag abouts" from Figure 7.6 represent an integral part of the multilevel measurement pyramid used to assess customer satisfaction at Walke-Parker (see Figure 7.7). Jim Black, vice president of Operations, explains that the ultimate goal of producing value for a customer group is at the apex and that value production is determined by measuring satisfaction of patients, physicians, employees, and payers as represented by the four basic "brag about" scores. The twenty-four "brag abouts" form the next layer. These indicators are, in turn, related to core cross-functional processes managed by clinical or administrative support QI teams (see Figure 7.2). The next level of measurement detail is the 400 functional (departmental)

Figure 7.6

Hospitalwide Customer Expectations

"A physician brags about Walke-Parker Medical Center when . . ."

- Available time is maximized.
- Scheduling needs are met.
- Nurses are responsive, informing, and accessible.
- Reports are timely.
- High-quality consultants are accessible.
- State-of-the-art equipment is available.
- Every employee is involved in quality improvement.
- Physicians are treated as valued customers by everyone.

"A patient brags about Walke-Parker Medical Center when . . ."

- The expected clinical outcome is achieved.
- Requests are responded to promptly and with TLC.
- Nurses are responsive, skilled, caring, and informing.
- Living arrangement needs are met.
- Billing and collections procedures are understandable, accurate, and efficient.
- Admission procedures are understandable, quick, and efficient.

"An employee brags about Walke-Parker Medical Center when . . ."

- Nurses are skilled, concerned, and caring.
- All departments work together to improve quality.
- Top leaders understand employee issues, communicate regularly, and recognize employee contributions.
- Corporate Office and Walke-Parker Medical Center have an image of high quality.
- New co-workers are highly qualified and will be long-term employees.
- Processes are sufficiently efficient to allow requirements to be met with budgeted staffing.

"A payer brags about Walke-Parker Medical Center when . . ."

- Employees brag about their care.
- His/her health costs are less than the competitors'.
- The hospital demonstrates efforts to reduce cost while improving quality.

Source: Walke-Parker Medical Center.

Figure 7.7   Measurement System Pyramid for Walke-Parker Medical Center

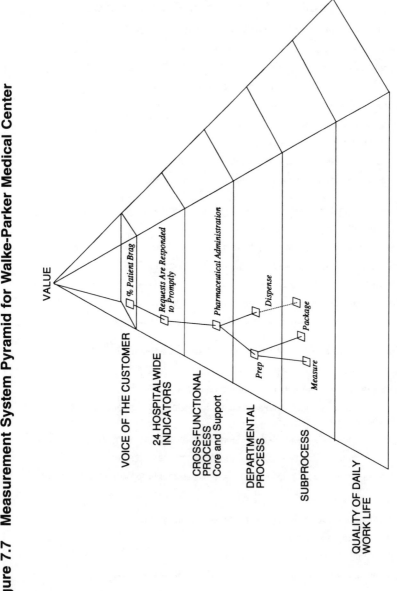

Source: Walke-Parker Medical Center.

processes. Each of these is related to a cross-functional process. The subprocesses (those that individual employees perform) form the last layer of the pyramid that is measured. As Black points out, the measurement system is significant because it establishes a link between customer satisfaction measures and the 400 process measures.

Quality Management Practice

Walke-Parker is an information-seeking system. Data, and new ways to use it, are not feared but sought out by its leadership. Christiansen notes that their measurement system has been called "better than Xerox's." Arnold Jefferson, vice president of Development, describes the monthly senior management meeting held in "Charles' data room," where graphed and flowcharted survey results "completely cover the walls." "Brag about" results are posted throughout the hospital in key places for employees, physicians, and the public to see—the physicians' lounge, the employees' cafeteria, the bridgeway connecting the physicians' office building to the hospital. In discussing the customer surveys, Black states:

> We believe that one reason for our success is our understanding very clearly what our customer wants. Now we have a mechanism for measuring that and, furthermore, to tell that we are improving. It has improved because of science that we are adding to the art of management that we've had before and some of these measurement systems that are out there that let us know that we are, in fact, on track with our efforts. We had no reliable, valid tool for measuring that before. We had some surveys that were of limited value in terms of validity. We had a difficult time in comparing ourselves to previous efforts to know that we were going in the right direction.

Like Henry Ford Health System, Walke-Parker uses a modified version of the Shewhart cycle. This approach is heavily dependent on process knowledge and data collection. It is used extensively both by cross-functional teams at WPMC and as a general management tool (e.g., to understand why some things take two months to initiate, and some take 14 months). Teams using such an approach start by developing a process map using data collected from numerous sources. A picture is "drawn" of the process through careful flowcharting of the steps from beginning to end. Figure 7.8 presents an excerpt from a flowchart developed by a clinical team

Figure 7.8

Flowchart for Repeat C-Section Process

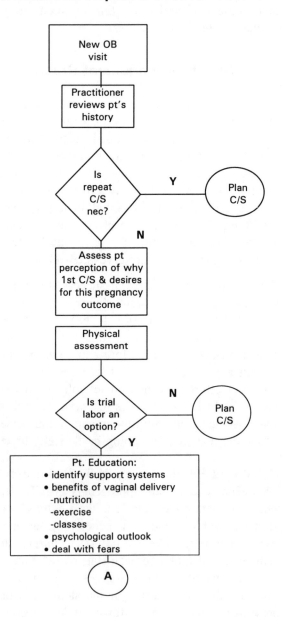

Continued

Figure 7.8   Continued

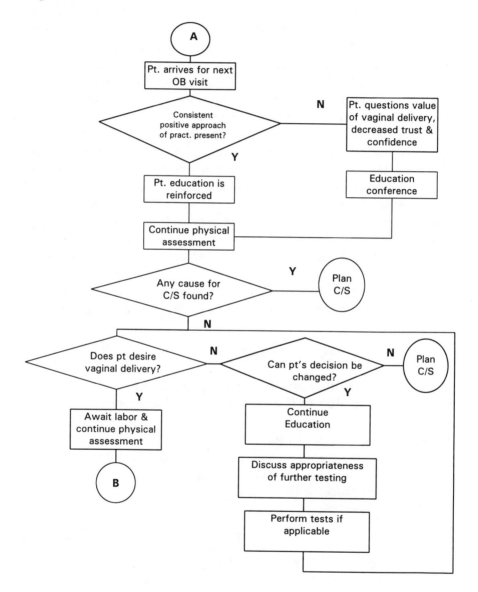

at Walke-Parker to describe the process that led to repeat cesarian sections. (Walke-Parker had earlier determined that C-sections were associated with decreased patient satisfaction with the birthing experience as well as potentially increased risk for patient mortality and morbidity.) This section of the process is of particular interest because the perceptions and desires of the patient regarding the procedure are addressed. A complete picture of the process would include the steps associated with labor, delivery, and follow-up.

After drawing the flowchart of the process, the team proposed a cause-and-effect diagram (Figure 7.9), identified the data necessary to answer their questions, and developed procedures to collect it. After the data on causes of repeat C-sections was collected, it was plotted (Figure 7.10) and discussed with the OB staff. The two most frequent causes were analyzed to understand the variation within them. Interventions were then developed and implemented for both of these, and data on C-section rate was again collected. Figure 7.11 shows the drop in C-sections from a 22 percent median rate in the 36 months before intervention to a 1989 median rate of 18 percent, a statistically significant change.

Measurement in the C-section case was handled manually, as is the majority of measurement. Even if Walke-Parker had a computer-based

Figure 7.9

Cause-and-Effect Diagram of the Decision to Perform a Repeat C-Section

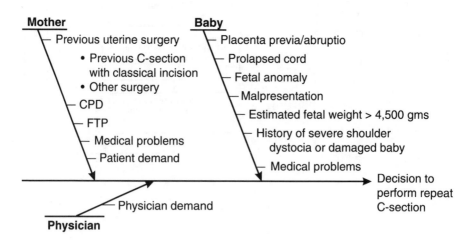

Figure 7.10

Causes of Repeat C-Sections

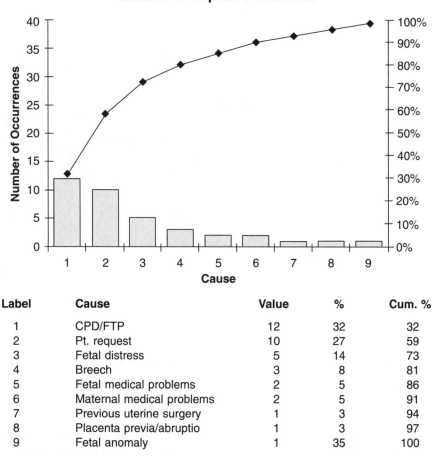

Label	Cause	Value	%	Cum. %
1	CPD/FTP	12	32	32
2	Pt. request	10	27	59
3	Fetal distress	5	14	73
4	Breech	3	8	81
5	Fetal medical problems	2	5	86
6	Maternal medical problems	2	5	91
7	Previous uterine surgery	1	3	94
8	Placenta previa/abruptio	1	3	97
9	Fetal anomaly	1	35	100

clinical information system, the indicators related to the C-section rate were not known until the process was analyzed, and so could not have been built into the system until after that step was completed. In general, this observation is true of the data elements needed by teams to research their specific areas of concern. Christiansen has reservations about further automation:

> People who spend that much creative energy trying to drive it in that direction will find themselves at process crossroads that will require

Figure 7.11

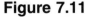

WPMC Cesarian Section Percentage by Month

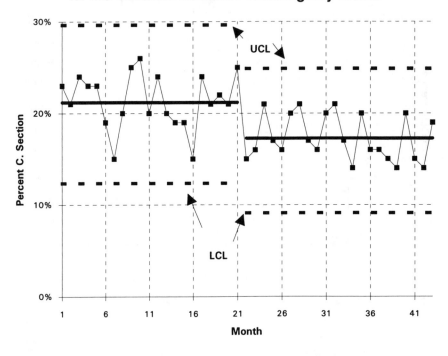

Notes: UCL = upper confidence level; LCL = lower confidence level.

them to change their information system unless it is so robust that it can handle any data point. And, I think that that kind of robustness is probably unaffordable." [On the other hand,] the ability of people to feel comfortable identifying and collecting data manually in painless ways is critical. And that is one of the barriers to departments enjoying process analysis. So we have to break through that barrier. How do we make data collection painless?

In fact, Christiansen notes that Walke-Parker has enough teams (probably 50–60) but that "our ability to break through the barriers to having people want to and enjoy working on process improvement continues to be our greatest struggle and challenge." He is currently in the midst of assessing the Walke-Parker culture, policies, procedures, and the organizational environment in general to determine what drivers are in place to create an environment where people are intrinsically motivated to work on improving their processes and what inhibitors and barriers exist.

The data needed for strategy deployment have been clearly identified and are collected on an ongoing basis. This part of the data system does not have as much complexity associated with it as that which meets departmental needs such as team data requirements. In general, measurements above the department level (including the satisfaction measures) are mostly automated.

According to Lorraine Smith (director, Quality Management), working together to figure out where data to answer questions exists and whether it is easy to retrieve has had the added benefit of improving communication between departments. At times it has proven easier to design prospective data collection systems than to try to retrieve data already in the system—and often the data is more accurate. When a local team is in charge of designing the collection instrument and determining how the data will be used, there is also less grumbling about collecting it. Even in this case, it is still important that the team representative for each group of staff involved in the collection communicate feedback and the importance of collection back to other members of the group.

The lack of an integrated computer-based information system is felt especially by the staff in Quality Management, and WPMC has hired a person for decision support. This person (Sue Carmina, Marketing Systems analyst) updates monthly an internal database that pulls key information from various systems.

The cross-checking and communication that occur now of necessity due to the nonlinking of various computer systems has shown that many times "identical" data does not match. For example, diagnostic codes assigned for reimbursement do not match those found on detailed chart review. This discrepancy reflects a general problem in the field; variation in coding occurs between coders and between facilities based on differing interpretations. Smith observes: "It's a bit scary, the only way most hospitals can have diagnosis and treatment data is via the coding—and the data is never any better than the coding. We have more systems for checking when data doesn't tell us what we expect than for consistently assessing data."

One example of quality management practice is explored further at the end of this chapter: the innovative application of Walke-Parker's philosophy of emphasizing and integrating customer focus, process focus, and measurement and improvement focus through intentional linkage of the overall hospital quality strategy with the long-range capital planning and allocation process.

Customer Awareness Development

Patient feedback regarding satisfaction and concerns about services is an important input into Walke-Parker's quality improvement plans. To gather feedback, they use a nationally available patient satisfaction survey. The survey questions have been carefully assessed for both reliability and validity, and care is taken to collect responses from an adequate number of patients. Figure 7.12 shows examples of survey items. Every third patient discharged is surveyed. Recently a similar "every third patient" survey was added for outpatient surgery. In addition, work is in progress on surveys for users of the emergency room and outpatient registration. Figure 7.13 shows results from the "brag about" Question 56.

Walke-Parker trends patient survey information for themselves; the corporate office gives feedback regarding how they stand relative to other System hospitals. Previous patient surveys have shown that care after discharge is a concern to patients. As part of exploring what the role of Walke-Parker Medical Center should be in this area, there are plans to more intensively explore patient satisfaction in certain categories of medical need (mental health, OB, diabetes, and oncology). It is likely that they will attempt to survey all patients in these categories upon discharge and add an "expected health status" survey three months postdischarge to determine the person's function (as related to what could be expected at that time) and their attitude.

Physicians appear to be satisfied with the hospital based on both survey results (see Figure 7.14) and from reports of other staff who work with them. The input from the "brag about" areas is used both to evaluate where the medical center stands today and to focus planning efforts related to physicians. The survey also has a great deal of specificity regarding identifying unmet needs and satisfaction with current services. Since the physician surveys are carried out at the quarterly medical staff meetings, there is some concern about the representativeness of the sample (some physicians may not attend the meetings and therefore, may never be surveyed); therefore, changes in this procedure for sampling are being considered.

The employee satisfaction survey has undergone recent modification. Attitudes and response rates had fallen off (see Figure 7.15); therefore, a

Figure 7.12

Patient Satisfaction Survey

Walke-Parker uses a survey developed and administered by its corporate office. It contains 68 questions on nine pages covering the following:

      Background on your hospital stay
      Admission: entering the hospital
      Your daily care in the hospital
      Keeping you informed
      Your nurses
      Your doctor
      Other hospital staff
      Living arrangements
      Discharge: leaving the hospital
      Billing by hospital
      Looking back on your care
      Overall satisfaction with hospital
      Your overall health status
      Recommendations and suggestions
      Facts about you

Most of the evaluative questions take the form of a declarative statement and an "agree-disagree" scale, such as the "brag about" questions:

The care I received at the hospital was so good that I have bragged about it to family and friends.	☐ Strongly Agree	☐ Somewhat Agree	☐ Somewhat Disagree	☐ Strongly Disagree

Source: Walke-Parker Medical Center.

QI team was formed and focus groups convened to discuss how to bring joy to work. Likes and dislikes about the survey were discussed. It became apparent that employees felt that the survey was too stiff and sterile, so some changes were made in wording and in some of the areas covered. Some consideration is now being given to weighting the various indicators to assist in setting priorities for changes.

Organization Quality Awareness Building

A number of quality awareness building elements have been mentioned earlier. The CEO and senior management actively participate on a ongoing

Figure 7.13

Patient Satisfaction Surveys, Walke-Parker: "Would you brag about your care to family and friends?"

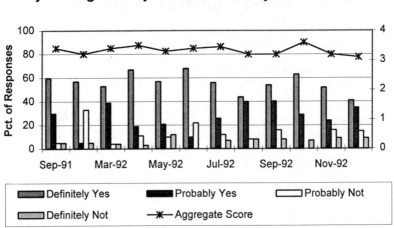

basis in quality orientation and training for employees, as well as in quality improvement team storyboard reviews. Numerous teams involving many employees have been in existence for several years. The storyboard reviews include specific references to a team's successes in their project and are viewed as part of the "celebration" reward of CQI. "Brag about" results are trended and posted in a number of places easily visible to employees, physicians, and the public using the facility. The "brag abouts" themselves are printed on a laminated card, with the facility mission statement and quality definition on the other side. These cards are shared with visitors to help them understand WPMC's QI policy. There is also a "QI Profile" in the employee newsletter and "High Q" employee recognition during national hospital week. "Caught Ya" cards are widely distributed throughout the hospital; patients, families, and co-workers are encouraged to complete these cards for individual acts of kindness and thoughtfulness. The best are recognized in the newsletter and with small awards.

Progress to Date and Future Direction

When asked if the quality improvement initiative had met his expectations to date, Arnold Jefferson replied that changing expectations are inherent in

Figure 7.14

Physician Satisfaction Surveys, Walke-Parker: "Would you use WPMC yourself if you needed care that it offers?"

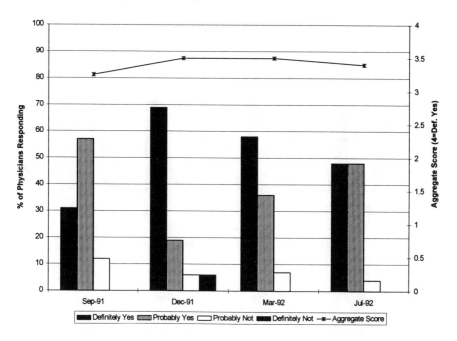

the QI philosophy and that of the expectations for last year, "some were met and some weren't. But that was last year and now I'm focused on next year. We will never get to the point where we say, 'Great! It's working. Our expectations are met. We don't have to worry about them.' "

It "delights" Jefferson that all department managers are tracking indicators (and doing so willingly). The framework for QI has been laid, and he feels it "probably exceeds most of our expectations." Several expectations haven't been met "with good reason." He explains:

> Much of the effort has been focused on laying the framework. We've got a number of initiatives now that will create innovations in the next three to six months. We're now set up to make those innovations more rapidly. Because we have these indicators on an ongoing basis, the work of the teams is a lot easier. For example, in food service, they have been measuring late trays for six months now. Now they've got a

Figure 7.15

Employee Satisfaction Surveys, Walke-Parker: "If you had to do it all over again, would you care to work for WPMC?"

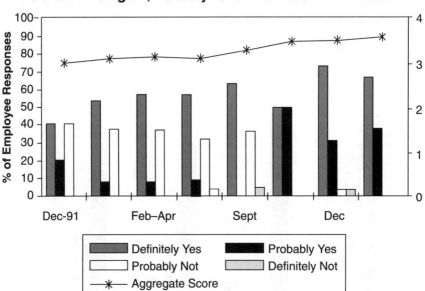

team. The data is already collected. All they have to do is examine the process, make improvements, and continue with the data collection."

In the clinical area, Jefferson feels:

A number of teams (for example, C-section, chest pain) have done great things. There are a number of areas that deserve and require the same attention. It's preliminary to ask here, because we've really just set expectations for the clinical area and they have to do with next year. It's a big part of where we are going. A key next step is to address the variation in clinical processes.

Christiansen observed that his expectations of what quality improvement can do for Walke-Parker have changed dramatically since 1987—that it has come to mean much more than some quality improvement tools such as Focus-PDCA.[3]

I believe that people have a sense of systemness and process. In a widespread way, I think that we have broken out of some paradigms that keep us from doing our best. I think people appreciate that quality is as much variation from the mean as it is the mean itself. I think the notion of empowerment is fairly widespread. I don't hold us out as an empowered workforce yet, so we haven't met my expectations in that regard, but I think that people in general know that without empowerment, we won't have achieved our desired end state.

Christiansen also comments on the role of CQI as a means to an end, and not the end itself:

I still believe it [CQI] is a tactic, a methodology to implement strategy. If you use a very sophisticated methodology to achieve the wrong things, you're going to fail. Given the right strategy, TQM accelerates achievement. . . . The fact that we decreased non-RN duties for RNs from 40 percent to 24 percent and that the operating room turnaround time has been reduced by 25 percent through the reduction of length of time in the holding area from 23 minutes to 16—these are only symptoms of what my expectations are. So, when I read the reports about all these teams that are working, I think people are getting trapped in the symptoms. We haven't pulled back to see the framework—the inner relationship to process. I didn't really appreciate that until a year or so ago.

Where is Walke-Parker headed with their quality initiative? Again Christiansen talks about a focus on process:

We will continue to move upstream in processes. We have pledged that our use of [quality improvement] tools to further measurements that exist in the quality data framework will just intensify. We're going now to more realization of the framework that was created in the last 18 months. The application of clinical process or health system process will become more widespread. It's almost building a more critical mass. I don't see the framework changing a lot.

To help illustrate his commitment to TQM, Christiansen shared a story. He had participated in a panel where a prominent health care leader was asked what he saw as future trends in health care. Christiansen remembers his response as, "For the first time in my 35-year career, I feel like I haven't the faintest idea." Christiansen's personal reaction was intensification of his resolve:

TQM is the only management strategy that I know of that can help you posture yourself to respond more rapidly to environmental events than your competitors. If you're in an environment that is increasingly unpredictable, then that intensified my resolve that I want to work in a place where we have this framework that if we need to change direction quickly, we're not driving a big cruise ship; we're driving a PT boat. All we have to do is say, "Look folks, we've got to go this way." And, two days later, we're organized to do that. People are physically at work. Whereas, an organization without TQM, you're talking about three months just to get your heads together—"OK, we've got to do this. What are we going to do next?"

Special Focus: Building a New Capital Budgeting System

The vision of Walke-Parker Medical Center to become "the best-value Southern City health system by 1996" requires a long-range capital planning and allocation process that emphasizes and increases the value perceived by customer groups (see Figure 7.16).

WPMC's measurement system pyramid (Figure 7.7) establishes a link between customer satisfaction measures and process measures, assisting strategic resource allocation decision making. For example, if the goal is to increase physician satisfaction, the hospital knows that it needs to improve

---

Figure 7.16

Statement of Purpose, Long-Range Capital Planning, Walke-Parker Medical Center

As part of the Hospital's overall quality strategy, a long-range capital planning process that emphasizes and increases value as perceived by our various customer groups is essential. The purpose of a long-range capital plan is to program, plan, and coordinate the allocation of limited capital resources in a way that supports the strategy goals of the hospital. The inputs to the process of long-range capital planning are many and varied, but will emphasize customer judgments and expectations of our existing capital equipment and facility as measured by quality indicators. Additional inputs will be provided by department managers, space planning, risk management, regulatory agencies, technology evolution and evaluation study, biomedical services, and conventional wisdom.

one of the hospitalwide indicators that relate to physicians (e.g., test reports are timely). As Black points out, the next step is to understand what processes influence a physician's perception of timely reports. Understanding and knowledge of the customer and the process involved will give a priority for investment.

Black also reminds us of the importance of employee education and training here:

> If all employees are not educated to our purpose and goals, it will be difficult to get clean data to support the capital allocation process. If employees are not customer minded, the capital requests may not be directed at increasing customer satisfaction. A group of customer-driven and intrinsically motivated people is the engine for innovation in seeking the "best bang for the buck" in an environment of competing demands for limited capital funds.

By late 1992, proposed capital investments at Walke-Parker were accepted or denied based on three criteria: net present value, customer feedback, and survival. The previous system had emphasized net present value but was not very good at predicting which investment created value for their customers. The WPMC leaders came to believe that maximizing ability to produce customer value with limited resources was the key to survival. Therefore, questions that prompt thinking about customers and value are at the heart of the capital allocation process. Figure 7.17 shows the annual capital budgeting process, beginning with a restatement of the vision. The initial steps tie the proposals explicitly to the QI measures rather than strictly financial criteria.

To the careful reader, Figure 7.17 suggests several important concepts:

1. Capital requests should probably be tied to one of the six sources at the top of the page.

2. Any capital request needs a champion who has mastered the request and its implications. This mastery is more than just filling out the request form. It is intimate knowledge of the process in question and its linkage to hospitalwide QI measures" (as seen in Figure 7.18).

3. Any request must meet one of four value criteria. These are clearly ranked in importance:

   a. "Increase quality while maintaining competitive cost."

   b. "Lower cost without adversely affecting quality."

Figure 7.17   Annual Capital Budgeting Process at Walke-Parker Medical Center

Goal: To distribute capital in a way that supports the hospital's goal of being the best-value health care system by 1996 and to be recognized as such.

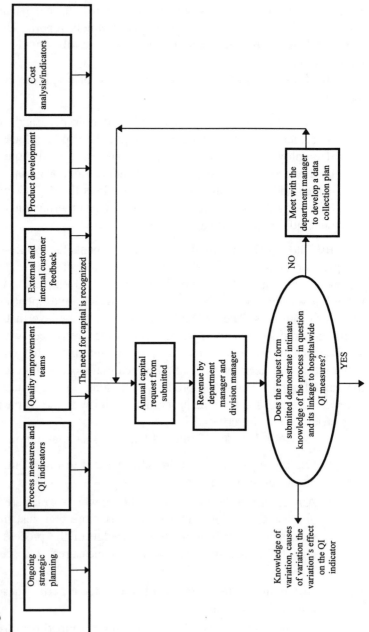

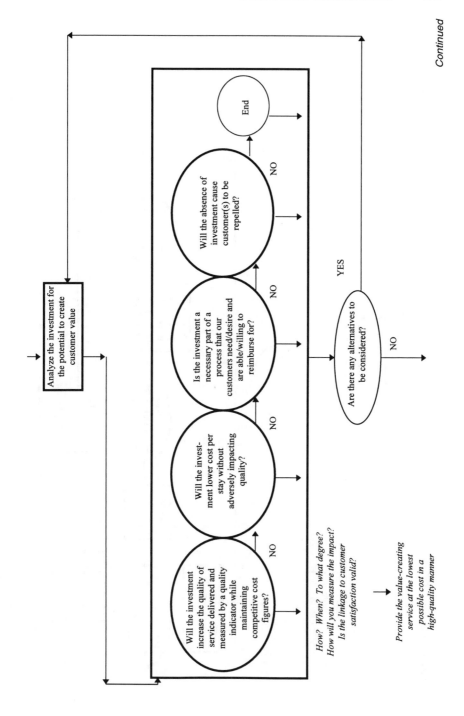

Continued

Figure 7.17 Continued

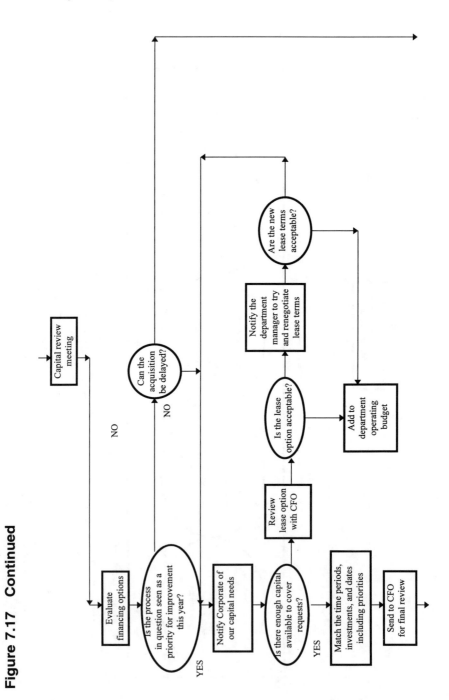

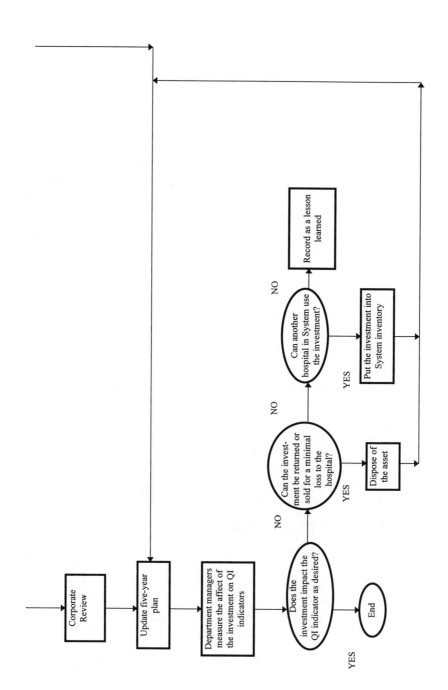

c. "Be a process customers need and are willing to reimburse for."

d. "Absence of investment causes customers to be repelled."

These four criteria match the textbook requirements, generally summarized as marketing, productivity, finance, and competition.

4. The project will be subject to competitive review at the capital review meeting. (Note that requests are submitted annually rather than when arising. The annual submission is essential to get competitive review.)

The request form itself functions as an educational tool and as an investment evaluation tool. Department directors completing the form are led to consider the fundamentals of Walke-Parker's CQI philosophy. For example, the request form (Figure 7.18) asks for a description of how the investment will add value in the form of process improvement or increased customer satisfaction and requires a flowchart of the process of which this investment will be a part.

Black concludes with a final step—the assignment of a staff member to compare the results of the investment with the hypothesis for the investment in order to make this process a learning opportunity for the organization: Did the investment actually have the intended effect? If not, what can we learn that will enable us to make better, more informed decisions in the future that will maximize value?

Notes

1. See the items listed in the Suggested Readings.
2. Senge, P. 1990. *The Fifth Discipline: The Art and Practice of the Learning Organization.* New York: Doubleday/Currency.
3. See *Quality Management in Health Care*, an Aspen quarterly publication that includes a tutorial section on tools for use in TQM/CQI in each issue.

References and Suggested Readings

American Hospital Association. 1991, 1992. *AHA Guide to the Health Care Field.* Chicago: AHA.

American Medical Association. 1992. *Physician Characteristics and Distribution in the United States.* Chicago: AMA.

Boyer, R., and D. Savageau. 1989. *Places Rated Almanac.* New York: Prentice-Hall.

Conroy, T. F., ed. 1992. *Markets of the U.S. for Business Planners*, Vol. 1. Detroit, MI: Omnigraphics, Inc.

Homer, E. R., ed. 1993. *Almanac of the States.* Palo Alto, CA: Information Publications.

The Universal Health Care Almanac. 1991. Phoenix, AZ: Silver and Cherner, Ltd.

Figure 7.18

Department Capital Request Form, Walke-Parker Medical Center

Expenditure name: _____ Date form completed: _____

Department:_____ Department number: _____

Requested by: _____ Total estimated cost

Vendor name: _____ (form pro forma):_____

Equipment category: _____ Is this a replacement? YES/NO

Is on the facility master plan? YES/NO

Equipment or expenditure description (include make, model, specifications, preferences, supplier, cost, labor ,etc.)

_____

_____

_____

For which customer(s) on your department does this investment create value (suppliers, physicians, employees, payers, outside auditors, and/or patients)?

_____

_____

_____

What data have you collected or will collect which will support the assertion that this investment is needed to improve customer satisfaction and/or a departmental quality indicator (for example, negative trends in rework, accuracy, downtime, increased costs, increased process variation, employee or customer feedback, etc.)?

_____

_____

_____

Please describe how this investment will add value in the form of process improvement or increased customer satisfaction. Attach a flowchart of the process of which this investment will be a part.

_____

_____

Please briefly list any alternative solutions considered for this problem and the reason(s) for discounting the option(s).

_____

_____

How will you measure the impact of the investment on customer satisfaction or process improvement (for example: cycle time, customer brag abouts, downtime, accuracy, etc.)?

_____

_____

_____

Is this investment an attempt to improve a departmental quality indicator? If so, which indicator(s)?

_____

_____

Economic cash flow information: Please provide a pro forma financial statement for both purchase and lease options (if applicable). To aid you in the development of pro formas, a step-by-step guide is included. Please briefly summarize the results below.

_____

_____

_____

_____

Submitted by:_____ Reviewed by: _____

8

Henry Ford Health System Case Study

The Henry Ford Health System (HFHS) is a vertically integrated regional health system (see Figure 8.1). Located in southeastern Michigan, it encompasses over 60 health care delivery sites in five southeastern Michigan counties within a 30-mile radius of the corporate offices in downtown Detroit. It includes Henry Ford Hospital (a 903-bed tertiary care hospital, education, and research facility in Detroit's New Center area), two acute care community hospitals in suburban areas east and southwest of Detroit (175-bed Cottage Hospital and 359-bed Wyandotte Hospital and Medical Center), Kingswood Hospital (a 100-bed psychiatric facility), and Maplegrove (a 50-bed inpatient/outpatient chemical dependency center). HFHS also participates in a joint venture with Mercy Health Services to manage four other hospitals in southeastern Michigan. The Henry Ford Medical Group (HFMG), with 850 physicians, is one of the country's largest group practices. Metro Medical Group (MMG), with 140 physicians, is also part of HFHS; both provide most of the care delivered by HFHS but are extensively complemented by community-based private practice medical staffs. Health Alliance Plan (HAP), a wholly owned mixed-model health maintenance organization with 450,000 members, is Michigan's largest managed care plan. HFHS currently has 9.6 percent of the southeastern Michigan inpatient health care market and 14.8 percent of the ambulatory care market. Figure 8.2 shows key trends for HFHS for 1971–1991.

Figure 8.1

HFHS Vertically Integrated Regional Health Care

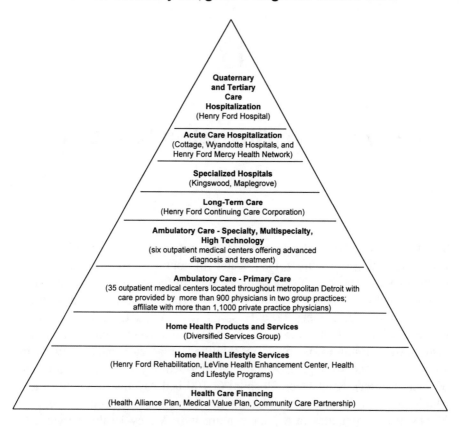

Quaternary and Tertiary Care Hospitalization
(Henry Ford Hospital)

Acute Care Hospitalization
(Cottage, Wyandotte Hospitals, and Henry Ford Mercy Health Network)

Specialized Hospitals
(Kingswood, Maplegrove)

Long-Term Care
(Henry Ford Continuing Care Corporation)

Ambulatory Care - Specialty, Multispecialty, High Technology
(six outpatient medical centers offering advanced diagnosis and treatment)

Ambulatory Care - Primary Care
(35 outpatient medical centers located throughout metropolitan Detroit with care provided by more than 900 physicians in two group practices; affiliate with more than 1,1000 private practice physicians)

Home Health Products and Services
(Diversified Services Group)

Home Health Lifestyle Services
(Henry Ford Rehabilitation, LeVine Health Enhancement Center, Health and Lifestyle Programs)

Health Care Financing
(Health Alliance Plan, Medical Value Plan, Community Care Partnership)

Organization Structure and Leadership

HFHS is governed by a board composed of prominent Detroit citizens, including several members of the Ford family. Three members of the medical group and one attending physician are also on the board. HFHS is managed through 11 operating divisions, each with a board of directors including leaders of their local communities and representatives of their medical staffs. Over 200 individuals are involved in governance. The HFHS CEO reports to the system board; all subsidiary organizations report through him.

Within the HFHS structure, HFMG has its own executive who reports to the system CEO. The physicians in HFMG elect a medical group board

Figure 8.2

HFHS Key Trends, 1971–1991

	1971	1980	1985	1990	1991
Ambulatory care	712,000	924,000	1,486,966	2,381,503	2,434,719
Ambulatory sites	1	6	14	32	35
Admissions	28,687	33,482	34,264	53,519	52,312*
Hospitals	1	1	4	4	4†
HMO enrollment	0	86,173	179,048	399,960	395,765‡
Salaried physicians (FTE)	210	N/A	400	990	903§
Employees (FTE)	3,500	N/A	6,181	13,373	13,622
External research grants (millions)	—	$3.7	$4.8	$14.3	$15.8
Net operating revenue (millions)	$65	$224.3	$497.0	$990.3	$1,210.0
Net margin (millions)	N/A	$4.5	$28.1	$67.3	$36.1

Notes: N/A = data not available.

* HFHS physicians have over 6,000 admissions annually in six other hospitals not owned by HFHS.

† In addition to the four wholly owned hospitals, HFHS jointly owns two hospitals in Macomb County with Mercy Health Services.

‡ HFHS also owns an HMO in Toledo, Ohio, with current enrollment of 40,000 members. This HMO was consolidated into HFHS HMO Health Alliance Plan in 1992.

§ In addition to full-time salaried medical staff, HFHS hospitals have approximately 1,000 community-based private practice physicians.

of governors, which meets every two months to address strategic and policy issues. It consists of 26 members, including the chairs of the Medicine and Surgery Departments, the vice president of Academic Affairs, and HFHS's COO on an ex officio basis. The board of governors appoints an Operations Committee, which meets monthly and is responsible for capital allocation, budgeting, and staffing for the medical group. It includes the chairs from the Medicine and Surgery Departments, the COO of the HFMG, the medical group chief administrative officer, the senior vice president of Medical Affairs, the vice president of Academic Affairs, the chair of the board of governors, two regional medical directors (from the ambulatory care centers), and the chairs of the four section committees (Medicine, Surgery, Hospital-Based Specialties, and Suburban Medical Centers).

The mission and vision statements are presented in Figure 8.3. The current statements evolved out of Board discussions early in the quality improvement process and were approved in 1990. They were given special emphasis in the most recent ten-year plan and are published both in the annual system report and in a small, easy-to-carry informational brochure, along with the statement of corporate values and quality guidelines. Gail Warden, CEO, stresses that the "vision and mission are incorporated into everything we do."

Unique Factors

Henry Ford was one of a group of prominent Detroit businessmen who initiated the development of a hospital in 1912. In 1914, when the project stalled, he stepped in, paid off the other donors, and took over its development. From then until 1987, the chair of Henry Ford Hospital's board was always a member of the Ford family. The salaried group practice instituted by Ford was modeled after the Mayo Clinic and continues as the Henry Ford Medical Group.

During the 1950s, Michigan auto companies spread enormous wealth among state workers and businesses. By 1960, the state had one of the world's highest per capita income levels. By 1980, the bottom seemed to have dropped out of its economy, as the serious national recession was aggravated by fierce international competition in the auto industry. Michigan led the United States in unemployment through the early 1980s and, in the late 1980s, remained among the states with the higher rates. The metropolitan Detroit area remains economically troubled because of automobile plant closings. On the positive side, private nonmanufacturing businesses are gaining modestly, and Detroit is a doorway to international trade with Canada. The southeast region remains the mainstay of the Michigan economy, employing 50 percent of the state total labor force.

Since the 1970 census, Wayne County (including the city of Detroit) has lost 20 percent of its population. This decline is projected to continue. The surrounding counties, on the other hand, have increased in population. In 1989, the area overall had relatively high hospital admission rates (128 per thousand, versus the state average of 119 and national average of 126) The number of community hospital beds per 1,000 was almost the same

Figure 8.3

HFHS Mission and Vision Statements (1990)

Mission

Henry Ford Health System is dedicated to developing and providing the highest quality, compassionate health care to serve the needs of the Southeastern Michigan community. The System's services will be the most comprehensive, efficient, and clinically effective in the region, supported by nationally recognized Henry Ford education and research programs.

Vision

Henry Ford Health System will:

- Evolve into the highest quality, most comprehensive and integrated health system in the region.

- Develop a Center for Health Sciences which will be engaged in leading edge tertiary care, research, and teaching.

- Provide virtually all of the health care needs of the population served, from primary care to highly specialized tertiary care.

- Offer a range of health insurance and managed care programs that meet the diverse needs of the population and payers.

- Think of itself as an entity to which the users of its services belong. Administrative systems will emphasize the ease and convenience of use by the members.

- Be a responsible member of the community and assume leadership in developing sound health care policies at the local, state, and national level.

as the national average (3.7 versus 3.8). The number of physicians per 100,000, however, is 11 percent higher than the national average (219 versus 198). In both cases, there is great variability between beds and providers and population base through the area, leaving the impression that location of medical care services is not well matched to current population locations. There are three other health care systems generally considered competitive with HFHS. The Detroit Medical Center, with the Wayne State

Medical School, serves the central and northern areas. The University of Michigan Medical Center is in the western suburbs, and William Beaumont Hospitals are in the northeast suburbs. Three other health systems also serve the area: Mercy Health System, St. John Health System, and Oakwood Health System.

Henry Ford Hospital's board made a commitment to remain in Detroit in the late 1960s when a large proportion of Detroit's more economically well-off population was streaming to the suburbs. Today, the Henry Ford Hospital and Ambulatory Care Building in downtown Detroit employs 4,000 people, 27 percent of all HFHS employees. The leadership at Henry Ford anticipated the direction in which health care services would move and, starting in the mid-1970s, added satellite clinics to offer primary, specialty, outpatient surgery, and emergency services in the suburban areas. Beginning in the 1980s, HFHS acquired three hospitals and developed joint ventures with several more. As a result, it is positioned to provide coverage to the three main counties of the metro area.

The average operating margin for all Michigan hospitals in 1988 was 0.9 percent. Average occupancy was 66 percent. Payment sources are increasingly restricted. In fiscal year 1985, Michigan Medicaid implemented DRG-based payment for inpatient care; in FY 1988 this was extended to certain outpatient procedures. Blue Cross and Blue Shield of Michigan began DRG payment with limited annual increases in 1988. It is the state's largest health insurer and has about two-thirds the private insurance market in southeast Michigan. Managed care programs have become popular with employers and insurers, and now serve about 25 percent of the metro population. There is a large uninsured population. In addition, Michigan medical liability costs are among the highest in the nation. Detroit area hospitals pay the highest liability rates in the country—five times the national average.

Initiating the Quality Vision

The specific focus on quality improvement at HFHS started in 1988. When Gail Warden arrived he brought with him an interest in quality management programs. He saw "quality improvement" as a way of introducing a common culture and developing a sense of system throughout the diverse set of relatively independently functioning operating entities. A quality focus could also serve as the driver for the strategic change that was going to be necessary.

Warden formed a task force in October 1989 under the leadership of the corporate vice president of Planning and Marketing, Vinod Sahney, to study and recommend how to initiate a quality program within the Henry Ford system. Three months were spent reading and discussing the concepts of Deming, Juran, and Crosby. Visits were made to companies that had instituted quality programs, including 3M, Ford, Chrysler, Rush Presbyterian St. Luke's Hospital in Chicago, Harvard Community Health Plan, and HCA. Advice was sought from other companies and consultants Donald Berwick, M.D., then of Harvard Community Health Plan, and Paul Batalden, M.D., of HCA.

The task force then prepared a document outlining the key concepts of TQM and keys for successful implementation. Their findings were presented to Warden and then to senior management. Warden was committed to implementing TQM, but there were a number among the senior management staff who raised questions: Could Henry Ford afford a new initiative? Was a quality initiative necessary? Should they wait three months until senior management had completed the budget planning cycle and could give the issue greater attention? Those that found the time to read the material that was circulated however became more and more convinced that they should go forward. Some of the reasons underlying the decision to proceed were the following:

- To develop a quality culture throughout HFHS with a focus on continuous quality improvement
- To improve service to HFHS patients
- To increase value for HFHS customers
- To improve productivity and control increases in the cost of health care
- To improve the work environment in order to maintain and attract a qualified workforce
- To improve organizational understanding of practice pattern variations
- To use benchmarking to compare performance and learn from the best practices

A request for proposal was developed and sent to 15 consulting organizations. Twelve detailed vendor proposals were submitted and reviewed using criteria specifically developed for this purpose:

1. Depth/breadth of experience with quality improvement engagements and specific improvement experience in health care, including inpatient and outpatient service and clinical components
2. Willingness and ability to modify approach for health care, particularly training materials
3. Improvement process structure and plan consistent with HFHS requirements
4. Type and degree of support provided in addition to basic implementation plan:
   • Willingness to assist HFHS in education program development
   • Willingness to provide service on-site
5. Professional level of consultant resources proposed:
   • Style, experience, sophistication, and credibility of proposed project team
   • Intensity of resource to be provided (i.e., consultant time and skill mix)
6. Pricing
7. Established, proven history
8. Exclusions and restrictions.

Paul Batalden and his Quality Resource Group at HCA were selected as the external consultant to guide the TQM process in its early stages. Batalden's background as a physician, the depth of his understanding of TQM, and his past experience in group practice and in implementing quality management in hospitals were all important factors in his selection, as was his underlying interest in changing the health care industry through TQM.

In order to clearly convey that the quality initiative was a process and not a program, it was named "Henry Ford Quality Management Process." The objective was stated:

> To develop and implement a total quality management process that can be followed throughout the organization to improve the quality of health care services provided to our customers. The goal of the process is to retain market leadership in health care delivery through quality.

Translating the Vision into Organizational Reality

Both Warden and Sahney recognized the importance of building ownership of the process across the system—quality management could not be viewed as a corporate-level or individual-driven process. For Warden, this belief was an outgrowth of his view that his role is to focus "on the vision for the future and getting us ready for the strategic aspects of things" and to let "my operating people manage the place." Sahney's criterion for success of the quality management process was "each one of the chief operating officers feeling that they are driving the process."

The principle of operating level responsibility has guided the implementation process. The initiative has been rolled out by levels across the system, rather than by divisions, in order to raise everyone's consciousness level and to anchor the process at each level before moving it a step lower in the organization. This Quality Management Process rollout includes five steps:

1. Quality management awareness and learning
2. Quality management framework development
3. Quality management practice
4. Customer awareness development
5. Organization quality awareness building.[1]

Step 1: Quality Management Awareness and Learning

Early on, two staff were hired to support the quality management efforts, but their role was (and is) to support learning and communication throughout the system, not to actually implement the process. As Patricia Stoltz, director of the Department of Health Care Quality Improvement Education and Research, notes, a large department staff is not a goal since the department expects to complement the resources in each of the line operating units within HFHS. In fact, keeping the unit small is seen as "key to the assumption of full responsibility for change within each of the operating units, including the offices of the top leadership of the HFHS."

Also early on, a Quality Technology Council (QTC) was formed to provide guidance to the staff resource group. This council included two representatives from each operating entity and staff group across the system. This diverse group included physicians, nurses, COOs, and human resource people. For the first three years, members of the QTC met every two weeks for two hours. They brought in speakers, discussed journal articles, shared information from conferences, and generally promoted cross-learning on quality management at a system level. Members of this group became the champions of the quality management process to the rest of the system.

Senior management formed a corporate-level Quality Steering Committee (QSC). In addition, each operating level unit formed its own QSC. The job of each committee is to guide the implementation of the quality management process within its operating group. Each unit also identified a coach (a member of the QTC) to act as an internal resource to itself.

Step 2: Quality Management Framework Development

In keeping with the principle of operating unit responsibility, each entity was charged with developing its own quality framework, including statements of mission, vision, quality definition, and quality guidelines.

At the system level, senior management and the board of trustees spent nine months finalizing the system quality framework. While senior management developed quality guidelines, the board formulated a ten-year strategic plan. The guidelines and strategy plan interacted synergistically, ultimately leading to revision of the mission and vision statements and inclusion of the quality guidelines "right up front" in the ten-year plan.

The operating units have proceeded at different rates on framework development. The medical group, which manages numerous ambulatory care locations, has had particular difficulty. While some regions within the medical group have developed their own vision statements, the overall group has not yet. There continue to be some concerns (especially among the physicians) as to how well the system vision and the aims of the medical group fit together.

Cottage Hospital and Henry Ford Hospital found they first needed to understand their individual operating units as systems. This understanding was then used to critique their vision statements and to set priorities for quality improvement. Gregory Vasse, president of Cottage Hospital, describes the first two to two and a half years as a rather long period of disjointed activity while people tried to figure out how to implement the process. The foundation of education and training had been laid, but by design, actual implementation at each site was up to the people there. It was not until the division managers found a way to focus their priorities that the process began to feel structured and less frustrating. Cottage Hospital's CQI history is presented in detail at the end of this chapter.

Using a system focus, Cottage Hospital's Quality Steering Committee critiqued their vision statement and developed five themes around which to build their quality improvement process. Individual departments were also encouraged to look at themselves as systems and to develop a vision for themselves. Vasse acknowledges the importance of support from the corporate level, including the consultant's assistance in helping them link an understanding of their hospital as a system to their strategic planning process: "The system umbrella gave us the building blocks—the philosophy, the intellectual understanding to get through the process." He also notes, however, that the decision to examine Cottage's core process and to understand the operation of the hospital as a system and, from there, to link to HFHS's strategic plan was "an independent decision out here."

Henry Ford Hospital (HFH) used a broad spectrum of its management to develop their quality management framework. Its leaders attacked it on their own using some of the tools that they had learned from the education and training sessions (e.g., brainstorming, multivoting) to identify the key issues they wanted to get across for each element of the framework. The members of its Quality Management Steering Committee were then asked to put more meat on the bare framework bones. The framework was taken to the rest of the management staff (over 250 people) for input. The input was collected, patterns noted, and final modifications made.

Initially, the road map for implementing the quality framework at HFH, the annual goals and objectives for the Hospital, and the rolling three-year strategic objectives for HFHS involved three separate planning processes. The planning process for 1992 combined the quality objectives and the hospital objectives into leadership strategies. As noted by HFH's group vice president, Stephen Velick, an outcome of this integration was the realization that "this is now part of how we function. This is our daily work. We have integrated it [quality improvement] into how we think." The planning process for 1993 integrated the three-year strategic planning process with the leadership strategies planning process. Where there were three, now there is one.

At both Cottage and HFH, a locally developed framework for managing quality has been integrated with the operating entity's strategic planning process. At both hospitals, a good deal of pride exists in both the "solution" and in the process carried out locally to get to it. And, both cases are considered successes by the system overall.

Step 3: Quality Management Practice

During the first year of implementation, 350 senior managers and physicians were trained in basic quality management concepts and methods. Quality steering committees with coaches were formed in each operating group.

Each operating group also developed a preliminary rollout plan for 1991. During the next two years, more than 1,300 additional HFHS members (top leadership to midlevel employees) completed the internal six-day basic workshop. On top of this, certain units such as Henry Ford Medical Group (HFMG) offered their own one-day courses for employees to accelerate exposure to some of the principles of quality. They put concepts into practice. Persons who worked within the system prior to 1989, in particular, have noted the increase in meeting skills (e.g., agendas, time keeping, stated objectives). Meetings are much more efficient. People are much more aware of work as a process and of its customer-driven nature.

David Griffenhagen, a HFMG administrator (and a member of the initial Quality Technology Council), pointed out the importance of tailoring the implementation of concepts to the specific group rather than rigidly following a recipe. For example, empowerment is a critical principle in quality management. When working with physicians (who are traditionally empowered), the issue becomes more how to harness the energy to use it positively and avoid putting up barriers, than how to engender it in the first place. As Griffenhagen noted: "If a physician wants to do something, he or she is going to do it. Chartering a team doesn't matter." Therefore, HFMG as an operating unit never felt it important to charter teams. This responsibility has been left to the work groups—for example, the medical departments at HFH and the various medical centers.

Understanding the role of information and being comfortable with statistical thinking are two critical components of a quality improvement process. Having accessible, relevant information is key to understanding processes and to designing and assessing changes. Statements from various operating units and working groups reflect the importance of measurement as a guiding principle to the implementation of the quality improvement process throughout HFHS (see Figure 8.4). These statements from various components of HFHS show a clear awareness of the need for information beyond the traditional data of operating margins, length of stay, and occupancy ratios. As HFHS moves further into quality improvement, the role of statistical thinking and the collection of information specific to quality-related questions is increasing. However, to quote Vasse of Cottage Hospital, "We will probably be a disappointment in terms of being able to show you a highly evolved data management system that is responsive to quality improvement efforts." Most data collection that is supportive of QI activities is manual. Structural measures and deficiency detection continue to dominate the information collected on a routine basis by the data management system (e.g., Is there an active ethics committee? Did the consultation happen within 24 hours? Do surgical wound infection rates exceed CDC-recommended limits?). This limitation results from the momentum from the past, which emphasizes QA requirements of regulatory and licensing agencies. The leaders of Cottage Hospital want to focus more on clinical outcomes and patient satisfaction and are taking steps to move in this direction. However, the data system is pretty much preoccupied by the prescriptive requirements of regulatory agencies.

The leaders of HFH realized that they had no mechanism for determining which of their currently collected databases were most important to the hospital as a team. They used nominal group and brainstorming techniques to put together a list of 16 administrative and clinical activity indicators:

Figure 8.4

Comparative Perspectives: Information and Quality Management

HFHS: All work units within the System are committed to using customer and process knowledge as an input to identify key quality indicators.

All work units will develop quality reports using the key quality indicators to monitor progress and to identify areas for improvement.

The System is committed to the process of competitive benchmarking as a means of improving its services.

Cottage Hospital: Cottage Hospital is committed to using customer and process knowledge to identify key quality indicators. Cottage Hospital will use competitive benchmarking as one means of improving its services. All services at Cottage Hospital are responsible for the monitoring of specific key quality indicators and identifying areas for improvement.

HFH: We will use customer feedback, data, and statistical methods to guide our decision making and to improve our processes. We seek to continuously improve our processes through reduction in variation.

General Internal Medicine: Decisions to charter QI teams and to provide resources (money, equipment, FTEs) will be data driven, based on cost effectiveness and will be part of the strategic goal for General Internal Medicine as a whole.

---

1. Patient days (actual and budget)
2. Admissions (actual and budget)
3. Outpatient clinic visits by region
4. Infection control surveillance reports
5. Hours "closed" in ER by category
6. ER patient registration by category
7. ER patient registration by shift
8. FTEs (actual and budget)
9. Inpatient pharmaceutical costs
10. Discharge delay days
11. Operative cases
12. Overnight patients in recovery room
13. Ten most common DRGs
14. OB deliveries
15. Employee injuries
16. Monthly inpatient falls.

These are now trended so that they can see where things are going. The next step, currently under way, is to develop criteria to determine when some action should be taken to improve the situation.

The medical group reports some movement toward clinical indicators in addition to the current standard (regulatory requirement based) outcomes data. Through its Center for Clinical Effectiveness, it is in the early stages of developing an outcomes studies group and is an active participant in an effort by the American Group Practice Association. On a team level, the group has done many projects including access improvement, total hip replacement, and chemotherapy. During the course of these efforts, they learned how difficult it could be when there is no ongoing system to automatically pick the information up as a quality monitor. As Mark Young, M.D. (associate chair, Department of Medicine, HFMG), notes, "We had to jury-rig all types of things, convince people that they could start measuring this as part of their job." They also learned the importance of being clear about what people can stop measuring and what human resources can be redirected toward clinical indicators that are meaningful. "If measurement is all seen as an add-on, it creates big time problems as far as having it routinely collected."

As part of an effort to instill an overall managed care focus, Health Alliance Plan is working to standardize data collection within all system providers. Much of HAP's efforts go into assessment of customer satisfaction and needs. To this end, it collects medical process data (e.g., immunization rates within the population served, compliance with mammography recommendations, C-section rates, transfer rates of members among physicians). The caregiving units (e.g., HFH, HFMG, Cottage), however, have tended to look at HAP as a financing and insurance entity and in the past have been reluctant to share data on clinical outcomes.

Step 4: Customer Awareness Development

The quality management initiative has increased the voiced sensitivity of operating units toward both internal and external customers. The units have been allowed to frame their own detailed statements, resulting in minor variations across the system (see Figure 8.5).

Figure 8.5

Comparative Perspectives:
Customer and Quality Improvement

HFHS: Quality patient care and service is a key principle for HFHS. HFHS is committed to continuously improving the quality of services to its internal and external customers, and to giving priority attention to their concerns.

Communication with customers is key to better understanding their needs and expectations, continuously improving processes, and building their trust.

HFH: We strive to continuously improve the quality and value of services to all our internal and external customers, dedicating ourselves to excellence in all that we do.

Cottage Hospital: Cottage Hospital is committed to continuously improving the quality of service to our customers including patients, medical staff, employees and all others with whom we work in following our mission. Customers are listened to and responded to in an efficient and individualized manner. Communication with all of our customers is key to better understanding their needs and expectations, continuously improving processes and building trust.

General Internal Medicine: The quality of the services we provide will be measured by how well we meet the needs of our customers, internal and external.

After being exposed to TQM ideas, Cottage used the concept of developing customer knowledge to assist in planning its Obstetrics Department. The resulting single-room mother-baby maternity care with cross-trained staff working 12-hour shifts was specifically designed to meet the customers' stated desire to interact with fewer staff and to receive more patient education.

Currently Cottage mails a questionnaire to all patients two weeks after their discharge to learn their satisfaction with their experience. It now has a stable set of indicators and 13 quarters of trended data. This data is increasingly used in decision making and in focusing the hospital's initiatives. One of its priorities is to get patient feedback on the "post healing" process. What happens to a patient after discharge is an area that Cottage feels it could improve on. One initiative for improvement in 1993 concerns following up with patients after discharge, that is 100 percent callback on ambulatory surgery patients, monitoring and support of breast-feeding mothers for up to six months after discharge to continuously improve successes here, and selected callback criteria for nursing units and the emergency room.

HFH is making a special effort to learn about the satisfaction levels of three of its customer groups—patients, physicians, and nonphysician employees. A patient feedback system designed to capture complaints and compliments is now being converted to electronic mail. Hospital staff enter the data and message other departments if their action is required. They have been pleased to discover that one-third of the responses have been compliments and are now working on ways to get this positive feedback back to the nursing assistant, doctor, nurse, or whomever should receive it. They expect to be able to identify patterns that indicate where processes should be changed or where QI teams should be directed.

Employees are also important customers, and one of HFH's leadership strategies for 1992 was to carry out a hospitalwide survey of employee satisfaction. The results were shared with employees, together with the plans to be taken to address identified issues.

The physician satisfaction survey in 1992 confirmed that physician satisfaction has fallen significantly during the last five years. Young described the situation as follows:

> Five years ago was at the peak of our growth, where we were continuously adding more doctors, building new buildings. [There was] a sense that this was a terrific place to be. Three years ago was when we

first started to deal with the organizational issues related to growth. It's no longer a couple of hundred doctors who all know each other. Today we're dealing with the overall health care environment in terms of all the host of issues that we're facing . . . [At the same time,] there hasn't been a sense of really having to meet the needs of [physician] customers. . . . The hospital sort of has their doctors sewn up. . . . At the same token, we take the hospital for granted. . . . Maybe we'd be incredibly worse off if we hadn't made the commitment to quality. . . . We have paid some price in that the system as a whole has gotten a lot of ink and good press on what we are doing. The doctors say, "Two years in, the CEO writes an article and people think we're famous. What difference has that made in my everyday life?' "

The discontent is being addressed directly by the HFH COO, Steve Velick. He has gone to the major clinical chairs and asked, "How can we meet your needs?" It is also being addressed by the leadership of the medical group through meeting with small groups of physicians to ask about their needs and expectations. This switch from an annual staff meeting of all 800 physicians is tied to the TQM principle of customer listening (getting direct input).

HAP uses a number of methods to measure client satisfaction. Each fall, for the last six or seven years, a telephone survey of members has been conducted by an external research group. These results are reported back to HAP management, HFMG, Metro Medical Group, corporate Marketing and Planning, and the corporate board. Overall consumer satisfaction is reported as relatively high (6 out of a possible 7 points today). There is also a mailed "report card" on which members rate HAP. The response rate is low, but the results are similar to the phone survey.

The annual phone survey pinpointed access to services as an important member concern. Under the direction of Elizabeth Anctil, director of Access and Quality Improvement for HFMG, data was collected using multiple inputs (i.e., HFHS and HAP board directives, extensive internal and external customer research regarding perception of access, lead time information reflecting appointment availability, and senior leadership input). First, internal focus groups (ten groups of 6–10 participants each—providers, support staff, and managers) were convened to explore HFMG staff perceptions of the greatest needs, expectations, and issues related to client access. Fourteen key issues were identified, validated, and ranked. General efforts made by service sites to compensate for or to overcome barriers were also explored with the focus groups, and access management strategies that had proven successful were identified.

Second, during March and April of 1992, the same research group that does the annual survey conducted a random sample phone survey of patients who had received care at the ambulatory care sites over the previous 4–6 weeks. A series of 14 access-focused questions related to the core process of an ambulatory visit were asked. Each of 82 HFHS points of service had 100 patients surveyed. Results were correlated to overall satisfaction to form a baseline for what is expected to be an annual survey. Figure 8.6 presents a summary of findings of the staff focus groups and patient surveys as they relate to the identified steps of the primary care visit process.

Ongoing lead time reports for sick, routine, well, and new specialty consultation appointments are a third source of data. For example, how far in the future is the third available appointment for a consultation? Three to four years of data are now available on specialty consultations (see Figure 8.6). The graphic display of data helps staff understand whether they have a stable process or not. Summary information is fed back to primary care providers on a monthly basis so that they can give patients accurate information about how long they can expect to wait for a specialty appointment, and the full report is updated quarterly. Making lead time data collection a local facility responsibility has helped with staff perception of data accuracy.

The information from the various input sources was then linked to specific corrective recommendations. Both local and system level efforts were identified as necessary to achieve access improvements. For example on a local level, HFMG established several priorities to be addressed during 1993:

- Enhance the after-hours on-call nurse program to accommodate after-hours emergency transfer for patients not at HFH
- Add physicians for access improvement at specified centers
- Implement a daytime nurse triage program at specified centers

These priorities were included as specific items in the 1993 HFMG strategic plan and budget along with their related assumptions regarding membership/revenue increases and itemized expense categories. As these steps are implemented, evaluation of satisfaction data and access monitors will be carried out and further resource allocation will be considered as required.

Figure 8.6

Customer Issues Regarding Access to HFMG Primary Care

Perceived Need For Service
• ER or Walk-in use is routine rather than primary care physician visit
• HAP Patients perceived as having unrealistic expectations for care

Telephone Access

Appointment Scheduling

• Existing telephone equipment not capable of accommodating demand
• Lack of Registered Nurse triage for appropriate appointment use
• Patient orientation to HFHS does not exist
• *Ease of getting through by telephone*
• *Amount of time "on hold"*
• *Being able to get medical information or advice*
• *How long spent on phone making appointment*

• Inadequate staff to handle appointment requests
• Physician scheduling practices present barriers to efficient access
• Appointment scheduling system and training measures are not adequate
• Appointment availability on Mondays and after holidays for sick care
• Unclear when to close a practice or what size a practice should be
• Same day holds are not used consistently
• The wait for an appointment with a specialist is excessive
• *Ease of scheduling appointments with the doctor of your choice*
• *Length of time waited between making appointment and day of visit*
• *Being able to see a specialist when needed*

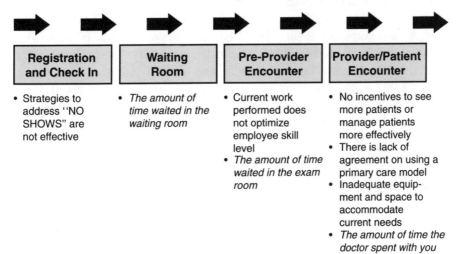

Registration and Check In

Waiting Room

Pre-Provider Encounter

Provider/Patient Encounter

• Strategies to address "NO SHOWS" are not effective

• *The amount of time waited in the waiting room*

• Current work performed does not optimize employee skill level
• *The amount of time waited in the exam room*

• No incentives to see more patients or manage patients more effectively
• There is lack of agreement on using a primary care model
• Inadequate equipment and space to accommodate current needs
• *The amount of time the doctor spent with you*

Continued

Figure 8.6   Continued

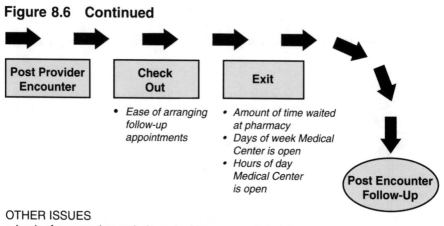

OTHER ISSUES
- Lack of access data to help make Management decisions
- Lack of opportunity for continuing education and sharing of successes

HAP also tracks and trends disenrollment data and member transfers between HAP primary care physicians. All calls to HAP (30,000 per month) are categorized into complaint/dissatisfaction categories, and the information is shared through HFHS as appropriate. In addition, HAP keeps in touch with group customers through account reps and surveys. It also contacts groups that are not HAP members to learn what they look for. HAP's COO, Roman Kulich, states, "It is my role to go out of my way to recognize and place priority on customer-focused improvements."

At the corporate level, HFHS has two main methods of obtaining information on its geographically defined community. First, for the Detroit area, the Greater Detroit Area Health Council publishes assessment information for each segment of the area (e.g., incidence of heart disease, number of "crack" babies). Second, the operating divisional boards function to represent their community's needs. These groups meet every two months and involve over 200 people. On a less structured basis, HFHS also meets periodically with the Detroit Health Department and benefit managers of the major employers. Information is also obtained from the customer marketing surveys (random digit dialing by an external agency annually; data are now available for several years) and the customer satisfaction surveys done specific to each product line (e.g., each hospital, the medical group, HMO).

Warden feels that even though HFHS is still working through its information requirements, it clearly has a balanced approach that relates to its broad set of customers and, therefore, has a pretty good understanding of the issues and problems.

Step 5: Organization Quality Awareness Building

Efforts are being made at HFHS to raise the general consciousness about quality improvement and to convey the sense that top management considers it important, including some kind of reporting of quality or customer satisfaction at every meeting of the executive committee. Senior managers are encouraged to participate in teaching the quality improvement training classes. Its informational brochure lists the quality definition and corporate values and quality guidelines alongside the HFHS mission and vision statements (see Figure 8.7).

Subsidiaries have also taken special measures to build environments that encourage quality awareness. For example, HFHS, HFH, and Cottage Hospital have adopted policy statements endorsing such action (see Figure 8.8).

At Cottage Hospital, Greg Vasse implemented a process in 1992 to talk at departmental meetings with all employees about the strategic plan. In those meetings, he links back to, "Where are we coming from? We've got this vision which is a statement of the intent of the board of trustees about this institution and here is what we are doing to try to get there." Because of these discussions, the vision statement has become very visible there.

At HFH, in addition to the formal system-sponsored training sessions of varying lengths that have reached down to the supervisor level, special effort has been made to reach all employees. Steve Velick and the executive vice president for HFH split the duties. Through 75 meetings (all shifts and all departments), they presented two hours of the key elements of quality management at HFH. Quality, from the standpoint of process, teamwork, and collaboration, was discussed as well as the role of statistical data and other key elements of HFH's customer-perspective approach. The quality management framework (mission and vision statements plus values and guiding principles) was also reviewed. There is an ongoing weekly newsletter for employees that talks about the quality effort; HFH also produces a quality management framework brochure that lists its mission and vision statements, values and guiding principles, and quality definition.

How to give appropriate recognition to employees was a specific focus area for HFH leadership during 1992. By the end of the year, a plan was developed that set forth both criteria for receiving recognition and guidelines regarding what constituted appropriate recognition. This plan was put into action in 1993. As another type of recognition activity, at the end of December 1992, HFH sponsored an internal Leadership Forum Day. For three and a half hours in the middle of the day, twenty teams

Figure 8.7

HFHS Corporate Values and Quality Guidelines

Quality is continuous improvement in patient care and service, education and research, and all other activities in which we are involved, in order to make the System a leading standard of excellence within the health care industry.

Henry Ford Health System embraces these basic values and quality guidelines and recognizes their role in its continued success.

1. Customer Focus
   - Quality patient care and service is a key principle for HFHS.
   - HFHS is committed to continuously improving the quality of services to its internal and external customers, and to giving priority attention to their concerns.
   - Communication with customers is key to better understanding their needs and expectations, continuously improving processes, and building their trust.

2. Management and Clinical Leadership
   - Leadership demonstrates commitment and behaves in a manner consistent with quality management concepts, including teamwork, continuous improvement, process focus, and statistical thinking.
   - Leadership accepts principal responsibility for creating an environment that encourages the involvement of all System employees and medical staff in continuous quality improvement.

3. Employee Focus
   - HFHS employees are an important asset and resource, and will be treated fairly, with dignity and respect.
   - Employees will be given an opportunity to develop their potential through education and training, including the use of tools and techniques of quality improvement.
   - Communication with all employees about the System's mission, strategy, plans, and objectives is key to building their understanding and trust.
   - Employees are an important source of knowledge about current processes and ideas for improvement.
   - Employees at every level will be active members of quality improvement teams.

4. Measurement
   - All work units within the System are committed to using customer and process knowledge as an input to identify key quality indicators.

Continued

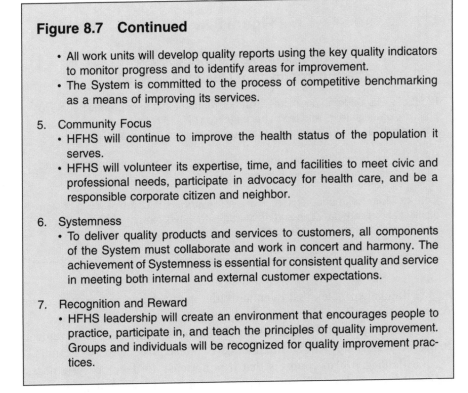

Figure 8.7 Continued

- All work units will develop quality reports using the key quality indicators to monitor progress and to identify areas for improvement.
- The System is committed to the process of competitive benchmarking as a means of improving its services.

5. Community Focus
- HFHS will continue to improve the health status of the population it serves.
- HFHS will volunteer its expertise, time, and facilities to meet civic and professional needs, participate in advocacy for health care, and be a responsible corporate citizen and neighbor.

6. Systemness
- To deliver quality products and services to customers, all components of the System must collaborate and work in concert and harmony. The achievement of Systemness is essential for consistent quality and service in meeting both internal and external customer expectations.

7. Recognition and Reward
- HFHS leadership will create an environment that encourages people to practice, participate in, and teach the principles of quality improvement. Groups and individuals will be recognized for quality improvement practices.

presented their work to their colleagues through storyboard presentations in a centrally located lobby. HFHS CEO, Gail Warden, participated in this celebration. In 1993 and 1994, a similar event was also held.

Progress to Date and Future Direction

General consensus among HFHS top management is that their expectations of the quality management and improvement process to date are being met. It is, however, not a process that can be implemented quickly. With this in mind, the Henry Ford representatives shared some insights. Young advises: "It is important to have a couple of areas where there is a champion who is really willing to do something in an accelerated fashion. To make it evident. To say, . . . here's an idea of how it can work. I think it would be almost impossible to have a sustained faith on 'it takes a long time.'"

Figure 8.8

Comparative Perspectives:
The Environment of Quality Awareness

HFHS: HFHS leadership will create an environment that encourages people to practice, participate in, and teach the principles of quality improvement. Groups and individuals will be recognized for quality improvement practices.

HFH: We will recognize efforts toward quality improvement and innovation and take time to celebrate our successes.

Cottage Hospital: Leadership provides an environment for the practice of high quality patient care services and encourages the involvement of all employees and members of the medical staff in continuous quality improvement.

Griffenhagen notes that eventually the medical group does expect to focus on some major initiatives such as clinical protocols for care. However, in the next few years the "biggest bang for the buck in process improvement [in the medical group] will be small things that take place in the work units."

Griffenhagen also counsels that it is not easy to develop systemness and, at the same time, empower different units to implement quality improvement processes in their own way. Some things will conflict. Finding the right balance between centralization and decentralization will be a challenge for HFHS in the next few years. Considering this issue on a more macro level, Vasse points out the difficult task for HFHS in the next years of balancing an efficiency-oriented, managed care approach with a customer satisfaction orientation.

Velick cautions that teams are a tool. By themselves they are not the answer to success in quality improvement. Success is based on a combination of things: an understanding by every employee of the principles underlying a quality perspective and an integration of these principles by each employee into their daily work, continued monitoring of relevant data, and leadership emphasis on the quality process as a way of future success. This quality emphasis has to be "a part of how we manage, how we look at things."

Kulich counsels against "too much religious evangelist approach to quality." This approach can hurt a program. He compares a cultural revolution led by outsiders who have no idea of the specific organization's history to a physician prescribing without examining the patient.

Some changes have occurred in the formal structure of the QI process since its inception, reflecting the changing needs of HFHS as an organization. The original Quality Technology Council has evolved into the Coach-Facilitator Forum, specifically focused on helping persons in those roles. The current corporate-level Quality Management Steering Committee (QMSC) includes the members of the Office of the President (the CEO; the senior vice presidents for Managed Care, Medical Affairs, Hospital Affairs; the senior vice president and chief financial officer; the senior vice president for Planning and Marketing); the chairs of the three senior leadership teams (Senior Operating Team, Senior Physician Leadership Team, and Senior Staff Team); the vice president for Health Care Quality; and the director of the Department of Health Care Quality Improvement Education and Research. A representative from the Coach-Facilitator Forum has recently been added to the working group of the QMSC. In addition, each operating entity has a quality management steering committee. Furthermore, discussions regarding the quality improvement process and its effect on intra- and interdepartmental affairs occur at the level of the departments within the operating entities.

Overall, the CEO and top management continue to be committed to quality improvement, and they plan to continue the rollout through the tiers of the organization. They believe they can permanently imbed CQI through the planning process. Wherever there is a group responsible for planning, quality improvement methods should inform this planning process.

The biggest disappointment noted by Warden is the amount of variation that exists between departments in the depth and speed of implementation of the quality management process. On the other hand, he feels that the biggest accomplishment is the interest and support from physicians for the initiative, which has surpassed his expectations. He suggests that one of the critical next steps is the search for the linkage between clinical quality assurance and QI in the development of practice guidelines, outcomes measurements, and critical pathways. He has encouraged a Quality Report Task Group, which reports directly to the board of trustees.

Sahney listed three specific "next step" activities that are now being implemented. The first is the merging systemwide of the strategic planning and quality improvement processes (as has already been done at HFH and Cottage Hospital). The second is the implementation of an annual standardized self-assessment tool (the "balanced scorecard") for operating entities to use to track their progress over time in the quality improvement process (see Figure 8.9). The third is the development of a systemwide quality report now being shared with the system board on a regular basis.

In many ways the future direction can be summed up in Vasse's words: "You really unleash an infinite process. There is no end point. It just keeps expanding. When you ask, 'Where is the organization going next?' We're just allowing that [process] to grow. Which is really the process of internal learning."

Special Focus: The Cottage Hospital Rollout

Greg Vasse, president of Cottage Hospital, describes the first two years of CQI as "long and disjointed." The leaders' initiation to CQI didn't stick. It wasn't clear how to establish priorities for quality improvement. Cottage Hospital's quality steering committee had a formal chartering process for teams and a lot of discussion overall about such things as the value of teams, who should be on them, and how much time people should take from their regular activities for team work. However, Cottage found itself in essentially passive response to every manager who proposed something concrete. This, in turn, had strained their available QI resources. Cottage had more teams than trained facilitators. The level of training among team members varied greatly, and the in-house support for such things as just-in-time training or preteam workup did not exist. A lot of frustration developed. "A lot of people wanted to do a lot of things and we were always kind of finding ourselves putting on the brakes, but not for the right reasons. We were putting on the brakes for resource limitations rather than because this was not a priority for us," Vasse says.

In its second year, Cottage Hospital's top management began to focus on the hospital as a system. They critically examined the vision statement. How applicable was it to the functioning of the hospital either today or in five years? Did the vision give specific guidance to the hospital's actions? Could it be used as the basis for improvement plans?

As a result, Cottage Hospital's mission and vision statements became shorter and more understandable (see Figure 8.10). A quality definition was added to point out that the trustees' perspective of quality was "meeting the expectations of the customer." New values and quality guidelines necessary to implement CQI permanently were delineated (see Figure 8.11). The

Figure 8.9

HFHS Balanced Scorecard Performance Measures

1. External Customer Satisfaction
   A. Percent of patients dissatisfied or very dissatisfied
   B. Percent of voluntary disenrollment
   C. Access indicators
   D. Physician satisfaction survey
   E. Business attitude evaluation

2. Clinical Process—Outcomes
   A. Accreditation and regulatory approvals
   B. Health status (SF-36)
   C. Number of claims and litigations
   D. Patient falls
   E. Nosocomial infection rates
   F. HCFA-derived disease-specific mortality rates

3. Financial Performance
   A. Net operating income
   B. Cost/enrollee or cost/case (case mix adjusted)
   C. Patient days/1,000 members
   D. DRG margin
   E. Bond rating

4. Philanthropy
   A. Total donations received (including commitments)
   B. Net philanthropic collections (net of expenses)
   C. Philanthropic expense ratio

5. Community Dividend
   A. Uncompensated care
   B. Contribution in voluntary efforts including such activities as community education (staff hours, $ value)

6. Growth
   A. Equivalent population served
   B. Market share

7. Business Strategic Advantage
   A. Cost leadership
   B. Distribution system

Continued

Figure 8.9   Continued

    C. Product offerings
    D. Process improvement teams—accomplishments

  8. Innovation
    A. Percentage revenue from new products
    B. Percentage revenue from new markets

  9. Internal Customer Satisfaction
    A. Employee satisfaction surveys
    B. Labor turnover
    C. Diversity goals

10. Academic (Education and Research)
    A. NIH grants received
    B. Total external funding
    C. Resident match results
    D. Student satisfaction with educational programs

vision statement became "a tool to drive into our system diagram, which was used as a tool to generate a big chunk of our strategic plan."

The critical self-evaluation took place at multiple levels within the hospital. Developing a system diagram became a learning exercise. Starting with identification of the hospital's core processes and three key questions (see Figure 8.12), the Quality Steering Committee used Batalden's framework to think about Cottage Hospital as a system. Cottage's vision was included as an integral part of the system diagram (see Figure 8.13). Each aspect of the core processes could then be further analyzed for greater understanding (Figure 8.14). Customer knowledge related to specific aspects of the core process became a critical input into its design and redesign.

Finally, the management team identified five QI theme areas:

- Emergency department patient assignment to on-call physician
- Psychiatry patient intake, assessment, and admission
- Ambulatory surgery patient intake, assessment, and admission
- Adult Med/Surg discharge
- Billing for hospital- and physician-directed services.

Figure 8.10

Cottage Hospital Mission and Vision Statements

Mission

Cottage Hospital is dedicated to providing patient care and service. A partnership of our hospital staff, physicians and the Henry Ford Health System will continue to establish higher standards of quality and value in the community and among health care providers.

Vision

I. Cottage Hospital's services demonstrate continuous improvement towards achieving benchmark levels of patient, physician, and employee satisfaction.

II. Its clinical programs reflect a dynamic definition of secondary level hospital care. High volume tertiary regional deployment in order to support improved access, market share, and cost. The hospital's clinical programs respond to the clinical and market preferences of its patients and physicians.

III. Its common use by Henry Ford Health System group practices and private practice physicians is a unique health care opportunity for Eastern Shores residents. Patient relationships with the hospital and its physicians are seamless and effective. These attributes serve all categories of physician practices and the mission of the Henry Ford Health System.

IV. Its governing body, management, and medical direction will be organizational elements of the Henry Ford Health System available to all of the System's providers in the Eastern Shores Region.

The objective for the third year became to make substantive improvement in the theme areas, in line with at least one area of the vision statement.

The knowledge gained was taken back to the individual departments by the respective managers. The departments, in turn, began to look at themselves as systems. Each examined its reason for existing and developed a vision. Questions were asked: What is the core business? Who are the customers? What is the core process and its key aspects? What are the things that need to be measured for each of the key aspects of the core

---

Figure 8.11

Cottage Hospital Values and Quality Guidelines

Cottage Hospital embraces these values and Quality Guidelines and recognizes their role in achieving success.

Customer Focus

- Cottage Hospital provides quality patient care and service.

- Cottage Hospital is committed to continuously improving the quality of service to our customers including patients, medical staff, employees, and all others with whom we work in following our mission.

- Customers are listened to and responded to in an efficient individualized manner.

- Attention is directed to the physical, emotional, and spiritual needs of our patients.

- Communication with all of our customers is key to better understanding their needs and expectations, continuously improving processes and building trust.

Leadership

- Leadership provides an environment for the practice of high quality patient care services and encourages the involvement of all employees and members of the medical staff in continuous quality improvement.

- Leadership demonstrates commitment and behavior consistent with quality management and continuous improvement concepts including teamwork, customer knowledge, process focus, and statistical thinking.

- Leadership communicates with employees and members of the medical staff and embraces their expectations as key elements of customer and process knowledge which are critical to our success.

---

process so that it can be determined whether or not it is working? What needs to be designed or redesigned? This process served to get people to learn the language related to the quality improvement program and to apply the skills necessary to focus on their core processes.

The more structured second round of CQI led to important changes in attitude and implementation. Vasse summarizes the hospital's QI work during 1992:

Figure 8.12

Building Knowledge of a System

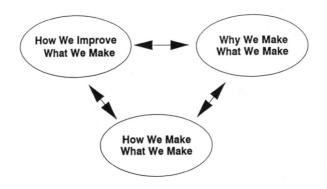

We haven't shut down. At any one time over the last year, we've had about a dozen teams running and they are still running, still pursuing their improvements. But, the point is, they represent kind of a broad shotgun approach to improvement, whereas I think the real substantive work in improvement at Cottage is now flowing through or within the parameters of our five initiatives. Which again are designed to support a specific piece of our vision.

Cottage's strategic plan spun off from this examination of the core process and resultant understanding of the operation of the hospital as a system. In 1993, the strategic plan included initiatives related to each key aspect of the core process. For example, "admitting patients to the hospital (with consideration for access and efficiency)" included the following: improve process for assignment of attending physician through ER, improve psychiatry admission process from intake to placement, and improve ambulatory surgery admission process including preadmission testing.

The integration of the quality program into Cottage Hospital's day-to-day routine was summed up by Vasse as follows: "You can't come in here and slice off the quality program. That's wrong. We shouldn't be there at this point. It's sort of all around us. It's into our strategic plan, our billing process. It's the way people focus on the short-term resolution of a problem."

Vinod Sahney, Ph.D., senior vice president for Planning and Strategic Development, summed up his experience:

Figure 8.13   Hospital System Diagram

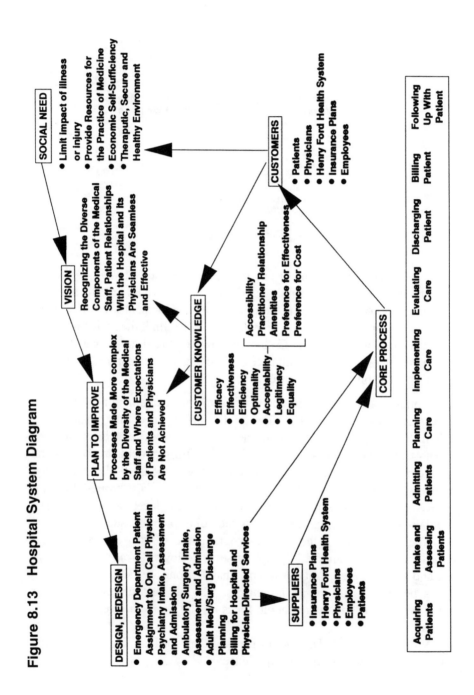

Figure 8.14 Cause-and-Effect Analysis

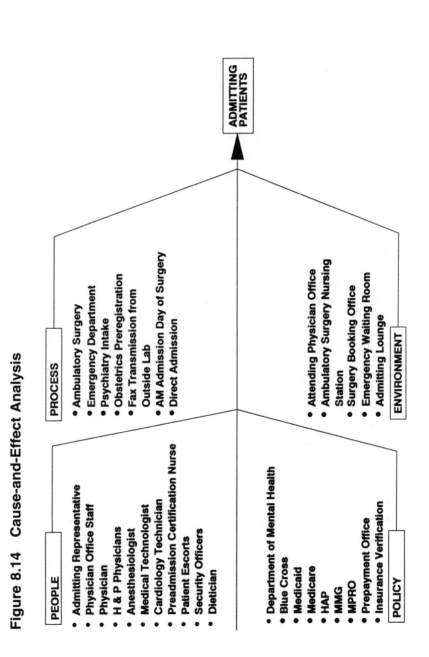

The Quality Management Process is now an integral part of the management tools within HFHS. It is at the same stage as other management tools like performance evaluation, budgeting, and management control. Managers who have taken the time to understand the concepts and used the concepts actively are reaping the benefits. There are many within the organization who are still not sure that the quality management process adds an important dimension in helping them manage. Each day, there are more believers and practitioners and we hear more successes.

Everyone would like the benefits of the Quality Management Process to be instantly achievable, but the reality is that the results come slowly and the organization's progress grows exponentially over time [see Figure 8.15]. The difference between expectations and the reality created an expectations gap, which if not managed can kill the quality initiative prematurely.

Note

1. Originally presented in Sahney, V. K., and G. L. Warden. 1991. "The Quest for Quality and Productivity in Health Services." *Frontiers of Health Services Management* 7 (4): 2–41.

References and Suggested Readings

American Medical Association. 1992. *Physician Characteristics and Distribution in the United States*. Chicago: AMA.

Facts about Hospitals and Health Care in Michigan. 1984–1989. Lansing, MI: Hospital Association and Michigan Health Care Institute.

Henry Ford Case Study. 1991. Chicago: APM, Inc.

Henry Ford Health System. 1992a. *Fact Sheet*. Detroit, MI: HFHS.

———. 1992b. *System Report*. Detroit, MI: HFHS.

Michigan in Brief: 1990–91 Issues Handbook. 1990. Lansing, MI: Public Sector Consultants.

The Universal Health Care Almanac. 1991. Phoenix, AZ: Silver and Cherner.

Figure 8.15

Barriers and Strategies for Staying on Track

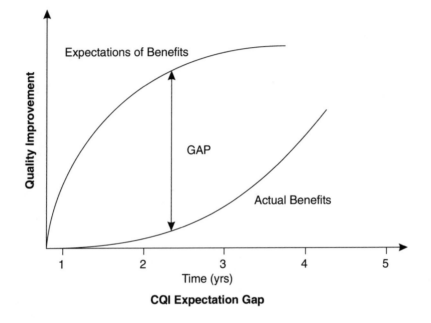

CQI Expectation Gap

Index